Anesthesia for Oral and Maxillofacial Surgery

Hong Jiang • Ming Xia
Editors

Anesthesia for Oral and Maxillofacial Surgery

Springer

Editors
Hong Jiang
Department of Anesthesiology
Shanghai Ninth People's Hospital
Affiliated to Shanghai Jiao Tong
University School of Medicine
Shanghai, China

Ming Xia
Department of Anesthesiology
Shanghai Ninth People's Hospital
Affiliated to Shanghai Jiao Tong
University School of Medicine
Shanghai, China

ISBN 978-981-19-7286-7 ISBN 978-981-19-7287-4 (eBook)
https://doi.org/10.1007/978-981-19-7287-4

This Springer imprint is published by the registered company Springer Nature Singapore Pte Ltd.
The registered company address is: 152 Beach Road, #21-01/04 Gateway East, Singapore 189721, Singapore

Contents

Contributors

Jian Cao Department of Oral and Craniomaxillofacial Surgery, Shanghai Ninth People's Hospital Affiliated to Shanghai Jiao Tong University School of Medicine, Shanghai, China

Shuang Cao Department of Anesthesiology, Shanghai Ninth People's Hospital Affiliated to Shanghai Jiao Tong University School of Medicine, Shanghai, China

Jie Chen Department of Anesthesiology, Shanghai Ninth People's Hospital Affiliated to Shanghai Jiao Tong University School of Medicine, Shanghai, China

Xi Chen Department of Anesthesiology, Shanghai Ninth People's Hospital Affiliated to Shanghai Jiao Tong University School of Medicine, Shanghai, China

Rong Hu Department of Anesthesiology, Shanghai Ninth People's Hospital Affiliated to Shanghai Jiao Tong University School of Medicine, Shanghai, China

Hong Jiang Department of Anesthesiology, Shanghai Ninth People's Hospital Affiliated to Shanghai Jiao Tong University School of Medicine, Shanghai, China

Jue Jiang Department of Anesthesiology, Shanghai Ninth People's Hospital Affiliated to Shanghai Jiao Tong University School of Medicine, Shanghai, China

Jingjie Li Department of Anesthesiology, Shanghai Ninth People's Hospital Affiliated to Shanghai Jiao Tong University School of Medicine, Shanghai, China

Yu Sun Department of Anesthesiology, Shanghai Ninth People's Hospital Affiliated to Shanghai Jiao Tong University School of Medicine, Shanghai, China

Ming Xia Department of Anesthesiology, Shanghai Ninth People's Hospital Affiliated to Shanghai Jiao Tong University School of Medicine, Shanghai, China

Yuelai Yang Department of Intensive Care Unit, Shanghai Ninth People's Hospital Affiliated to Shanghai Jiao Tong University School of Medicine, Shanghai, China

1 History of Oral and Maxillofacial Anesthesia

Hong Jiang

1.1 History of Oral Anesthesia

Published discussions about anesthesia for oral and maxillofacial surgery have been rare in recent years. However, dental anesthesia was an important subject as the history of anesthesia was almost overlapped with the development of oral anesthesia. Therefore, in this chapter, the author will systematically introduce the history of anesthesia for oral and maxillofacial surgery.

The pain in the mouth and head has tortured human beings since their existence. That pain may be caused by tooth decay or surgery in oral and maxillofacial region. Before anesthesia techniques were invented, it was common to pull out bad teeth without any form of analgesia or anesthesia, and avoiding the suffer of pulling teeth has been attempted all the time. For example, alcohol, hemp, poppy, henbane, and mandrake have been used to alleviate pain [1]. However, with contemporary knowledge, we knew that all these chemicals or herbs were poisonous and could barely alleviate pain. As more scientific advances were achieved, techniques such as using cold, pressure, and hypnotism were embraced. Some of them have been used till today. Yet, these were not anesthesia and could never replace people's demand for all kinds of anesthesia.

H. Jiang (✉)
Department of Anesthesiology, Shanghai Ninth People's Hospital Affiliated to Shanghai Jiao Tong University School of Medicine, Shanghai, China

Anesthesia did not emerge until the modern medicine began to develop. The discovery of surgical anesthetics in the modern era was originally linked to inhaled anesthetics [2]. By the end of the eighteenth century, a number of gases had been identified and could be produced relatively reliably. Scientist Joseph Priestley had identified nitrous oxide in 1773. Humphry Davy, his apprentice, was interested in that gas as well, yet he failed to publicize the beneficial quality of the gas.

By the mid-eighteenth century, as chemistry progressed, "modern" anesthesia dawned. The American dentist Horace Wells in 1844 noticed and suggested that volatile gases, such as nitrous oxide, could be inhaled and used for medical and dental anesthesia [3]. He tested the effect himself and found that while extracting a tooth with the inhalation of nitrous oxide, he did not feel any pain. However, when he chose to demonstrate the anesthetic efficacy of nitrous oxide, he failed. Later, William Thomas Green Morton learned from Wells and also Charles T. Jackson, a chemist and physician. After successfully anesthetized a pet dog by giving it ether, he found an opportunity to publicly demonstrate his findings on 16 October, 1846 by using ether anesthesia in the auditorium of the Massachusetts General Hospital to help Collins Warren, the chief surgeon, to remove a patient's submaxillary gland tumors painlessly. It was a well-known and successful demonstration. The term "anesthesia"

H. Jiang, M. Xia (eds.), *Anesthesia for Oral and Maxillofacial Surgery*,
https://doi.org/10.1007/978-981-19-7287-4_1

was suggested by another Boston physician, Oliver Wendell Holmes, in a letter to Morton on 21 November, 1846 [4]. The name was adopted, announcing the beginning of anesthetic age.

Early anesthetics came into use in different areas. Whereas, early anesthesia was unpleasant and unpredictable for the patient. Early anesthesia provided pain relief for the patient, but there were greater risks associated with dosage and treatment issues. A sponge was placed in a glass vessel, into which ether was dripped, and then held it to the patient's face. The evaporation of the ether caused a decrease in the temperature of the glass and thus a risk of burning the skin.

In late 1847, an Edinburgh obstetrician, James Young Simpson, successfully used chloroform for the relief of labor pain. In 1855, the German chemist Gaedicke extracted Erythroxylon from coca leaves. Four years later, the Austrian chemist Niemann purified and refined cocaine. Because of its good anesthetic effect and penetration, cocaine was used in clinical anesthesia by Dr. William Holsted in 1885 [5]. In the nineteenth century, general anesthesia was no longer the only option for oral surgery, with the introduction of cocaine, procaine, cinchocaine, and lidocaine. Although local anesthesia was not widespread in the USA and the United Kingdom at the time, general anesthesia, such as nitrous oxide and ether, which had been used earlier in dental surgery, was gradually replaced by local anesthesia for tooth extraction or oral surgery. However, due to the lack of sedation in local anesthesia, there was still a high risk of patient fainting or cerebral infarction or sudden heart attack during surgery, so there was still a need to find a drug or method that addresses both analgesia and sedation.

Both ether and chloroform were risky to use and need to be given under the supervision of a surgeon or doctors who practiced anesthesia. Nitrous oxide was relatively simple and safe to use, so it became the biggest contributor to the spread of anesthesia. By the late nineteenth century, the role of the anesthetist was taken up by a full-time physician practitioner in order to reduce the risk of accidents, providing a solid step toward specialization in the discipline of anesthesia.

Ivan Magill revolutionized head and neck surgery, and his contribution to the field of oral anesthesia can be seen in the comment that he "made the ventilator more like the present ventilator, the laryngoscope more like the present laryngoscope, and anesthesia more like the present anesthesia" [6]. He invented the Magill apparatus and the Magill laryngoscope, and successfully introduced tracheal intubation and laryngoscopy into everyday surgical anesthesia, solving the problem of not having free access to the face and mouth during surgery. Since then, tracheal intubation has been widely used in complex surgery, effectively improving the safety and operability of surgery.

The introduction of barbiturates, benzodiazepines and synthetic opioids in the 1830s further reduced the risks of anesthesia. The early twentieth century saw the rapid development of inhalation anesthesia, which was highly dependent on the expertise of the physician and involved many uncontrollable risks. The introduction of intravenous anesthetic drugs increased the physician's control over anesthetic drugs.

Robert Macintosh was the first professor of anesthesia outside the USA and developed academic training for anesthetists. He had been devoted to make anesthesia safer and simpler. He invented a laryngoscope, named after himself—the Macintosh laryngoscope, which was still widely used today. It was fair to say that the rapid expansion of anesthesia during the Second World War was made possible by a combination of rapid growth in medical cases, increased training opportunities for doctors and the development and production of new drugs and equipment.

The establishment of the National Health Service (NHS) in the UK and the creation of a specialist department at the Royal College of Surgeons in London and the appointment of senior anesthetists as consultants led to substantial progress in the recruitment of specialist anesthetists and the advancement of the anesthetic profession as a whole. The abundance of staff boosted anesthetic research and the development of drugs and techniques, such as muscle relaxants, lidocaine, and other new inhalants to meet the need for sedation in surgical anesthesia. The anesthetists no longer worked for the surgeons and their duties were divided. By keeping the patient's airway open, but also away from the surgical area, they worked alongside the surgeons to reduce morbidity and mortality during surgery and to provide a more effective and safe procedure for the patient.

Victor Goldman, along with Stanley Drumond-Jackson and Adrian Hubell, introduced Hexabarbital to intravenous anesthesia in clinical oral surgery [7]. The use of general anesthesia was regulated in the 1970s due to the side effects and risks associated with general anesthesia. In 1998, the General Dental Council issued guidelines banning the use of general anesthesia for some procedures. By 1999 the number of general anesthesia was further reduced to a minimum and by the end of 2001 the use of general anesthesia in dental surgery had been completely eliminated.

Today, anesthesia for oral surgery is strictly controlled and is only allowed to be performed by experienced anesthetists with a full range of equipment and facilities. Popular anesthetic drugs such as nitrous oxide and halothane are almost no longer used and have been replaced by sevoflurane and isoproterenol. A wide range of alternative drugs have been developed to reduce side effects, provide sedation and analgesia, and ensure a smooth operation.

Nowadays, from routine tooth extractions to complex reconstructive craniofacial surgery, the range of treatment that is covered in oral and maxillofacial (OMF) surgery has expanded in recent years. Since 1844, when two physicians founded Baltimore's first school of dentistry, this surgical specialty has emerged and evolved from the formal practice of dentistry. Societies belonging to this specialty sprung up, with the American Society of Exodontists established in 1918 being the first. In 1921, the society changed its name as the American Society of Oral Surgeons and Exodontists, and in 1946 changed again as the American Society of Oral Surgeons. In 1977, the "maxillofacial" became part of the society's name, manifesting its designation at the moment, while reflecting its wide range of directions this specialty intend to explore and serve [8].

1.2 History of Oral Anesthesia in China

As an integral part of surgery, anesthesia encompasses the preparation, treatment, and monitoring of the entire perioperative period. Modern anesthesia is a comprehensive discipline that can be divided into clinical anesthesiology, resuscitation and intensive monitoring and treatment, pain management, and among others. With a short history of about 160 years, modern oral anesthesia, as an emerging discipline, has had an even shorter history of development in China. During these decades, oral anesthesiology and oral and maxillofacial surgery have complemented each other and developed together, and through generations of researchers' dedication in the discipline, oral anesthesiology has made great progress in China, and the team of talents in the relevant fields has grown day by day.

Western medicine was introduced to China with the sprout of foreign churches' hospitals and medical schools in China, the earliest being the Boji Medical Hall in Guangzhou (1866), the Tong Ren Hospital in Shanghai (1879), the Bo Xi Hospital in Suzhou (1883), and the Peking Union Medical College (1903). The Tianjin Medical College and the Peking University Hall of Medicine in Beijing were established by the Qing government in 1881 and in 1903, respectively. After the Revolution of 1911, medical schools with hospitals were established one after another in various places. These hospitals did not have separate anesthesia departments at the time of their establishment, and major operations could only be performed in city's general hospitals, where the anesthetic equipment was rudimentary and the technique was unsophisticated.

It was only in the early twentieth century that the first dental clinic was established in China, followed by the opening of specialist dental hospitals in Beijing, Shanghai and Wuhan one after another. Local anesthesia during surgery was undertaken by stomatologists. The professional dental anesthesia in China was not formed until the 1940s, when Wu Jue, Shang Deyan, Li Xingfang, and others returned to China, bringing foreign dental anesthesia techniques back and carrying out teaching and scientific researches in clinical anesthesia. At that time, anesthesiology was in its infancy, and the equipment, staff management and anesthesia methods were not sophisticated. Constrained by the poor health and medical condition at that time, clinical anesthesia practice in China could only adopt simple anesthesia methods such as open drop ether anesthesia and tracheal intubation inhalation anesthesia.

In the late 1950s, some hospitals in China set up post anesthesia care unit, and in the 1970s, research on pain mechanisms was carried out. In the 1980s, intensive care units (ICUs) were commonly established in hospitals, which played an important role in the treatment of critically ill patients. In 1988, the Law on Licensed Doctors of the People's Republic of China further classified the use of sedative drugs in general anesthesia surgery and the monitoring of intraoperative care as the functions of anesthesiologists. In 1989, the Chinese Ministry of Health recognized the Department of Anesthesia as a Class I clinical department and a Class II discipline, and at the same time defined its field of work and functional areas, which laid a solid foundation for the subsequent development of anesthesiology.

In 1992, Division of Anesthesiology, Chinese Society of Oral and Maxillofacial Surgery was established, and a national academic conference on oral anesthesia was held every four years. In 2007, the Society joined hands with the Japanese and Korean Dental Anesthesia Societies to form the Federation of Asian Dental Anesthesia Societies (FADAS). Conferences such as the 11th International Conference on Oral Anesthesia held in Yokohama, Japan in 2007, the First Summit Forum on Oral Anesthesiology in Shanghai in 2008 and the First and Second Meetings of Federation of Asian Dental Anesthesiology societies, and the 2008 Annual Meeting of Chinese Stemmatological Society of Anesthesiology were held. In 2008, the Chinese Society of Anesthesiology was formally established under the support of the Chinese Stomatological Association. These conferences have enhanced academic exchanges and cooperation at home and abroad, and continuously consolidated the important role of Chinese oral anesthesiology in Asia and even in the world.

1.3 Anesthesia for Oral and Maxillofacial Surgery

Anesthesiology has developed into a comprehensive discipline that is closely related to surgery. In addition to anesthesia, analgesia, and pain management, its field of study also encompasses perioperative anesthesia preparation and treatment, the monitoring and regulation of the patient's physiological functions during surgery, and the treatment and resuscitation of critically ill patients. The main responsibilities of the Department of Oral Anesthesia include guaranteeing the smooth performance of oral and maxillofacial surgery, such as safety, painlessness, muscle relaxation, and reasonable stress regulation; ensuring patient safety and prevention of complications in the preoperative, intraoperative, and postoperative phases; the establishment and management of postanesthesia care unit and intensive care units; emergency and resuscitation treatment; oral and maxillofacial pain management; and education and scientific research in oral anesthesiology. Specifically, oral procedures ranging from simple tooth extraction to complicated reconstructive carniofacial surgery require anesthesia techniques such as the application of local anesthetics, titration of intravenous sedation, and the administration of general anesthesia [9]. Skilled airway management technique and sophisticated invasive blood pressure monitoring technique are needed in successfully performing anesthesia. In order to successfully complete the above-mentioned oral anesthesia tasks, its supporting discipline construction has been improved gradually from the following aspects:

1. The number of oral anesthesiologists and other staff should be enough to ensure the smooth development of medical, scientific research, and teaching work;
2. In addition to the clinical medicine knowledge already mastered, practitioners should insist on improving their techniques through learning theories and practicing systemically;
3. The hospital should be equipped with adequate drugs, instruments, and equipment to ensure the safety of patients during the perioperative period;

4. A sound organization of the oral anesthesia department should include an anesthesia clinic, clinical anesthesia, postanesthesia care unit (PACU), intensive care unit (ICU), etc.

Craniomaxillofacial surgery is an interdiscipline consisting of plastic surgery, oral and maxillofacial surgery, neurosurgery, and ear, nose, and throat surgery. As craniomaxillofacial surgery is extensive, invasive, long, bleeding, and the surgical site is close to the airway and central nerves, this raises the risk and difficulty of the operation and places higher demands on the perioperative anesthetic management. In 1964, French plastic surgeon Paul Tessier first used a combined intracranial-extracranial approach to treat congenital orbital widening, and his successful experience confirmed important basic theories of craniofacial surgery. Firstly, the cranial or facial bones can be amputated free in large pieces and rearranged without osteonecrosis; secondly, the orbital skeleton in and around the eye can be moved up, down, left and right and fixed in a wide range without affecting vision; thirdly, the combined intracranial-extracranial surgical access ensures the repositioning or reconstruction of the orbital-cranial bones. These three theories formed the basis of modern craniofacial surgery.

Inspired by Paul Tessier's combined intracranial and extracranial pathway surgery, Professor Zhang Disheng of the Department of Plastic Surgery at the Ninth People's Hospital in Shanghai in 1978 completed the first case of orbital distance widening correction surgery in China, becoming the founder of craniofacial surgery in China. Since the 1950s, the development of oral and maxillofacial surgery in China has been rapid, with the yearly increasing number of anesthesia personnel, gradual improvement in anesthesia theory and clinical practice, maturity in the construction of anesthesiology, and the emergence of anesthetic drugs. In addition to general dental surgery, the scope of oral and maxillofacial surgery also includes the repair of cleft lip and palate in infants and children, correction of craniomaxillofacial deformities, fracture repositioning of the upper and lower jaws, removal and repair of oral tumors, and comprehensive treatment of maxillofacial hemangiomas or vascular malformations, i.e. the treatment of various craniomaxillofacial deformities, trauma and tumors, and other problems. As the surgical fields of oral and maxillofacial surgery and craniomaxillofacial surgery involve the oral cavity, head, face, and neck, general anesthesia with endotracheal intubation should be the more ideal choice. With the development and use of various new anesthetic drugs, the anesthesia methods and approaches have also evolved, becoming more relevant to the situation. The anesthesia induction depends on the patient's actual condition and past medical history, especially whether there being intubation difficulties. In principle, awake intubation should be considered for all patients with anticipated airway difficulties or critical conditions.

Commonly used anesthesia methods in craniomaxillofacial surgery are local and general anesthesia. Local anesthesia is suitable for short intraoral, maxillofacial, and superficial craniofacial and cervical procedures during which patients have a good degree of cooperation. Local anesthesia is simple to perform, requires no special preoperative preparation or equipment and has a low impact on the physiological function of the body. Commonly used local anesthetic methods include local infiltration anesthesia and nerve block anesthesia. General anesthesia is required for medium to major surgical procedures in craniofacial surgery, for patients who are unable to cooperate or who have difficulty maintaining a patent airway. Different anesthetic methods and drugs are chosen and combined according to different surgical sites. The advantage of the combined anesthesia is that it can complement the strengths and weaknesses of the single anesthesia method. On the one hand, it generates better anesthetic effect. On the other hand, it helps to reduce the side effects and complications caused by the anesthetic drugs.

From the use of open drop ether anesthesia to the current sophisticated closed circuit inhalation anesthesia and combined intravenous and inhalation anesthesia, the oral anesthesia in China has progressed all the time. The treatment techniques for cleft lip and palate deformities and temporomandibular joint diseases, and combined cranio-maxillofacial resection for oral and maxillofacial malignant tumors are world class. The research and development of new general anesthetic drugs and science and technology have led to the improvement of intravenous anesthesia techniques, which are widely used in oral and maxillofacial surgery. In recent decades, new drugs such as propofol, midazolam, remifentanil, and sevoflurane have been introduced to achieve targeted therapy, which reduces the adverse reactions caused by the use of a single drug, achieves better intraoperative analgesia and sedation effects, and ensures the quality of surgery and patient safety.

1.4 Summary and Prospect

Throughout its development, oral anesthesia has been closely intertwined with the history of anesthesia as a whole. Modern oral anesthesia and oral surgery are complementary, working together to ensure patients' safety throughout the perioperative and recovery periods. Anesthesia is a highly specialized and challenging high-risk discipline. Thus, while performing it, patient's safety must always be of priority. Dental Anesthesiology only embraces short history. Therefore, further efforts should be made in cultivating anesthesia professions and inventing devices and equipment.

The development of oral anesthesia should keep up with the times and be prepared to face challenges while grasping opportunities. As the standard of medical care in China steadily improves, its demographic structure, medical model, and disease types are all in a state of flux. The growing material abundance has brought many new diseases and oral problems while satisfying people's needs. The development of laryngoscopes, anesthetic drugs, etc. has helped to improve the controllability of surgery. This is the dividend of technology and the result of the tireless exploration of dental practitioners. While we enjoy the scientific achievements made by our predecessors and acquired professional knowledge, we must pursue higher goals by standing on the shoulders of our predecessors, striving to improve our medical standards and scientific research, and creating a safer and more reliable surgical environment for our patients. In the twenty-first century, we have wider channels and platforms to acquire new information and knowledge and learn how to operate new devices and equipment. The online platforms allow for the timely exchange of the latest scientific findings. With the development of science and technology, it helps to promote the development of dental anesthesia and oral surgery, and indeed the entire medical system, making its fair share of contribution to improving the quality of people's life, especially in recent years when artificial intelligence has taken root in the medical field and has a promising application in the field of dentistry and anesthesiology.

References

1. Shaw I, Kumar C, Dodds C. Oxford textbook of Anaesthesia for Oral and maxillofacial surgery. Oxford University Press; Jun 2010.
2. The History of Anesthesia | Anesthesia Key (aneskey.com).
3. Office-Based Anesthesia Provided by the Oral and Maxillofacial Surgeon. American Association of Oral and Maxillofacial Surgeons. Retrieved from advocacy_office_based_anesthesia_whitepaper.pdf (aaoms.org). Sept 3rd, 2021.
4. Orr DL 2nd. The development of anesthesiology in oral and maxillofacial surgery. Oral Maxillofac Surg Clin North Am. 2013 Aug;25(3):341–55. https://doi.org/10.1016/j.coms.2013.04.003.
5. López-Valverde A, De Vicente J, Cutando A. The surgeons Halsted and hall, cocaine and the discovery of dental anaesthesia by nerve blocking. Br Dent J. 2011;211(10):485–7. https://doi.org/10.1038/sj.bdj.2011.961.
6. Szmuk P, Ezri T, Evron S, Roth Y, Katz J. A brief history of tracheostomy and tracheal intubation, from the bronze age to the space age. Intensive Care Med. 2008;34(2):222–8. https://doi.org/10.1007/s00134-007-0931-5. Epub 2007 Nov 13
7. Gopakumar A, Gopakumar V. Stanley L Drummond-Jackson. Pioneer of intravenous anaesthesia in dentistry. SAAD Dig. 2011;27:61–5.
8. Krohner RG. Anesthetic considerations and techniques for oral and maxillofacial surgery. Int Anesthesiol Clin. 2003;41(3):67–89. https://doi.org/10.1097/00004311-200341030-00007.
9. Abdelmalak B, Riad I. Chapter 1 evolution of anesthesiology as a clinical discipline: a lesson in developing professionalism. In: Longnecker DE, Brown DL, Newman MF, Zapol WM, editors. Anesthesiology. New York: McGraw Hill; 2012.

2 Oral and Maxillofacial Anatomy

Ming Xia

2.1 Systematic Anatomy of Oral Cavity

2.1.1 The Bones

Human skull lies above the spine and consists of 23 bones. The skull is divided into two parts: the viscerocranium and the neurocranium. There are eight cranial bones, including paired temporal bones and parietal bones, unpaired frontal bone, sphenoid bone, ethmoid bone, and occipital bone, together forming the cranial cavity and accommodating the brain tissue. There are 15 bones of facial cranium, including paired nasal bones, lacrimal bones, maxillary bones, palatine bones, inferior nasal bones, and unpaired mandible, vomer, and hyoid bone, forming a facial framework, among which the mandibles and paired temporal bones form a movable mandibular joint, enabling the mandible to function in complex oral physiological motions [1, 9]. In this chapter, only bones of facial cranium and bones like sphenoid bone, temporal bones, etc. that are closely related to the oral surgery shall be concerned.

2.1.1.1 The Maxilla

At the middle of face lies maxilla, one is on the left and the other is on the right. The two maxillary bones are fused at the intermaxillary suture, forming the anterior nasal spine to support the midface. Maxilla consists of five parts, including the body of the maxilla and four processes (frontal, zygomatic, palatine, and alveolar). The body has four surfaces. The upper face is opposite to the orbital cavity and contains the infraorbital canal, which is attached posteriorly to the infraorbital sulcus and leads forward to the infraorbital foramen; the posterior face is opposite to the inferior temporal fossa, also called the infratemporal, with its lower elevation, called the maxillary tubercle; the medial face is also called the nasal face, through which the air-containing cavity in the maxilla, the maxillary sinus, is visible; the anterior face is opposite to the face with the infraorbital foramen. In the maxilla, the frontal process extends upwards from the anterior medial side to join the frontal bone, medially to the nasal bone and laterally to the lacrimal bone; the alveolar process extends downwards with a socket for the roots of the teeth; the zygomatic process extends outwards to join the zygomatic bone; and the horizontal palatal process extends medially, with the palatal processes of both maxillae joining to form the anterior part of the hard palate, the posterior edge of which meets the horizontal plate of the palate [2].

There is a cavity in the maxillary body, namely the maxillary sinus. Each maxillary sinus leads to the middle nasal meatus of the nasal cavity, the opening of which is the maxillary hiatus. Like the

M. Xia (✉)
Department of Anesthesiology, Shanghai Ninth People's Hospital Affiliated to Shanghai Jiao Tong University School of Medicine, Shanghai, China
e-mail: xiaming1980@xzhmu.edu.cn

H. Jiang, M. Xia (eds.), *Anesthesia for Oral and Maxillofacial Surgery*,
https://doi.org/10.1007/978-981-19-7287-4_2

maxillary bone, the maxillary sinuses are pyramid-shaped with the apex extending toward the zygomatic bone. Inflammation and infection of the maxillary sinuses is not an uncommon condition, for the bone wall at the bottom of the maxillary sinus is thin and very close to the radix dentis of the posterior teeth. The infection of the root apex might spread upward, resulting in odontogenic maxillary sinusitis. Tumors and other lesions in the maxillary sinus can sometimes present with symptoms such as tooth pain and loosening. Sometimes careless tooth extraction might even have oral cavity and maxillary sinus perforated or broken radix dentis fracture pushed into the maxillary sinus. Therefore, these anatomical features and clinical significances should be noted.

The upper part of maxilla takes part in the formation of the borders of the inferior orbital fissure in the floor of the orbit, while the lower part of it and some other bones shall form the roof of oral cavity. The orbital fissure transmits several vessels and nerves, including the maxillary nerve or its continuation, the infraorbital nerve. The infraorbital nerve proceeds anteriorly to enter the face through the infraorbital foramen. The infraorbital foramen, an opening in the maxilla inferior to the orbit, allows passage of the infraorbital blood vessels and nerve, a branch of the maxillary division of the trigeminal nerve. Another prominent foramen in the maxilla is the incisive foramen just posterior to the incisor teeth. It transmits branches of the greater palatine blood vessels and nasopalatine nerve. A final structure associated with the maxilla and sphenoid bone is the inferior orbital fissure, located between the greater wing of the sphenoid and the maxilla. These specific bone landmarks should be especially paid attention to.

2.1.1.2 The Mandible

The mandible sits beneath the maxilla, is the largest bone in the human skull, and is the only mobile bone of the skull, which also supports the lower teeth. Mandible can be divided into two parts: a body and two rami. The body of mandible is the anterior portion of the mandible and is grafted to the ramus on each side.

Structurally, the body of mandible comprises of two surfaces and two borders. The two surfaces are external surface and internal surface. The external surface consists of symphysis menti, mental foramen, oblique line, and incisive fossa. Symphysis menti lies in the median of the external surface, below which there exists two mental tubercles. Between the premolar teeth or below the second molar, slightly above the upper and lower margins of the mandibular body, there is the mental foramen. The external oblique line is the bone crest runs from the mental tubercle through the mental foramen posteriorly up to the anterior margin of the mandibular ramus, where the depressor labii inferioris muscle and depressor anguli oris muscle attach. On the internal surfaces, near the midline, there are two pairs of protrusions, called the upper and lower mandible spines respectively. From below the mandible spines, the bone crest slopes upwards posteriorly and corresponds to the external oblique line, called the internal oblique line, where the mylohyoid muscle attaches. Above the internal oblique line lies the sublingual fossa. Below the internal oblique line, on either side of the midline near the inferior border of the mandibular body, there is the digastric fossa, which is the beginning of the anterior digastric muscle. Posteriorly and inferiorly to the digastric fossa there is the submandibular fossa [3].

The mandibular branch, also called the mandibular ramus, is the second largest part of the mandible after the mandible body and has two surfaces, four borders, and two processes. Two surfaces refer to the lateral (external) surface and medial (internal) surface. Four borders include superior border, inferior border, posterior border, and anterior border. And two processes are coronoid and condyloid processes. On the internal surface near the middle is a funnel-shaped opening called the mandibular foramen, through which the mandibular canal can be accessed, and the canal curves forward and downward through the mandibular body to the mental foramen. On the anterior medial side of the mandibular foramen is a thin triangular piece of bone called the mandibular lingula, where the sphenomandibular ligament attaches. Posteriorly above the foramen is the mandibular nerve sulcus, which is positioned approximately 1 cm above the mandibular molars plane. Anteriorly above the foramen is the torus mandibularis, a bony crest where the coronoid process and the condyle process converge. The surface of this torus is lined from anterior to posterior by the buccal, lingual, and inferior alveolar nerves. Descending anteriorly from the backside of mandibular lingula is the mylohyoid groove, which contains the mylohyoideus. Posteriorly below the mandibular lingula there is the pterygoid tuberosity, to which the medial pterygoid attaches. On the anterior part of the internal surface, a bony prominence develops from the medial of the coronoid process and diverges in two anteriorly and inferiorly to the posterior edge of the alveolus, called the buccinator crest. The triangle enclosed by the buccinator crest and the posterior edge of the alveolus is called the retromolar triangle. The angle of the mandible, also known as the gonial angle, is where the body of mandible and the rami intersect.

2.1.1.3 The Palatine Bone

The palatine bone is a thin paired bone that shapes like an "L," which participates in the formation of the nasal and oral cavities, as well as the pterygopalatine fossa. The palatine bone consists of two plates—horizontal plate and perpendicular plate.

2.1.1.4 The Sphenoid Bone

The sphenoid bone makes up most of the middle part of the base of the skull and contributes to the floor of the middle cranial fossa of the skull. The sphenoid bone consists of four parts: a body, two greater wings, two lesser wings, and pterygoid processes. The greater wings contain two important openings near their roots: the foramen rotundum and the foramen ovale. The foramen rotundum transmits the maxillary nerve, while the foramen ovale allows the passage of the mandibular nerve, accessory meningeal artery, lesser petrosal nerve, and emissary vein. The pterygoid processes contain the starting point of the extension of internal pterygoid muscle and ectopterygoid.

2.1.1.5 The Temporal Bone

The temporal bones are paired bones that sit between the occipital bone and the parietal bone and help make up the sides and base of the skull. Each temporal bone is composed of five parts: the squama, the petrous, mastoid, and tympanic parts.

2.1.2 The Temporomandibular Joint

2.1.2.1 The Formation

The temporomandibular joint (TMJ) is the articulation of the mandible and the temporal bone of the cranium, which is composed of mandibular condyle, articular surface of temporal bone, articular disk located in between and joint capsule and ligaments surrounding the joint [4].

2.1.2.2 The Movements

The movements of the joint are dominated by the muscles of mastication, and the hyoid muscles. According to the basic function, the temporomandibular joint movements can be divided into three categories: the anterior and posterior movements; the opening and closing; the lateral deviation. These three basic movements are achieved by rotation and translation of the joint.

2.1.3 The Muscles

The muscles of the oral, maxillofacial, and cervical regions are composed of four parts: the muscles of facial expression, the muscles of mastication, cervical muscle, and palatine muscles.

2.1.3.1 The Muscles of Facial Expression

The muscles of facial expression are flat and thin cutaneous muscles, most of which are originated from the bony surface of the skull or fascia and ending at the skin. Those muscles can deliver expressions of joy, anger, sadness, and happiness when moving in concert. The muscles of facial expression can broadly be divided into five groups: the orbital, nasal, oral, aural, and cranial (Table 2.1) [5].

Table 2.1 The sections of muscles and corresponding nomenclature

Groups	Nomenclature
Muscles of the mouth (buccolabial group)	Superficial layer: Levator labii superioris alaeque nasi, levator labii superioris, zygomaticus major, zygomaticus minor muscles, risorius, levator anguli oris, depressor anguli oris Deep layer: Levator anguli oris, depressor labii inferioris, buccinator muscle
Muscles of the eyelid (orbital group)	Orbicularis oculi, corrugator supercilii muscle
Muscles of the nose (nasal group)	Nasalis, compressor naris, musculi dilator naris, musculus depressor septi nasi, musculus procerus
Muscles of the external ear (auricular group)	Auricularis superior, auricularis anterior muscle, auricularis posterior
Muscles of the cranium (epicranial group)	Occipitofrontalis, temporoparietalis

2.1.3.2 The Masticatory Muscles

Although various muscles in the head and neck participate in the masticatory movement, generally the masticatory muscles simply refer to masseter muscle, temporal muscle, lateral pterygoid muscle, and medial pterygoid muscle. Its specific functions are elevation and protrusion of the mandible, as well as providing support to the articular capsule of the temporomandibular joint when speaking or chewing [6]. The origin and end, blood supply, and innervation of the masticatory muscles can be seen in Table 2.2.

2.1.3.3 The Muscles of Neck

Based on the position of muscles in the neck, the muscles of the neck are composed of three major muscle groups: the superficial neck muscles, the suprahyoid and infrahyoid muscles in the anterior cervical area, and prevertebral muscles of the neck.

2.1.3.4 The Muscular Palate and Muscles of Pharynx

The soft palate is composed of five pairs of muscles that enable it to move: The tensor veli palatine, levator veli palatine, palatoglossus muscles, palatopharyngeus muscles, and musculus uvulae. The function of the palate is to open and close the nasopharynx or eustachian tube. The muscles of pharynx consist of six groups: the superior pharyngeal constrictor muscle, middle pharyngeal constrictor muscle, inferior pharyngeal constrictor muscle, palatopharyngeus muscle, salpingopharyngeus muscle, and stylopharyngeus muscle. The function of the pharyngeal constrictor muscles is to elevate the larynx, shorten the pharynx, and push the food bolus down from the oral cavity and into the esophagus, while the other muscle groups act on the elevation of the pharynx and closing of the laryngeal aperture.

2.1.4 The Salivary Gland

2.1.4.1 The Parotid Glands

The parotid glands are the largest paired salivary glands, which are situated in the preauricular area on each side of the face, below the zygomatic arch, in the anterior lower part of the external auditory canal, mostly in the fossa retromandibularis, and is cuneiform and wrapped in fascia. The parotid glands weigh around 15–30 grams each. Each gland is irregular and divided into a superficial and a deep lobe by traversing by the facial nerve. The saliva secreted by the parotid gland is serosity in nature, flowing through stensen duct to the buccal mucosa of the vestibulum oris [7].

2.1.4.2 The Submandibular Glands

The submandibular glands are flat-oval-shaped glands that are situated in the submandibular triangle, located underneath the medial mandible, between the hyoglossus and styloglossus. The submandibular gland's excretory duct originates at the submandibular gland hilum and runs along the gland, eventually opening into the oral cavity at the sublingual caruncula [7].

2.1.4.3 The Sublingual Glands

The sublingual glands are the smallest of the three major pairs of head salivary glands, which look like apricot pit and weigh about 3 g each.

Table 2.2 Origin and end, blood supply, and innervation of masticatory muscles

Nomenclature	Origin point	Ending point	Blood supply	Innervation	Function
Masseter muscle	The maxillary process of the zygomatic bone and the inferior border of the zygomatic arch	The ramus of mandible and lateral gonial angle	A branch of the maxillary artery	The masseteric nerve	Elevation and protrusion of mandible
Temporal muscle	Temporal fossa (up to inferior temporal line) and temporal fascia	The coronoid process and the anterior border of the ramus of mandible	Deep temporal branches of maxillary artery, middle temporal branches from superficial temporal artery	Deep temporal branches of the anterior trunk of the mandibular nerve.	Elevation, retrusion, and side-to-side movements of mandible
Medial pterygoid muscle	The medial surface of the lateral pterygoid plate of sphenoid bone, the pyramidal process of palatine bone and the maxillary tuberosity	The ramus of mandible and medial mandible	The pterygoid and buccal branches of maxillary artery	The medial pterygoid branches of mandibular nerve.	Elevation and side-to-side movements of the mandible
Lateral pterygoid muscle	The infratemporal surface and infratemporal crest of the greater wing of sphenoid bone, and the lateral surface of the lateral pterygoid plate of sphenoid bone	The superior head: The anteromedial part of the articular capsule and articular disc of the temporomandibular joint. The inferior head: The pterygoid fovea on the neck of the condyloid process of mandible	The pterygoid branches of the maxillary artery	The nerve to lateral pterygoid muscle	Pull the mandibular condyle and articular disc anteriorly, achieving protrusion and depression of the mandible; participate in the side-to-side movements of the jaw

The sublingual glands lie bilaterally in the floor of the mouth and within the sublingual folds, close to sublingual gland fossa. The saliva secreted by sublingual glands are mucous saliva. There are 8–12 ducts secreting saliva along the margin of the sublingual folds, whereas the other part of saliva opens into the sublingual meatus through the major sublingual duct [7].

2.1.5 The Vessel

2.1.5.1 The Artery

The arterial blood supply to the maxillofacial region mainly comes from the external carotid artery, which is a branch of the common carotid artery. The minor part of the arterial blood supply from the branch of the arteria clavicularis.

The Common Carotid Artery

The common carotid artery is divided into internal and external carotid arteries at the height of the thyroid cartilage. There are two specialized structures at the bifurcation of the common carotid artery: (1) the carotid sinus, which is an enlarged part of the beginning of the internal carotid artery, and there are specific baroreceptors on the sinus wall. When blood pressure rises, it can reflexively slow down the heart rate and reduce blood pressure when being stimulated by pressure; (2) the carotid body, which is brown in a shape of flat oval, is connected to the posterior wall of the bifurcation of the common carotid artery by connective tissue. The carotid body is a chemoreceptor, which senses the content of carbon dioxide in the blood. When the concentration of carbon dioxide in the blood increases, it reflexively deepens and fastens the respiration [8].

The External Carotid Artery

The external carotid artery originates from the bifurcation of the common carotid artery, starting first on the medial side of the internal carotid artery, passing through the posterior biventer and the deep stylohyoid muscle, penetrates the parenchyma of the parotid gland, and travels to the inner posterior part of the mandibular condyle in the neck. The external carotid artery gives off several side branches that can be subdivided into three groups: the anterior, posterior, and medial branches. The anterior branches include the superior thyroid, lingual and facial arteries; the posterior branches include occipital and posterior auricular arteries; the medial branch is ascending pharyngeal artery. The terminal branches of the external carotid artery are the superficial temporal artery and the maxillary artery. The external carotid arteries shall supply blood to the face and neck regions via these eight branches.

Among the branches, the lingual, facial, maxillary, and superficial temporal arteries are the main ones that are frequently involved in clinical practices. The lingual artery is the anteriorly directed branch of the external carotid artery and is the main blood supply artery to the tongue and also supplies the floor of the mouth. The facial artery usually passes through the deep surface of the mandibular marginal branch of the facial nerve, travels in a tortuous line superiorly to the medial canthus via the corners of the mouth and the lateral aspect of the nose, and changes to the medial canthal artery. At the intersection of the inferior border of the mandible and the anterior border of the occlusal muscle, the pulsation of the facial artery can be palpated, and this can be compressed to stop bleeding in case of superficial facial bleeding. The maxillary artery, also known as the internal maxillary artery, is one of the two terminal branches of the external carotid artery and is mainly located in the oral cavity, nasal cavity, teeth, masticatory muscles, and dura mater. It begins at the deep surface of the mandibular neck, and enters the orbit through the superficial surface of the extrapontine muscles via the pterygopalatine fossa from the inferior orbital fissure, renamed the infraorbital artery. The superficial temporal artery runs anteriorly up the external auditory meatus, over the root of the zygomatic arch to the frontal subcutis, branching to the parotid gland and the soft tissues of the frontal, temporal, and apical areas. In vivo, the pulsation of the superficial temporal artery can be felt above the anterior part of the external auditory meatus and at the root of the zygomatic arch, where it can be compressed to stop bleeding in the anterior part of the scalp.

The Internal Carotid Artery

The internal carotid artery is a major branch of the common carotid artery, supplying blood for several parts of the head, especially the brain. The internal carotid artery originates from the common carotid artery of fossa carotica, travel through the carotid sheath in a superior direction along the neck, and enter the skull through the external opening of carotid canal. Along its course, the internal carotid artery gives rise to ophthalmic arteries, anterior cerebral arteries, and middle cerebral arteries.

The Subclavian Artery

Depending on the side of the body, the subclavian arteries have two origins: the aortic arch on the left and the brachiocephalic trunk on the right. Both sides come from the anteromedial aspect of the apex pulmonis to the upper opening of the thorax, to the root of neck. The cervical part of both the arteries has similar course. They arche laterally across the anterior surface of the cervical pleura to the first rib posterior to the scalenus anterior muscle. At the outer border of the first rib, it continues as axillary artery. The main branches are vertebral artery, thyroid axis, and the truncus costocervicalis.

The Arterial Anastomosis in Head and Neck

Perioral artery circle: the superior and inferior labial arteries given rise to by facial arteries.

The floor of the mouth: the sublingual arteries given rise to by lingual arteries and the submental arteries given rise to by facial arteries.

The mentum: the arteries given rise to by inferior alveolar arteries and the inferior labial arteries given rise to by facial arteries.

The malar surface: the transverse facial arteries and facial arteries given rise to by superficial temporal arteries and the infraorbital arteries.

The orbital region: the bifurcation of angular artery and ophthalmic artery.

The vertexal region: both sides of superficial temporal arteries.

Intra-thyroid area: the superior thyroid artery of the external carotid artery and the inferior thyroid artery originated from subclavian artery.

The occiput: the occipital artery and deep and transverse cervical artery.

2.1.5.2 The Veins

The oral and maxillofacial veins can be roughly divided into two networks of deep and superficial veins. Facial veins are characterized by few venous valves, blood is prone to reflux infection, and infection in the danger triangle can easily cause cavernous sinus thrombophlebitis.

The Superficial Veins in the Oral and Maxillofacial Region

The anterior facial vein: being originated from angular veins, the anterior facial vein merges with the anterior branch of the retromandibular vein to form the common facial vein at the anterior inferior part of gonial angle, which joins the internal jugular vein.

The superficial temporal vein: is a blood vessel that arises from the plexus of veins that anastomose across the scalp. The superficial temporal vein descends along the auricular anterior surface, joining with the maxillary vein at the level of mandibular neck to continues further as the retromandibular vein, which drains into the internal or external jugular vein.

The Deep Vein of Oral and Maxillofacial Region

The pterygoid plexus: also called pterygoid venous plexus, is located in the infratemporal fossa, distributed in the venous plexus among the temporalis and the medial and lateral pterygoid muscles, and finally converges into the maxillary vein.

The maxillary vein: also known as internal maxillary vein, is located in the infratemporal fossa collecting blood from the pterygoid plexus, and converges into the retromandibular vein.

The retromandibular vein: also called the posterior facial vein, is located in the parenchyma of the parotid gland behind the mandibular condyle, and is formed by the superficial temporal vein and the maxillary vein. It passes through the lower pole of the parotid gland and descends to the angle of the mandible where it divides into two branches, the anterior and the posterior. The anterior branch merges with the facial vein to form the common facial vein, and the posterior branch merges with the posterior auricular vein to form the external jugular vein.

The common facial vein: is located in the carotid triangle and formed by the confluence of the facial vein and the anterior branch of the retromandibular vein, which crosses the hypoglossal nerve and the internal and external jugular veins posteriorly and merges into the internal jugular vein at the deep surface of the sternocleidomastoid muscle at the large angle of the flat hyoid bone. The common facial vein can also remerge into the internal jugular vein through the external jugular vein.

Superficial Jugular Veins

External jugular vein: is located in the deep surface of the platysma and formed by the confluence of the posterior branch of the retromandibular vein and the posterior auricular vein at the angle of the mandible in the parotid gland. The external jugular vein passes through the superficial layer of the deep cervical fascia to the deep and merges into the subclavian vein or the internal jugular vein.

The anterior jugular vein is originated from the superficial vein at the hyoid bone in the anterior neck, goes down the anterior midline of the neck to the lower part of the neck, turns outward, and merges into the external jugular vein through the deep surface of the sternocleidomastoid muscle.

Deep Jugular Veins

The internal jugular vein: is the main course of the venous return in the head and neck. It is located in the posterior and lateral side of the internal carotid artery, and travels in the carotid sheath along the lateral side of the common carotid artery to merge with the subclavian vein to form the brachiocephalic vein.

The subclavian vein: starts from the axillary vein and joins with internal jugular vein in the posterior part of sternoclavicular joint to form the brachiocephalic vein. The angle between the subclavian vein and the internal jugular vein is the jugular venous angle.

2.1.6 The Lymph Node and Lymphatic Vessel

The lymphatics of the head and neck shall be divided into two groups: the annular groups and the vertical groups, which are listed in Tables 2.3 and 2.4.

2.1.7 The Nerve

2.1.7.1 The Trigeminal Nerve

The trigeminal nerves (CN V) are the largest paired cranial nerves. While being the main sensory nerve of the oral maxillofacial region, it also mingles in the realm of motor supply to control mastication. It has four nuclei that send fibers to form its tracts and three sensory nerve branches—the ophthalmic nerve (CN V1 or Va), the maxillary nerve (CN V2 or Vb), and the mandibular nerve (CN V3 or Vc), which shall converge in the trigeminal nerve at an area called the trigeminal ganglion to bring sensory information into the brain.

The Ophthalmic Nerve

The ophthalmic branch is the first division of the trigeminal nerve. It branches out the frontal nerve, the lacrimal nerve, and the nasociliary nerve, which further split out small branches and all of them are situated in and around the eye, nose, forehead, and scalp. Before joining the

Table 2.3 The annular lymphatic groups

Structure	Location	The influenced area	Regions drained
Occipital lymph nodes	Start of the occipital bone at the cucullaris	Occipital region	Superficial cervical and accessory nodes
Retroauricular lymph nodes	Near the superior point of sternocleidomastoid muscle	Parietotemporal and retroauricular region	Superficial and deep cervical nodes
Parotid lymph nodes	Inside the parotid glands	Parotid glands and their proximity	Superior deep cervical nodes
Facial lymph nodes	Buccal region	Facial region	Submandibular lymph nodes
Submandibular lymph nodes	Submaxillary triangle	Intraoral region, floor of the mouth and nearby regions	Superior deep cervical nodes
Submental lymph nodes	Submental triangle	Labium and mentum, etc.	Submandibular lymph nodes and superior deep cervical nodes

Table 2.4 The vertical lymphatic groups

Structure	Location	The influenced area	Regions drained
Retropharyngeal lymph nodes	Retropharyngeal space	Pharynx and its surrounding lymph	Superior deep cervical nodes
Perivisceral lymph nodes	Around the neck organs	Cervical organ lymph	Deep cervical nodes
Superior deep cervical nodes	Above the omohyoid, along the internal jugular vein	Lymphatic efferent duct of annular groups	Inferior deep cervical nodes and jugular lymphatic trunk
Inferior deep cervical nodes	Below the omohyoid, along the internal jugular vein	All the lymphatic efferent duct of vertical groups	Jugular lymphatic trunk
Accessory nodes	Along the accessory nerve	Occipital lateral cervical lymph	Inferior deep cervical nodes
Supraclavicular lymph nodes	Along transverse cervical vessel	Subclavian lymphatic efferent duct	Inferior deep cervical nodes
Inferior cervical nodes	Below the hyoid bone and around the anterior jugular vein	Anterior cervical skin and muscle	Inferior deep cervical nodes
Superficial cervical nodes	Around the external jugular vein superficial to the sternocleidomastoid muscle	Annular lymph nodes passing through the lateral skin	Superior deep cervical nodes

main branch of the trigeminal nerve, the ophthalmic nerve stretches to the skull through a small opening, namely the superior orbital fissure.

The Maxillary Nerve

The maxillary division of the trigeminal nerve (CN V2) starts from the anterolateral trigeminal ganglion and enters into the skull through an opening called the foramen rotundum. The maxillary nerve detects sensation in the middle part of the face, and this sensory area is often described as V2. The maxillary nerve has five main branches: the middle meningeal nerve, zygomatic nerve, sphenopalatine nerve, Pterygopalatine nerves, posterior superior alveolar nerves, and infraorbital nerve.

The Mandibular Nerve

The mandibular division is the largest component of the trigeminal nerve, which carries both sensory and motor stimuli. The sensory information is carried from the lower third of the face which includes the lower lip, the jaw, the preauricular area, the temporal area, and the meninges of the anterior and middle cranial fossa. Meanwhile, the mandibular nerve also in charge of the motor innervation of the muscles of mastication, the mylohyoid, tensor tympani, tensor veli palatini muscles, and the anterior belly of the digastric muscle.

The mandible nerve and its branches run past the ear and the temporomandibular joint, then spread out through the lower part of face. The main branches stemming from the mandibular nerve include medial pterygoid nerve (motor), lateral pterygoid nerve (motor), masseteric nerve (motor), deep temporal nerve (motor), meningeal branch (sensory), buccal nerve (sensory), auriculotemporal nerve (sensory), and lingual nerve (sensory). The motor components as marked above run as a single, slender, nerve fiber along with the larger sensory fibers. They pass through the external opening of the foramen ovale and head toward Meckel's cave. Before breaking in the trigeminal ganglion, the mandible nerve obtains the recurrent meningeal nerve carrying afferent stimuli from the dura.

2.1.7.2 The Facial Nerve

The facial nerve is a kind of mixed nerve with three types of fiber component— motor, sensory, and autonomic fibers. Among these nerves of various function, the motor nerve is responsible for facial expression muscles, posterior belly of digastric muscle, stylohyoid muscle, and stapedius muscle; the special sensory contributes to the taste from anterior two-thirds of the tongue; the Parasympathetic innervates the submandibular gland, sublingual gland, and lacrimal glands.

The facial nerve is originated from pons of the brainstem and can be divided into facial nerve canal segment and the extracranial segment, bounded by the intracranial branches consist of greater petrosal nerve, communicating branch with otic ganglion, nerve to stapedius and chorda tympani. The extracranial branches include posterior auricular nerve, branch to posterior digastric belly, branch to stylohyoid muscle, temporal branch, zygomatic branch, buccal branch, marginal mandibular branch, and cervical branch.

2.1.7.3 The Glossopharyngeal Nerve

The glossopharyngeal nerve is originated from the brainstem and exits the cranium from the jugular foramen, giving rises to the following main branches: the tympanic nerve, carotid sinus nerve, pharyngeal nerves, muscular branch to stylopharyngeus, tonsilar branch, and lingual nerves.

The glossopharyngeal nerve is a sort of mixed type that consists both of the motor and sensory fibers. There are four neuronal fibers of this nerve: the somatic sensory, visceral sensory, special sensory, parasympathetic and motor fibers. The somatic sensory fibers provide the sensory input from the posterior one-third of the tongue, palatine tonsils, oropharynx, mucosa of the middle ear, pharyngotympanic tube, and the mastoid air cells; the visceral sensory fibers carry the sensory information from the carotid body; the parasympathetic fibers innervate the salivary parotid gland; the motor fibers innervate the stylopharyngeus muscle and the superior pharyngeal constrictor muscle from the third pharyngeal arch.

2.1.7.4 The Vagus Nerve

Among all those cranial nerves, the vagus nerve has the longest path and is the most widely distributed mixed nerve. The branches of the vagus nerve in the neck are: (a) pharyngeal branch, which innervates the pharyngeal constrictor muscle and soft palate muscle; (b) superior laryngeal branch, which innervates the mucosal sensation of cricothyroid muscle and that near the root of tongue and the glottic fissure; and c. recurrent laryngeal nerves, which innervate the laryngeal muscle and mucosal sensation below the glottic fissure.

The vagus nerve gives off the recurrent laryngeal nerve, which originates from the thoracic segment of the vagus trunk but immediately returns to the neck and is the main motor nerve of the laryngeal muscle, divided into the left and right recurrent laryngeal nerves.

In addition to the recurrent laryngeal nerve, the other major motor nerve in the vagus branch is the superior laryngeal nerve. The superior laryngeal nerve is divided into inner and outer branches at a height equivalent to the greater horn of the hyoid bone. The external branch is mainly a motor nerve and the internal branch is mainly a sensory nerve.

2.1.7.5 The Hypoglossal Nerve

The hypoglossal nerve is the motor nerve of the tongue, which innervates extrinsic tongue muscles and geniohyoid muscle. It originates from hypoglossal nucleus in medulla oblongata and gives rises to meningeal branch, superior root of the ansa cervicalis, and terminal lingual nerves. Once there is hypoglossal nerve injury on one side, the tip of tongue will tilt to the injured side when it is extended.

2.1.7.6 The Accessory Nerve

The accessory nerve is motor nerve. The cranial division of it originates from the medulla oblongata of the brainstem and exits the cranium through the jugular foramen. The accessory nerve innervates the muscle of sternocleidomastoid, trapezius, and larynx.

2.1.7.7 The Cervical Plexus and Cervical Sympathetic Trunk

The Cervical Plexus

The cervical plexus is a conglomeration of cervical nerves formed by the anterior rami of 1st–

fourth cervical nerves. The cervical plexus is located on the anterior side of the mediscalenus and the levator scapulae muscle, deep to the sternocleidomastoid muscle. Two branches are given off by cervical plexus—the superficial branch and the deep branch. The superficial branches are sensory branches, which can be divided into four parts: the lesser occipital nerve, great auricular nerve, transverse cervical nerve, and supraclavicular nerve. The deep branches are motor branches, which passes superficially and medially down the scalenus anterior muscle, through the subclavian artery and vein to the thoracic cavity, and finally innervates the diaphragm muscle.

The Cervical Sympathetic Trunk

The cervical sympathetic trunk has three ganglia: superior, middle, and inferior ganglia, which is located in front of the cervical transverse and on the deep surface of prevertebral fascia. Once the cervical sympathetic trunk gets injured, Horner's sign might appear.

2.2 The Regional Anatomy of the Oral Cavity

2.2.1 The Oral Cavity

2.2.1.1 The Realm and Distribution of Oral Cavity

The oral cavity is the beginning of digestive system, leading upwards to the outside of human body through the oral fissure enclosed by the upper and lower lips and backward to connect to the pharynx by the oropharyngeal isthmus, hence completing eating procedure and mechanical digestion. Inside the oral cavity are salivary glands that also participate in food digestion by secreting enzymes that start the digestion of carbohydrates. These glands are the parotid, submandibular, and sublingual glands [10].

The cavity is separated into anterior and posterior parts by the teeth, gingiva, and mucosa of alveolar process. The anterior part—the oral vestibule, lies anteriorly to the teeth and behind the lips, whereas the posterior part—the oral cavity proper, refers to the area behind the teeth.

Oral Vestibule

The oral vestibule is the horseshoe-like shaped area bounded externally by the lips and cheeks and internally by the teeth and gingiva and the inner aspect of the cheeks. It connects the external environment with the oral cavity proper.

Oral Cavity Proper

The oral cavity proper is the area behind the teeth. The oral cavity proper extends from the maxilla's and mandible's alveolar arches to the entry into the oral part of the pharynx (oropharynx) posteriorly. The oral cavity proper contains the tongue, soft and hard palate, and three pairs of salivary glands such as parotid, sublingual, and submandibular glands. The tongue fills the oral cavity proper.

2.2.1.2 The Lips

The realm of lips: The lip anatomy consists of two parts—the upper and lower body. The upper lip's superior border goes along the nasal septum base while the lower lips along the mentolabial groove. Both lips are laterally connected in the place called oral or lateral commissures forming the corners of the lips, and these two lateral angle are the two sides of the lips. The lips define the boundary, namely the vermillion border, that separate both lip bodies from the facial skin.

The surface marker of the lips: the vermilion of the lip, vermilion border of lip, cupid bow, philtrum notch, Glogau-Klein points, the labial tubercle, philtrum, and philtrum column.

The lips can be divided into five layers from the shallower to the deeper: the skin, superficial fascia, muscularis, submucosa, and mucosa.

2.2.1.3 The Cheeks

The realm of cheeks: the superior border is the lower margin of the zygomatic bone and zygomatic arch, the inferior border is the lower margin of the mandibular bone, the anteromedial border of the mandibular bone, and the posterior border is the anterior margin of the masseter.

The cheeks can be divided into six layers from the shallower to the deeper: the skin, subcutaneous tissue, buccal fascia, buccinators, submucosa, and mucosa.

2.2.1.4 The Teeth

The teeth are a structure found in many vertebrates, and teeth are the hardest organ in the human body.

Each tooth is divided into three parts: the crown, the root, and the neck. The crown is the part of the tooth that is exposed outside the gums and is white and shiny; the root is embedded in the socket and is firmly connected to the alveolar bone by the periodontium, and there is a hole at the tip of the root, called the apical foramen, which is connected to the crown cavity by the root canal and contains blood vessels, nerves, and lymphatic vessels. The periodontium, alveolar bone and gingiva are together called periodontal tissue, which protects, fixes, and nourishes the tooth.

The structure of the tooth is mainly composed of dentin, enamel, bone, and pulp. The dense and hard dentin, which forms the main body of the tooth, is located inside the tooth. At the root of the tooth, the dentin is wrapped with a layer of bonded material (bone), while at the surface of the crown there is white, shiny, hard enamel. The enamel is the most calcified and is the hardest tissue in the body. The crown cavity and the root canal together are called the cavity, which is filled with blood vessels, nerves, lymphatic vessels, and connective tissue called the pulp. Lactobacillus in the oral cavity can make sugar fermentation and acid production, resulting in enamel decalcification and cavity, which is called dental caries clinically. If the cavity deepens continuously and affects the nerve of the pulp, it can cause severe pain.

According to the different forms and functions of teeth, permanent teeth can be divided into incisors, cuspids, premolars, and molars. Milk teeth are divided into incisors, cuspids and molars.

Incisors are single-rooted teeth with flat, chisel-shaped crowns, mainly used for biting and cutting food; cuspids are also single-rooted teeth with vertebral-shaped crowns, used for biting and tearing food; premolars are also generally single-rooted teeth with nearly square crowns, used to assist the molars in grinding food; molars generally have three roots in the maxilla and two roots in the mandible, with square crowns, used to grind food.

2.2.1.5 The Gingiva

The gingiva refers to the mucosa covering alveolar arches of the maxilla and mandible, which has a pink color. There is no submucosa in the gingiva and the tunica propria is directly connected to the periosteum, which helps chewing in the oral cavity.

2.2.1.6 The Palate

The palate forms the superior wall of the oral cavity proper, which also separates the nasal from the oral cavity. The palate consists of two parts—the hard palate anterior and the soft palate posterior.

The Hard Palate

The hard palate dome-shaped, based on the bony palate and covered by a layer of mucous membrane tissue.

The hard palate composes two-thirds of the total palate area, which provides space for the tongue to move freely and supplies a rigid floor to the nasal cavity so that pressures within the mouth do not close off the nasal passage.

The surface marker of the hard palate: the median palatine suture, incisive papilla, palatine folds, hard area of the maxillary, maxillary process, and greater palatine foramen.

The Soft Palate

The soft palate is a mobile fold of soft tissue attached to the posterior margin of the hard palate, it is about 1 cm thick, and separates the oral cavity from the pharynx incompletely.

The surface marker of the soft palate: the foveola palatina, velum palatinum, palatine uvula, palatoglossal arch, palatopharyngeal arch, tonsillar fossa, and oropharyngeal isthmus.

Lying between the oral and nasal cavities, the soft palate composes one-third of the total palate area and features the oral and nasal surfaces. The soft palate forms the roof of the fauces, an area connecting the oral cavity and the pharynx. Two arches bind the palate to the tongue and pharynx; the palatoglossal arches anteriorly and the palatopharyngeal arches posteriorly.

The soft palate can be divided into four layers from the superficial to the deep: the mucosa, submucosa, palatine aponeurosis, and palatine muscle. The core of the soft palate consists of the palatine aponeurosis and five muscles of the soft palate, which are the musculus uvulae, tensor veli palatini, levator veli palatini, palatopharyngeus, and palatoglossus muscles.

2.2.1.7 The Pharynx

The pharynx is a hollow structure lined with moist tissue, which starts behind the nose, goes down the neck, and ends at the top of the trachea and esophagus. As a whole, the pharynx is about 5 cm in length and consists of three parts: the nasopharynx, oropharynx, and hypopharynx. The pharynx allows the air through the respiratory tract, and both circular constrictive muscles and longitudinal muscles surrounding the pharynx work together to send food and drink down to the esophagus.

The pharyngeal wall from the inside out into mucous layer, fibrous membrane, muscular layer, and outer membrane. The posterior pharyngeal tissue flap is formed by the first three layers.

2.2.1.8 The Tongue

The tongue is a mobile muscular organ that lies in the bottom of oral cavity and partly extends into the upper throat, which assists in the procedure of eating, tasting, swallowing, pronouncing, etc.

Tongue Morphology

The tongue has two sides, the curved upper surface is called dorsum, which can be divided into the posterior 2/3 of the tongue body and the back 1/3 of the tongue root with the V-shaped groove as terminal sulcus. The tongue may be further divided into right and left halves by the midline groove and just beneath the groove's surface lies the fibrous lingual septum. There is a foramen cecum at the tip of the sulcus, which is a remnant of the thyroglossal canal in embryonic life.

The lingual frenulum is the large midline fold of mucosa. The lower surface of the tongue is shorter than the dorsum of the tongue and its mucosa is smooth and floppy and converges with the mucosa of the floor of the mouth, facilitating the tongue tip to move freely. The posterior third of the tongue is the lingual root, which is located low in the mouth, near the throat, the position of which is comparatively fixed. Moreover, it is attached to the hyoid bone and the mandible (lower jaw) and quite near the hyoid and lingual muscles.

The Periglottis

The tongue is covered with moist, pink tissue called mucosa. Tiny bumps called papillae give the tongue its rough texture. These bumps vary in shape and location and are associated with taste buds. The muscles within and surrounding the tongue control its movement. There are four types of papillae—the vallate papillae, folate papillae, papillae, and fungiform papillae. Among these papillae, the last three types contain receptors for taste within taste buds. Filiform papillae are of the largest amount and only responsible for general sensation. The underside of the tongue is covered with a thin, transparent mucous membrane through which one can see the underlying veins.

The Muscles

The muscles of the tongue consist of intrinsic muscles and extrinsic muscles. The intrinsic muscles include the superior longitudinal, inferior longitudinal, transverse, and vertical muscles. The extrinsic muscles are composed of the genioglossus, hyoglossus, styloglossus, and palatoglossus.

The Nerves and Blood Supply of the Tongue

Our tongue can move, feel, and taste various flavors, which is possible because of nerves. The hypoglossal nerve is the most critical motor nerve to human's tongue, controlling almost all the muscles of the tongue, except for the palatoglossus muscle innervated by a branch of the pharyngeal plexus. The anterior two-thirds of the tongue's surface is in charge of sensation such as touch and feeling the temperature. Such function is supplied by the lingual nerve. A special sensation, taste is supplied by the chorda tympani nerve, a branch of the facial nerve. The back a third of the tongue can also supply sensation, but is controlled by the branch of the glossopharyngeal nerve. There is a small patch of the tongue in front of the epiglottis which gets its special sensation from the internal laryngeal nerve, branching from the vagus nerve.

The blood supply to the tongue comes mainly from the lingual artery, which is originated from the external carotid artery. The posterior third of the tongue has branches of the ascending pharyngeal artery. Venous drainage occurs in the accompanying veins of the lingual artery and the hypoglossal nerve. In the elderly, the sublingual veins may be enlarged and tortuous (varicose) but do not bleed, so such changes are deemed as clinically significant.

2.2.2 The Parotideomasseteric Region and Deep Lateral Aspect of Face

2.2.2.1 The Parotideomasseteric Region

The Realm

The anterior border of the parotideomasseteric region is the anterior margin masseter; the posterior border is the porus acousticus externus and mastoid process; the superior border is the acrus zygomaticus; the inferior border is the base of the mandible.

The Layers

From the superficial to the deep, this area can be divided into five layers: the skin, subcutaneous layer, superficial fascia, deep fascia, and spatium parotideum.

(a) **Skin** thick, hairy in men; innervated by auriculotemporal branch and great auricular branch from cervical plexus;
(b) **Subcutaneous layer** fat; superficial temporal artery, vein, and lymph nodes;
(c) **Superficial fascia** thin; not connected to bone;
(d) **Deep fascia** connected to zygomatic arch; covers the parotid gland;
(e) **Spatium parotideum** superficial muscles: masseter, medial pterygoid, and sternocleidomastoid; deep fascia; neurovascular bundles around the parotid gland: the posterior auricular nerve, the auricular branch facial nerve, parotid duct, transverse facial artery and vein, facial nerve, retromandibular, and carotid bifurcation.

2.2.2.2 The Deep Lateral Aspect of Face

The Realm

The anterior border lies at the back of maxilla, the posterior border is the parotid sheath, the inner border is the external pterygoid plate, and the outer border is the mandibular branch, which is the infratemporal space and the pterygomandibular space.

The Position Relation

Taking the lateral pterygoid muscle as a reference, the important surrounding blood vessels and nerves are as follows:

(a) Superficial surface of the lateral pterygoid muscle: the internal maxillary artery and its branches, pterygoid plexus.
(b) Superior margin of the lateral pterygoid muscle: deep temporal nerve and masseteric nerve.
(c) Between the superior and inferior heads of the lateral pterygoid muscle: the second segment of the buccal nerve and internal maxillary artery and the muscle branch that it gives rise to.
(d) Inferior margin of the lateral pterygoid muscle: the lingual nerve, inferior alveolar nerve, and auriculotemporal nerve.
(e) Deep surface of the lateral pterygoid muscle: the mandibular nerve and its branches.

2.2.3 Oral Maxillofacial Loose Connective Tissue Interspace

The oral and maxillofacial loose connective tissue interspace refers to the potential gaps located between fascia and muscle, muscle and periosteum, as well as between periosteum and periosteum. The loose connective tissue passes from one interspace to another, accompanied by neurovascular bundles, to make adjacent spaces open to each other.

2.2.3.1 The Infraorbital Space

The infraorbital space is located below the anterior part of the orbit, with the infraorbital margin as the superior border, the exognathion as the inferior border, the nasal lateral margin as the medial border, the zygomatic muscle as the lateral border, and the base is at the anterior maxillary wall centered with the canine fossa, with the superficial surface covered by facial expression muscles. The buccal cavity can be reached posteriorly, and there are facial veins and facial arteries passing through it.

The Buccal Cavity

The buccal cavity situated between the buccinator and masseter and is shaped like an inverted cone, with the front margin of buccinators as the anterior border and the front margin of ramus of mandible and temporalis as the back margin. Inside the space are buccal nerve, buccal artery, deep facial vein, and adipose tissue. This interspace is adjacent to the molars and is connected to the pterygomandibular, masseteric, infraorbital, infratemporal, and temporal space [11].

The Masseteric Space

The masseteric space located between masseter and ramus of mandible, with the front margin of masseter as the anterior border, the back margin of ramus of mandible or parotid tissues as the posterior border, the lower margin of zygomatic arch as the superior border and the portion attached to masseter as the inferior border. This space is open to pterygomandibular, buccal, temporal, and infratemporal space.

The Pterygomandibular Space

The pterygomandibular space located between the medial surface of the ramus of mandible and the medial pterygoid muscle. The anterior border is the temporalis and buccinators; the posterior border is parotid gland; the superior border is the lower margin of the lateral pterygoid muscle, and the inferior border is the portion of medial pterygoid muscle attached to the ramus of mandible. There is lingual nerve, inferior alveolar nerve, and vessel. This space is open to parapharyngeal, masseteric, sublingual, submandibular, and infratemporal space.

2.2.4 The Neck

2.2.4.1 The Border and Distribution

Triangles of the Neck

Neck triangles are spaces bordered by the neck muscles. There are two main triangles—the anterior and the posterior triangles of the neck.

The anterior triangle of the neck is made by the anterior border of the sternocleidomastoid muscle, the inferior border of the mandible, and the midline of the neck. The superior border of anterior triangle is the inferior margin of mandible, the medial border is the midline of neck and the lateral border is the anterior margin of sternocleidomastoid muscle. This triangle can be further divided into the submandibular triangle, submental triangle, muscular triangle, and carotid triangle.

Similarly, the posterior triangle is bounded by the posterior border of the sternocleidomastoid muscle, the anterior border of the trapezius muscle, and the middle third of the clavicle. The anterior border of the posterior triangle is the posterior edge of sternocleidomastoid muscle, the posterior border is the anterior edge of trapezius muscle, and inferiorly it is the middle one-third of clavicle. The posterior triangle can be subdivided into the occipital triangle and the omoclavicular triangle.

Additionally, in light of the position to the hyoid bone, the anterior triangle muscles are categorized as the suprahyoid and infrahyoid muscles. The posterior triangle connects with the upper limb; thus, muscles related to this area are sternocleidomastoid, trapezius, splenius capitis, levator scapulae, omohyoid, as well as the anterior, middle, and posterior scalene muscles.

2.2.4.2 Body Surface Symbol

The Hyoid Bone
The hyoid bone is a small horseshoe-shaped bone located in the front of your neck. It sits between the chin and the thyroid cartilage and is instrumental in the function of swallowing and tongue movements.

The Prominentia Laryngea
The prominentia laryngea located below the hyoid bone, especially in male. There is superior notch of thyroid cartilage at its upper margin.

The Cricoid Cartilage
The cricoid cartilage unpaired hyaline cartilage located in the larynx at C6 vertebral level. It sits on a level plane just below the thyroid gland and thyroid cartilage.

The Cervical Trachea
The cervical trachea located below cricoid cartilage, passing the anterior midline downwards to the superior margin of sternal manubrium.

The Sternocleidomastoid Muscle
The sternocleidomastoid muscle situated in the lateral part of the neck, starting from the sternoclavicular joint and the medial end of the clavicle and ending at the mastoid process obliquely and posteriorly. The anterior border is crossed by the external carotid artery, the internal carotid artery, and the internal jugular vein; the midpoint of the posterior border is where the cervical plexus concentrated superficially. There is external jugular vein crossing by in its superficial surface and the muscle is crossed by the accessory nerve. In the deep surface are common carotid artery, vagus nerve, and internal jugular vein.

The Supraclavicular Fossa
The supraclavicular fossa located above the middle 1/3 of the clavicle, and the pulsation of the subclavian artery can be palpated at its superior clavicular border.

The Suprasternal Fossa
The suprasternal fossa situated in the depression above the jugular vein incision of the sternum, and the trachea can be palpated.

2.2.4.3 The Cervical Fascia and Fascial Spaces
From the superficial to the deep, the cervical fascia can be divided into five layers. The human structures making up the neck are surrounded by a layer of subcutaneous tissue called the superficial cervical fascia, and are compartmentalized by a second group of fasciae referred to as deep cervical fascia, which also consists of three fascial layers: the investing layer of deep cervical fascia, pretracheal layer of deep cervical fascia, and prevertebral layer of deep cervical fascia.

Superficial Cervical Fascia
The superficial cervical fascia is a thin layer of subcutaneous connective tissue existing between the dermis of the skin and the investing layer of deep cervical fascia. Its unique feature is thin although it embraces the platysma muscle and coats the cutaneous nerves, blood and lymphatic vessels, superficial lymph nodes, and variable amounts of fat. It is divided into two layers in the submandibular triangle and the parotid area, which surround the submandibular and parotid glands, respectively, forming the fascial sheaths of both glands [12].

Deep Cervical Fascia
The deep cervical fascia is located on the deeper surface of the superficial fascia and the broad neck muscles, which surround the muscles, blood vessels, nerves, and organs of the neck, forming three layers: superficial, middle, and deep. The organs of the neck are separated from each other by it, with interstitial spaces filled with loose connective tissue, called fascial spaces. These layers also function to support the internal organs of the neck (such as the thyroid gland), the muscles, blood and lymphatic vessels, and the deep lymph nodes. Moreover, they form the carotid

sheath, which wraps around vessels such as the common carotid arteries, the internal jugular veins, and the vagus nerves. Importantly, they act as landmarks and natural planes through which tissues can be separated during surgery.

The Investing Layer of Deep Cervical Fascia

The investing layer of the deep cervical fascia refers to the superfacial layer of the deep cervical fascia. It surrounds the neck and attaches posteriorly to the ligamentum nuchae and the spinous process of the cervical vertebrae. Laterally and anteriorly, it first wraps around the trapezius and sternocleidomastoid muscles, and then covers the infrahyoid muscles from surface to the median line where it fuses with the opposite side, forming the cervical white line.

It attaches above to the neck line of the occipital bone and mastoid process and surrounds the parotid gland to form the parotid sheath; then below the mandible, it divides into two layers, wraps around the submandibular gland and attaches to the mandible, forming the submandibular sheath.

Below, it attaches to the acromion, clavicle, and manubrium sterni. Above the incisura jugularis, it splits into two layers, superficial and deep layers, which attach to the anterior and posterior edges of the incision, respectively. The gap between them is called the suprasternal space where the jugular arch and lymph nodes exist.

Pretracheal Layer of Deep Cervical Fascia

The pretracheal layer can be divided into the visceral layer and parietal layer. The visceral layer is thin and loose and wraps around the organs of the neck such as the larynx, trachea, thyroid, pharynx, and esophagus. The parietal layer is denser and lies in front of the organs of the neck, behind the infrahyoid muscles, and forms a carotid sheath on either side, encircling the common carotid artery, internal jugular vein, and vagus nerve.

The pretracheal space is formed between the visceral and parietal layers and contains loose connective tissue. The left and right inferior thyroid veins constitute the unpaired thyroid venous plexus that lies within the space. In young children, the lower part of the pretracheal space includes the upper thymus gland, which leads down to the anterior part of the upper mediastinum. Therefore, if there is an infection or bleeding in the anterior cervical tracheal space, it may travel down this space to the anterior mediastinum. If there is an emphysema in the anterior mediastinum, it can also extend up to the neck along this space.

The Prevertebral Layer of Deep Cervical Fascia

This layer surrounds the anterior vertebral muscles, anterior and middle scalene muscles, levator scapulae, brachial plexus, and subclavian veins, forming the base of the lateral triangle of the neck and extending outwards and downwards to cover the subclavian arteries and veins and the brachial plexus and connect with the axillary sheath. It attaches upwards to the base of the skull and fuses downwards with the anterior longitudinal ligament of the spine.

Between the prevertebral fascia and the posterior pharyngeal wall is the retropharyngeal space. The abscess in this space may bulge into the pharyngeal cavity causing difficulty to the patient's swallowing and articulating. In case of infection, it may extend down into the posterior mediastinum. There is an anterior vertebral space between the prevertebral fascia and the cervical part of the spine, where abscess or pus of the cervical spine tuberculosis accumulate or spread downwards to the posterior mediastinum or two laterals of the neck, or penetrate the prevertebral fascia into the posterior pharyngeal space.

2.2.4.4 The Submandibular Triangle

The submandibular triangle, also known as digastric triangle, is located superior to the hyoid bone [13].

The Borders

The lateral border of the submandibular triangle is the sternocleidomastoid muscle; the superior border is the inferior margin of the mandible; the medial border is the anterior midline of the neck. The roof of the triangle is formed by the skin, the superficial cervical fascia, the platysma, and the deep cervical fascia. The branches of the facial nerve and transverse cutaneous cervical nerves also pass over the roof of the triangle.

The Layers

From the superficial to the deep, the submandibular triangle can be basically divided into three layers: the skin, superficial cervical fascia, and deep cervical fascia.

The Contents

The submandibular triangle contains the submandibular gland, submandibular lymph nodes, the external maxillary artery, the anterior facial vein (posterior superior and superficial to the gland), the lingual nerve, the sublingual nerve (deep and inferior to the gland), and the submandibular duct.

2.2.4.5 The Cervical Part of Trachea

Cervical trachea, also named as cervical windpipe, belongs to a 10–11 cm long fibrocartilaginous tube of the lower respiratory tract. The cervical trachea is about 6.5 cm (6–8 tracheal cartilages) and lies inside the anterior visceral (pretracheal) layer of the neck. It starts at the lower edge of the larynx (cricoid cartilage) at the level of the C6 vertebrae and ends at the level of the jugular notch of the sternum, marking the upper border of the superior mediastinum [14].

From deep to superficial, the cervical part of trachea is covered anteriorly by several structures, including: the visceral cervical fascia, isthmus of thyroid gland, pretracheal lymph nodes, sternohyoid and sternothyroid muscles, and jugular venous arch.

Between the middle layer of the deep cervical fascia and the anterior tracheocervical segment, there is an anterior tracheal space containing unpaired thyroid venous plexus, the inferior thyroid vein, and sometimes the arteria thyroidea ima. There is an isthmus of thyroid gland which crosses the trachea between the second and fourth tracheal cartilages. The inferior thyroid arteries are located superior to the isthmus. The pretracheal fascia, inferior thyroid veins and thymus are located inferior to the isthmus.

2.2.4.6 The Carotid Triangle

The contents of the carotid triangle are made up of arteries, veins, and nerves.

The Arteries

The common carotid artery is the main artery of the triangle. It branches into the internal and external carotid arteries in the upper corner of the triangle. Other arterial branches that can be observed in this space are branches of the external carotid artery. Specifically, they are the superior thyroid artery, the lingual artery, the facial artery, the occipital artery, and the ascending pharyngeal artery [15].

The Veins

All the branches of veins correspond to a previously mentioned artery where they all drain into the internal jugular vein. The internal jugular vein runs laterally to the common carotid artery. These branches are: the superior thyroid vein, lingual veins, common facial vein, occipital vein, and ascending pharyngeal vein.

The Nerves

There is a carotid sheath formed by the middle cervical fascia where it encompasses the vagus nerve as well as the internal jugular vein, the common carotid artery, and deep cervical lymph nodes. Superficial to the carotid sheath, the hypoglossal nerve (CN XII) also descends within the triangle, as does the accessory nerve (CN XI), and the ansa cervicalis profunda. The hypoglossal nerve enters the carotid triangle through the deep posterior belly of digastric muscles, crossing the surface of the internal and external jugular vein. The superior laryngeal nerve originates from the vagus nerve and is divided downwards into medial and lateral branches that run obliquely down the deep surface of the internal and external carotid arteries.

The Posterior Belly of Digastric Muscles

At its deep surface to the inferior margin, from the posterior to the anterior, there are accessory nerve, internal jugular vein, hypoglossal nerve, internal carotid artery, external carotid artery, and external maxillary artery.

2.2.4.7 The Sternocleidomastoid Region

The sternocleidomastoid region corresponds to the site occupied by the sternocleidomastoid muscle and the area it covers.

The Realm

Being separated by sternocleidomastoid muscle, each half of the neck contains a triangle: the anterior and posterior one. The anterior, posterior, and superior boundaries of the anterior triangle are the mid line, anterior border of sternocleidomastoid, and the lower border of mandible, respectively. Accordingly, the posterior triangle is defined by posterior border of sternocleidomastoid, anterior border of trapezius, and middle third of clavicle (inferior).

The Layers

From superficial to the deep, the sternocleidomastoid region is composed of the skin, the superficial lamina of deep cervical fascia, sternocleidomastoid muscle and its sheath. Within the superficial lamina of deep cervical fascia, there are cervical plexus, external jugular vein, and cervical superficial lymph nodes.

The Structures

Superficial fascia contains fiber m. platysma. Under the fascia are the nerves of the cervical plexus, coming out from behind the rear edge of the sternocleidomastoid muscle: n. cutaneus colli, n. auricularis magnus, n. occipitalis minor, nn. supraclaviculares. The middle third stretch muscles crosses below external jugular vein. Own fascia neck forms a case for sternocleidomastoid muscle. At the bottom of the muscle behind it, sandwiches third fascia neck with the formation of the blind bags. Between the sheets fourth fascia is the main neurovascular bundle neck. This fascia not only fits the beam on the periphery, but also separated from each other by its components: the common carotid artery, internal jugular vein and the vagus nerve. Over the fascial sheath on the front wall of the common carotid artery passes in an oblique direction, ramus superior ansae cervicalis connecting with branches of I–III cervical nerves [16].

2.2.4.8 The Posterior Neck Triangle

The posterior triangle of the neck lies posteriorly at the sternocleidomastoid region.

The Borders

The borders include the trapezius muscle posteriorly, the sternocleidomastoid muscle anteriorly, and the middle one-third of the clavicle inferiorly.

The Layers

The posterior neck triangle is covered superficially to deeply by the skin, superficial and deep cervical fascia, and the platysma muscle.

The Contents

Within the posterior triangle of the neck, there are mainly paraspinal lymph nodes, spinal accessory nerve, transverse cervical artery, supraclavicular lymph nodes, and subclavian arteries and veins. There is brachial plexus on the deep surface of the prevertebral fascia [17].

References

1. Sadrameli M, Mupparapu M. Oral and maxillofacial anatomy. Radiol Clin N Am. 2018;56(1):13–29. https://doi.org/10.1016/j.rcl.2017.08.002. Epub 2017 Oct 10
2. Ogle OE, Weinstock RJ, Friedman E. Surgical anatomy of the nasal cavity and paranasal sinuses. Oral Maxillofac Surg Clin North Am. 2012;24(2):155–66 vii. https://doi.org/10.1016/j.coms.2012.01.011. Epub 2012 Mar 2
3. Vasil'ev Y, Paulsen F, Dydykin S, Bogoyavlenskaya T, Kashtanov A. Structural features of the anterior region of the mandible. Ann Anat. 2021;233:151589. https://doi.org/10.1016/j.aanat.2020.151589. Epub 2020 Sep 3
4. Ottria L, Candotto V, Guzzo F, Gargari M, Barlattani A. Temporomandibular joint and related structures: anatomical and histological aspects. J Biol Regul Homeost Agents. 2018;32(2 Suppl. 1):203–7.
5. Hou C, Chang S, Lin J, Song D. Anatomy, classification, and nomenclature. In: Surgical atlas of perforator flaps. Dordrecht: Springer; 2015. https://doi.org/10.1007/978-94-017-9834-1_2.
6. Isola G, Anastasi GP, Matarese G, Williams RC, Cutroneo G, Bracco P, Piancino MG. Functional and molecular outcomes of the human masticatory muscles. Oral Dis. 2018;24(8):1428–41. https://doi.org/10.1111/odi.12806. Epub 2017 Dec 27
7. Porcheri C, Mitsiadis TA. Physiology, pathology and regeneration of salivary glands. Cell. 2019;8(9):976. https://doi.org/10.3390/cells8090976.

8. Nakamoto T, Suei Y, Konishi M, Kanda T, Verdonschot RG, Kakimoto N. Abnormal positioning of the common carotid artery clinically diagnosed as a submandibular mass. Oral Radiol. 2019;35(3):331–4. https://doi.org/10.1007/s11282-018-0355-7. Epub 2018 Oct 30
9. Iwanaga J, Tubbs RS. Bones of the head and neck. In: Atlas of oral and maxillofacial anatomy. Cham: Springer; 2021. https://doi.org/10.1007/978-3-030-78327-3_2.
10. Iwanaga J, Tubbs RS. Anatomy of the oral cavity. In: Atlas of oral and maxillofacial anatomy. Cham: Springer; 2021. https://doi.org/10.1007/978-3-030-78327-3_3.
11. Iwanaga J, Tubbs RS. Buccal nerve dissection via an intraoral approach: correcting an error regarding buccal nerve blockade. J Oral Maxillofac Surg. 2019;77(6):1154–e1.
12. Iwanaga J, Tubbs RS. Anatomy of the superficial face. In: Atlas of oral and maxillofacial anatomy. Cham: Springer; 2021. https://doi.org/10.1007/978-3-030-78327-3_1.
13. Casale J, Varacallo M. Anatomy, head and neck, submandibular triangle 2021. Treasure Island (FL): StatPearls Publishing; 2022.
14. Joseph J. The larynx and cervical part of the trachea. In: A textbook of regional anatomy. London: Palgrave; 1982. https://doi.org/10.1007/978-1-349-16831-6_23.
15. Lucev N, Bobinac D, Maric I, Drescik I. Variations of the great arteries in the carotid triangle. Otolaryngol Head Neck Surg. 2000;122(4):590–1. https://doi.org/10.1067/mhn.2000.97982.
16. Lucioni M. Laterocervical region (sternocleidomastoid region: Robbins levels II, III, and IV. In: Practical guide to neck dissection. Springer, Berlin: Heidelberg; 2013.
17. Ihnatsenka B, Boezaart AP. Applied sonoanatomy of the posterior triangle of the neck. Int J Shoulder Surg. 2010;4(3):63–74. https://doi.org/10.4103/0973-6042.76963.

3 Characteristics of Patients Undergoing Oral and Maxillofacial Surgery

Ming Xia

3.1 Common Oral and Maxillofacial Diseases

Oral and maxillofacial diseases can be seen in all ages, including infants and elder people. According to the statistics of Shanghai Ninth People's Hospital affiliated to Shanghai Jiao Tong University School of Medicine, the youngest patient was a hard palate teratoma patient who was only 5-day-old, while the oldest patient was a 96-year-old patient who has a primary carcinoma of tongue. Both of them went through perioperative period safely.

3.1.1 Morbidity and Characteristics of Pediatric Patients

According to the 50-year in hospital surgery statistics of Shanghai Ninth People's Hospital, pediatric patients (under 13 years old) took up 30.7% of the total patients' number. Among pediatric patients, those who had cheilopalatoschisis malformation or birth defect were dominant, and the most common diseases were cheilopalatoschisis, tumors, and salivary gland diseases.

Congenial craniomaxillofacial anomalies, such as cleft lip, craniostenosis, and among others are recommended to be repaired when patients are under 1-year-old, to improve craniomaxillofacial forms and functions, reduce complications, and obtain better postoperative development. The anatomical and physiological characteristics of the pediatric patients change with age and cannot simply be seen as a microcosm of the adult. The younger the patient is, the greater the differences. In the perioperative period, this group of patients must be taken good care of to minimize the adverse effects of surgical anesthesia and maintain the homeostasis by using appropriate techniques.

3.1.2 Morbidity and Characteristics of Elderly Patients

According to the same statistics as mentioned above, elderly patients (over 60 years old) accounted for 11.6% of the total patients' number. The most common diseases in this population were tumors, salivary gland diseases, and infection, differing from pediatric patients' disease structure.

As getting older, the body structure and physiological functions of the elderly inevitably undergo degenerative changes, manifested in the atrophy of internal organs and tissues, cellular senescence and reduced regenerative functions,

M. Xia (✉)
Department of Anesthesiology, Shanghai Ninth People's Hospital Affiliated to Shanghai Jiao Tong University School of Medicine, Shanghai, China
e-mail: xiaming1980@xzhmu.edu.cn

H. Jiang, M. Xia (eds.), *Anesthesia for Oral and Maxillofacial Surgery*,
https://doi.org/10.1007/978-981-19-7287-4_3

and consequently, reduced function, decreased immune function, low resistance, and the body's ability to respond to the surrounding environment. Not only are they often accompanied by various other system and organ diseases, especially cardiovascular diseases, followed by respiratory diseases, digestive diseases as well as diabetes and hematological diseases, thus making the body significantly less resistant and tolerant to treatments such as surgery, but they are also prone to infections and complications. On the other hand, with the development of surgical techniques, elderly patients expect longer postoperative survival time and higher quality of life. Many elderly tumor patients not only receive radical resection for tumor, but need a certain degree of repair of large tissue defects and dysfunctions after radical resection. These increase the complexity and danger of surgical treatment for elderly patients, as well as the perioperative anesthesia risk and management.

3.2 Common Syndromes in Oral and Maxillofacial Surgery

There is a wide spectrum of syndromes that contain dental, oral, and craniofacial abnormalities, the range of which encompasses over 1/3 of all congenital malformations [1].

3.2.1 Common Syndromes in Oral and Maxillofacial Surgery

1. Syndromes in which maxillary hypoplasia is the main symptom, such as Crouzon syndrome, Apert syndrome, and Pfeiffer syndrome.
2. Syndromes in which maxillary hypoplasia is the main symptom, such as Pierre Robin syndrome, Treacher Collin syndrome, Goldenhar syndrome, Nager syndrome, and Stickler syndrome.
3. Syndromes relating to cleft lip and palate. Congenital cleft lip and palate is often the most common congenital anomaly and is associated with 150 syndromes. The incidence of cleft lip alone is 1/1000, and cleft palate alone is 1/2500. Syndromes related to cleft lip and palate include lethal alcohol syndrome, Shprintzen syndrome, and Van der Woude syndrome, in addition to Apert syndrome, Crouze syndrome, Robin syndrome, Treacher Collin syndrome, and Stickler syndrome mentioned above. More than 75% of the individuals have cleft palate or palatal anomalies and specific facial characteristics like hypertelorism [2].

3.2.2 Syndromes with Abnormal Development of Internal Vital Organs

Some congenital malformation, except for maxillofacial anomalies and deformed limbs may accompany with vital organ anomaly. Taking cleft lip and palate—the congenital malformation, for example, the incidence of congenital heart disease related to it is as high as 3–7%, commonly seen as atrial septal defect and ventricular septal defect. In Shprintzen syndrome patients, 80% has a variety of cardiac anomalies, such as ventricular septal defect (65%), right aortic arch (35%), tetralogy of Fallot (20%), and anomalous left subclavian artery (20%). Decreased compensatory function of vital organs damages children's tolerance of anesthesia.

3.2.3 Syndromes Related to Upper Airway Obstruction

Obvious craniofacial anomalies or disproportions are often closely associated with upper airway obstruction. For example, micrognathia and tongue collapse in Pierre Robin syndrome, recession of the maxilla and atresia of choana in Crouzon syndrome, plump tongue in Down syndrome and micrognathia and atresia of choana caused by achondroplasia in Treacher Collin syndrome are the main causes of upper airway obstruction. In some pediatric patients, the obstruction is already evident before surgery and may even lead to obstructive sleep apnea syndrome, which can also lead to chronic hypoxia and carbon dioxide accumulation, resulting in impaired cardiopulmonary function and systemic failure. Therefore, whether patients with congenital malformations have intubation difficulties or not, anesthetists should be alert to the potential risk of perioperative airway management difficulties and prepare intubation plans. Maintaining spontaneous breathing is recommended in most cases under such circumstances.

3.2.4 Syndromes Accompanied with Mental Retardation

Some syndromes are also associated with mental retardation, such as palato-cardiac-facial syndrome (Shprintzen syndrome), which is characterized by cleft palate, cardiovascular defects, specific facial features and mental retardation, and Hurler syndrome, which is also accompanied with severe mental retardation. Syndromes associated with upper airway obstruction, manifesting as obstructive sleep apnea, can seriously affect the growth and intellectual development of children. Therefore, the anesthetist should observe children's intellectual development through direct communication with children and inquiring their learning situation before administering anesthesia. At the same time, communicating with parents is also very important, helping them understanding their children's intellectual development and the impact of the syndrome on the children's intelligence to avoid unnecessary medical disputes.

3.2.5 Syndromes Involving Gingivodental Tissues

Features of gingivodental syndromes are shown though dental manifestations such as gingival hyperplasia. Neurofibromatosis type 1 (NF1) is a tumor predisposing syndrome. When affected, patients may have symptoms such as macrocephaly, short mandible, maxilla, cranial base, and low face height [3, 4]. Among all the NF1 patients, nearly 20% of them have an enlargement of the mandibular canal [5]. The common symptom intra-orally is unilateral swelling of the gingiva, which may appear as additional diffuse enlargements, or gingiva enlargement in certain cases [6].

3.2.6 Syndromes Involving Branchial Arches

The branchial arches syndrome usually refers to the first and second branchial arch syndrome, the classical symptom of which is craniofacial deformities [7]. The deformities can be complicated and various. Therefore, it may be referred by different researchers as Goldenhar syndrome (GS), oculo-auriculo-vertebral dysplasia (OVAD), hemifacial macrosomia (HFM), Treacher Collins (TCS) (subdivided into three types), Möbius Syndrome (MBS), and among others. In the following passages, they will be introduced in detail.

The branchial arches syndrome is the most frequent craniofacial condition after cleft lip palate (CLP) and affects 1 in 4000–5600 live births [8]. It is shown that 47 out of 51 patients have uni- or bilateral (24/23) ear abnormalities that were related to hearing loss [9]. HFM was present in 90% of the patients whose condition often accompanies facial nerve palsy (FNP). Apart from the mandibular condyle hypoplasia and the soft tissue discrepancy, FNP affects the craniofacial growth asymmetry as well [10]. The most commonly present characteristics of HFM are hypoplasia of the zygomatic, mandibular and maxillary bones, and facial muscle hypoplasia [9]. Through cephalometric analysis, it can be noticed that HFM patients present an upward cant of the occlusal plane and their mandibular body and ramus of the affected side turn to be smaller [11–13]. Accordingly, their gonial angles are inclined to be large and steep, their mandibles retrognathic, and their faces slightly convex [14–16]. Their retrognathic mandibles have no relation to mandibular growth rate since the rate is similar to that of the normal ones [17].

Moreover, colobomas of the upper eyelids are frequently seen. Sometimes, HFM may cause malformation of other facial structures, including the orbit, eye, nose, cranium, and neck. Normally, only one side of the above structure may be affected, whereas there are cases that involve the whole face. Though observing and comparing the oral and dental features, researchers found that in deciduous and permanent dentition, the mesio-distal dimensions of all molars are smaller than in control individuals, manifesting the opinion that HFM is a bilateral rather than a unilateral condition [14]. Nevertheless, the difference is most significant in the mandibular permanent first molar on the affected side. While it is reported that the development of the mandibular is deviating, the size of canines and the incisors are regular, no matter in the deciduous or the permanent dentition [14, 16].

The incidence of tooth agenesis (TA) in HFM patients is higher than in the control group, and reaches nearly to 25%, while the most affected are the mandibular second premolar and second molars [18, 19]. Patients with HFM have delayed tooth development when comparing with the controlled individuals, and only in the most severe cases where there are absent mandibular ramus and glenoid fossa, the affected side develops pronouncedly more delayed than the non-affected side [16, 19]. A feature prone to be overlooked is mild tongue dysmorphology, though it is shown on approximately half of the HFM children [20]. Besides, among patients with HFM, 10% of them present CLP [21]. Moreover, unilateral craniofacial microsomia is also reported to be an underestimated reason of obstructive sleep apnea, the incidence of which in patients with UCM is ten times higher than that in the normal population [22].

Treacher Collins Syndrome (TCS) is a congenital hypoplasia of zygomatic bone and mandible, with a penetrance of up to 90% and variable expressivity, and 1 out of 50,000 live births were affected [23]. Bilateral and symmetric downslanting palpebral fissures, malar hypoplasia, micrognathia, and external ear abnormalities are commonly shown features of the syndrome.

So far, researchers have identified three genes in TCS, namely, *TCOF1*, *POLR1D*, and *POLR1C* that may play scientific and effective role in diagnosis of the syndrome. Clinical trials were conducted in 146 patients with TCS [24]. Researchers proved that symptoms such as craniofacial and comprised downward-slanting palpebral fissures (in 100% of the patients); malar hypoplasia (in 99%); conductive deafness (in 91%); mandibular hypoplasia (in 87%); atresia of external ear canal (in 72%), microtia (in 71%); coloboma of the lower eyelid (in 65%); facial asymmetry (in 53%), and projection of scalp hair onto the lateral cheek (in 48%) were the most common features observed in patients with TCS with mutations in *TCOF1* [24].

In another study, it is reported that over half of the pediatric patients with TCS present with narrow arched palates, and hypoplasia of the maxilla, mandible, and facial soft tissue [25]. The complex abnormalities in the temporomandibular joint may result in the limitation of mouth opening [25, 26] and the anterior open bite of different severity [25, 27]. There are studies revealed the presence of cleft palate with or without cleft lip [25, 27, 28].

In a prospective case study that included 19 patients who received genetic testing, medical and dental examinations, and polysomnography, disturbed respiration was detected in all participating patients, among whom 18 met the diagnostic criteria for obstructive sleep apnea syndrome [29].

Similar to HFM, TA is the most frequent anomaly and it most commonly affects the mandibular second premolars, followed by maxillary second premolars, lateral incisors, and maxillary canines in patients with TCS [28]. Approximately 60% of the children with TCS have been found to have dental anomalies. Additionally, there have been reports of impacted maxillary supernumerary teeth, hypoplastic, and malpositioned maxillary central incisors, and ectopic eruption of the maxillary first molars [28].

3.2.7 Syndromes Involving Orofacial Clefts

Syndromes in this group are all related to the development of cleft lip and/or palate. Apart from that they also include a highly variable spectrum of clinical features, such as ectrodactyly, ectodermal anomalies, musculoskeletal problems, hypogonadism, mental retardation, and hearing loss. The 22q11.2 deletion syndrome (22q11.2DS), EEC-syndrome (Ectrodactyly–ectodermal dysplasia–cleft syndrome), Kabuki syndrome, Kallmann syndrome, Pierre Robin sequence, and Van der Woude syndrome are included in this category.

3.2.8 Syndromes with Unusual Faces

Syndromes belonging to this category include Coffin-Lowry syndrome (CLS), Opitz GBBB syndrome, and Smith-Lemli-Opitz syndrome.

Like other oral and maxillofacial syndromes, CLS is also caused by mutation of genes. However, its incidence is lower, about 1 in 50,000–100,000 [30]. Female are prone to be affected more severely than male, and the severity of the disorder varies greatly. Specifically, affected newborns usually have symptoms related to joint hyperlaxity and hypotonia. For example, their hands may be broad with soft, stubby, and tapering fingers, which may be observed when they were born and regarded as solid diagnostic features. Since the early age, affected children present delayed physical growth and psychomotor development. Other typical symptoms include short stature (95%), pectus deformity (80%), sensorineural hearing loss, paroxysmal movement disorders, and kyphosis and/or scoliosis [31].

For craniofacial abnormalities, children with CLS will not show specific symptoms until they were 2 years old when the typical facial features of the syndrome become obvious. Features contain prominent forehead, hypertelorism, flat nasal bridge, downward sloping of palpebral fissures, large and prominent ears, and a whole mouth with full lips, all of which progress gradually along with their increasing ages [31, 32]. Moreover, malocclusions and narrow palate are frequently present [33].

Hypodontia is another commonly encountered symptom of children with CLS. Peg shaped or absent upper lateral incisors, with a wide upper interincisal diastema, or a lingual midline fissure are also present in CLS [32, 33]. It is reported that detachment and disorganization of the periodontal ligament and alveolar bone loss with age are significantly associated with cementum hypoplasia and Rsk2 deficiency [34].

The Optiz GBBB syndrome is genetically heterogeneous, but signs and symptoms of different patient populations are in general the same. Although common general features of the syndrome are laryngo-tracheo-esophageal abnormalities, and urogenital defects like hypospadias, cryptorchidism, and bifid scrotum in males and splayed labia majora in females, imperforate anus, and congenital heart defects [35–41], distinct craniofacial features can also be observed in this disorder, including a prominent forehead, with a widow's peak hairline, hypertelorism, a flat nasal bridge, a thin upper lip, and low-set ears [42]. Cleft lip and/or palate is shown in approximately half of the affected population [36, 40–43].

As a developmental disorder, smith-lemli-opitz syndrome (SLOS) may influence more than one part of the body. Unlike the Optiz GBBB, the signs and symptoms of SLOS vary intensively, the range of which may cover from slightly affected patients with minor learning and behavioral abnormalities and physical deviations to severely tortured patients with life-threatening conditions. Manifested on craniofacial, microcephaly, bitemporal narrowing, ptosis, short nose with anteverted nares, low-set and retroversed ears, ocular problems and hypertelorism, a small chin, and micrognathia are usually present [44–46]. What is more, cleft palate or bifid uvula have been detected clinically. Cleft palate has been reported in 40–50% of the patients [45, 47, 48], while cleft lip is uncommon [49]. The oral and dental symptoms in SLOS patients are oligodontia or supernumerary teeth, broad alveolar ridges, enamel hypoplasia, protrusion of the maxillary front teeth, lip incompetence, and an anterior open bite [44, 46].

In conclusion, while performing anesthesia on these patients, the anesthetists should be very careful because of their complex pathophysiological conditions induced by congenital malformations. The anesthetists should be fully aware that not only are there oral and maxillofacial malformations, but there may also be other important organ malformations and serious complications arising from these defects. Therefore, a comprehensive consideration from anatomy, physiology, and pathology should be done before anesthesia.

3.3 Systemic and Vital Viscera Complications

Systemic diseases may have more prominent oral and maxillofacial manifestations. In oral and maxillofacial surgery patients, there may often be an underlying cause of systemic disorders. For example, Kaposi's sarcomas occur in about 34–35% of AIDS patients, and 77% of Kaposi's sarcomas occur in the maxilla, usually without other clinical symptoms. In addition, rheumatoid arthritis has symptom of temporomandibular joint disorders in the oral and maxillofacial region, with some patients requiring arthroplasty for joint ankylosis. It may cause jaw abnormality to children. This shows that it is important for the anesthetist to establish a systemic concept of the patient for oral and maxillofacial surgery. All information from the medical history, physical examination and laboratory tests should be reviewed carefully prior to anesthesia, with a thorough consideration of the correlation between their local lesions and systemic diseases, and further investigations to exclude suspectable diseases in some patients if necessary. A thorough pre-anesthetic examination will help to properly understand and assess the patient's condition and the impact of underlying diseases, select the appropriate anesthetic methods, formulate perioperative preventive measures and determine the complications associated with anesthesia.

Oral and maxillofacial diseases coexist with certain important organ dysfunctions. Unlike young adults, most elderly people suffer from other chronic diseases while they suffer from surgical diseases. According to the study [50], the prevalence of hypertension, diabetes mellitus and hypercholesterolemia in Chinese residents aged ≥60 years was 58.3%, 19.4% and 10.5% respectively, with 75.8% of the population suffering from one or more chronic diseases. The nature and severity of these comorbidities will have a direct impact on the choice of surgery or anesthesia methods and the safety of the patient throughout the perioperative period. A number of cases of perioperative death due to compensatory insufficiency from serious circulatory and respiratory diseases have also been reported in the past. In conclusion, a variety of factors complicate the condition and perioperative management of oral and maxillofacial surgery patients, and the anesthetist should make every possible preoperative adjustment to the patient's physical status to reduce the perioperative and anesthesia risks.

Even surgery with minimal risk such as dental and alveolar surgery can lead to serious complications and even life-threatening conditions for patients with systemic diseases, especially cardiovascular disease. Experience has shown that patients whose heart failure is NYHA Class I–III (the classification is attached in the following section) can tolerate tooth extraction and minor surgery, but patients whose heart failure is NYHA Class II–III should preferably receive surgery under cardiac monitoring. Patients with severe cardiac failure (NYHA Class IV), along with orthopnea, cyanosis, jugular vein distention, lower limb edema, etc., should not accept tooth extraction and other surgery, regardless of their heart disease types, and should be treated and receive surgery under cardiac monitoring after their symptoms have significantly improved.

3.4 Combined Modality Therapy

3.4.1 Combined Modality Therapy for Oral and Maxillofacial Tumors

Currently, oral and maxillofacial tumors tends to be treated with combined modality therapy, i.e. a multidisciplinary or multi-modal treatment, which is accomplished by oral and maxillofacial surgeons, radiologists, chemotherapists, traditional Chinese physicians and anesthetists. The anesthetists are in charge of the perioperative management. Normally, for patients suffering from oral and maxillofacial tumors, accepting chemotherapy and radiotherapy preoperatively may shrink tumors and reduce the viability of the tumor cells, creating the conditions for radical surgical treatment. However, chemotherapy and radiotherapy have adverse effects such as suppressing the body's hematopoietic function, reducing immune function and affecting gastrointestinal and liver functions, which may cause significant changes in the patient's regulation of physiological functions and drug metabolism during the perioperative period. In addition, preoperative radiotherapy may also cause extensive adhesions and fixation of oropharyngeal tissues in some patients, bringing difficulties to tracheal intubation after induction of anesthesia. Therefore, when encountering patients who have received radiotherapy or chemotherapy before surgery, anesthetists should assess their systemic and vital organ functions before administration of anesthesia and anticipate whether there is difficult airway to avoid accidents.

3.4.2 Combined Modality Therapy for Congenital Malformations

3.4.2.1 Cleft Lip and Palate

Cleft lip and palate is the most common congenital malformation of the oral and maxillofacial region, and is often associated with nasal cartilage anomaly and alveolar cleft. Therefore, it is impossible to repair the malformation through one operation. These associated anomalies need to be considered as a whole and treated in sequence. In light of sequence therapy, children should receive different repair surgery at different ages. For example, the appropriate age for cleft lip surgery is between 3 and 6 months old; for cleft palate surgery, between 12 and 18 months old; for bone grafting for alveolar cleft, between 8 and 9 years old; and for nasal cartilage surgery, at 12 years old.

Currently, in some countries, sequence therapy team for cleft lip and palate has been established. The team consists of an oral and maxillofacial surgeon, an orthodontist, an anesthetist and an ENT surgeon, each with their own role to play. The main responsibility of anesthetists is to guarantee the success of surgeries at each stage. Specifically, before the surgery, they should complete the preoperative examination, assess patients' tolerance of anesthesia, adjust anemia and nutrition, control infection, and treat cardiopulmonary complications. During the surgery, they are in charge of performing anesthesia, monitoring and maintaining the stability of patients' physiological functions and preparing for emergencies. After the surgery, treating the anesthesia complications is also their task. Besides, creating an anesthetic history for each patient enables the anesthetists to learn patients' previous surgeries, and consequently improves the safety of perioperative management and the implementation of the sequence therapy for congenital malformation.

3.4.2.2 Congenital Craniofacial Malformation

Repair surgery for congenital craniofacial malformation is also a complex procedure. Many craniofacial anomalies often require 2 or 3 stages of surgery. For example, patients with Crouzon syndrome may receive forehead bone flap transplantation at 2–4 months old, orbitofrontal advancement at 4 months to 2 years old, Le Fort I osteotomy, Le Fort II osteotomy and Le Fort III osteotomy after 6 years old to improve mid facial hypoplasia and occlusion. The treatment of difficult craniofacial anomalies also requires a multidisciplinary surgeon team. The successful management of children with craniofacial anomalies through multiple stages of surgery depends on the combined efforts of all disciplines.

3.5 Characteristics of Oral and Maxillofacial Injury Patients

The characteristics of oral and maxillofacial injuries are closely related to their anatomical and physiological features.

3.5.1 Rich Blood Circulation in the Oral and Maxillofacial Region and Related Effects

The oral and maxillofacial region bleeds more after the injury, easily forming hematomas and edema rapidly and severely. If the hematomas and edema occur at the floor of the mouth and the root of the tongue, they may obstruct the patents' airway and even cause asphyxia. On the other hand, due to the rich blood flow, the oral and maxillofacial tissues are more resistant to infection and have a stronger capacity for tissue repair and regeneration, so the wounds heal more quickly.

3.5.2 The Influence of Teeth

Oral and maxillofacial injuries are often accompanied by dental injuries, and if the strike is heavy, the teeth may suffer secondary injuries. Besides, two rows of teeth form an occlusion, the condition of which serves not only as an important diagnostic basis but also as the main criteria for the treatment of fractures of jaw.

3.5.3 Easy to Cause Complications Such as Craniocerebral and Neck Injury

As the maxillofacial surface is connected to the cranium, serious trauma to the middle part of the face is often accompanied by craniocerebral injury. As the maxillofacial region is connected to the neck, severe trauma to the lower part of the face may be associated with neck injury.

3.5.4 Prone to Cause Asphyxia

The oral and maxillofacial region is at the upper end of the respiratory tract. Injuries may affect breathing or cause asphyxia due to tissue displacement, swelling, posterior tongue drop, blood clots and blockage of secretions.

3.5.5 Affecting Eating and Oral Hygiene

The oral cavity is the entrance to the gastrointestinal tract, the injury of which often undermines the opening of the mouth, chewing and swallowing functions, thus seriously affecting patient's eating and nutrition condition. In addition, masticatory dysfunction weakens the self-cleaning of the oral cavity, thus seriously affecting oral hygiene.

3.5.6 Wound Contamination

In oral and maxillofacial region, there are many cavities and sinuses which accommodate a large number of bacteria. If the wounds overlap with them, contamination may break out.

Injury of special tissues and organs of the maxillofacial region, such as salivary glands, facial nerves and trigeminal nerves, will induce certain symptoms and signs, and should be treated promptly.

3.5.7 Facial Malformations

The oral and maxillofacial area occupies large part of human face. Therefore, if the orbital, lip and cheek, nose and other parts suffer open injuries and are not treated properly, scar contracture may appear after the wound heals, leading to displacement and deformation of normal tissues and organs and seriously affecting the patient's appearance and psychology. Consequently, while treating oral and maxillofacial injury, clinicians should also consider esthetic aspects.

Patients who bear oral and maxillofacial injury may also have physiological problems. With the achievements of psychology, perioperative psychological changes received high attention. Many oral and maxillofacial surgical disorders are often associated with psychosocial factors, such as tumors, primary temporomandibular joint muscle group spasm, oral and maxillofacial anomalies, psychogenic dental pain, psychogenic trigeminal neuralgia, various pains in the oral and maxillofacial region associated with menopause in women, abnormal salivation, and foreign body sensation in the mouth. Some of these disorders can be caused by psychological factors and may also lead to varying degrees of psychological disorders. Oral and maxillofacial diseases and psychological disorders are dialectical unity.

3.6 Preoperative Anesthesia Evaluation and Optimization

3.6.1 Preoperative Anesthesia Evaluation and Optimization of Patients Undergoing Oral and Maxillofacial Surgery

The goal of preoperative anesthesia evaluation is to ascertain whether the patient can tolerate the insult of the surgical procedure as well as the anesthetic techniques. The anesthetists care of the patient starts with an evaluation of the patient's medical history, including questions about precious surgical and anesthetic experience, physical examination and other examinations, with emphasis on the vital organs' functions such as heart, lung, brain, liver and kidney.

The anesthetist should make a comprehensive assessment of the patient's clinical diagnosis, the proposed operation, anesthesia techniques, anesthesia risks and the advantages and disadvantages of surgical anesthesia. Besides, several assessment tools are sought to assist the evaluation, such as ASA Physical Status Classification System. The purpose of the ASA classification is to assess the patient's ability to tolerate surgery and the risk of anesthesia, so that the anesthetist and surgeon can prepare for the risks in the perioperative period. When a patient with ASA III or above is encountered, the patient should be reported to a more senior physician as required; based on the report, the department head may communicate with the department head of the relevant departments or hold a consultation if necessary, and after thorough discussion, make adjustments to the patient's systemic status and treatment or report to the medical department.

A retrospective study of adverse events in Australia showed that one in ten reported perioperative accidents were related to inadequate preoperative assessment and preparation. The three most common factors were inadequate airway assessment, poor communication and failure to improve the anesthetic plan based on the assessment results. Respondents indicated that 57% of the accidents could have been prevented. The American Society of Anesthesiologists guidelines recommend that the pre-anesthesia visit and assessment should include communication with patients or their custodians, medical history, previous exposure to anesthetic drugs, medication, physical examination, test results and ASA classification.

Evidence-based medicine is used in pre-anesthetic assessment and decision-making, combining the best clinical research evidence with clinical practice and the actual situation (needs, psychology, concerns) of the patient. Anesthesia should be centered on the "patient-oriented" concept and ideology to implement and improve clinical practice. The choice and preparation of anesthesia should take into account the technical quality of the anesthetist, the hospital's equipment, the collaboration between departments, as well as the specific situation of each patient, in order to carry out scientific, rational and precise medical treatment. For example, one anesthesia case for a maxillofacial deformity may be common in one hospital, while difficult in another. Even in the same hospital, the difficulty of the same anesthesia may also vary greatly between anesthetists. Thus, the pre-anesthetic assessment and preparation should be personalized.

3.6.1.1 Assessment of the Patient's General Condition

The assessment of systemic conditions for anesthesia risk generally refers to the American Society of Anesthesiologists (ASA) physical status classification system (Table 3.1).

It is important to note that the ASA VI has now been added according to the 2016 ASA Physical Status Classification System, which defines a patient who has been declared brain

Table 3.1 ASA physical status classification system

ASA physical status classification	Definition	Adult examples, including but not limited to	Pediatric examples, including but not limited to	Obstetric examples, including but not limited to	Perioperative mortality (%)
ASA I	A normal healthy patient	Healthy, non-smoking, no or minimal alcohol use	Healthy (no acute or chronic disease), normal BMI percentile for age		0.06–0.08
ASA II	A patient with mild systemic disease	Mild diseases only without substantive functional limitations. Current smoker, social alcohol drinker, pregnancy, obesity (30 < BMI < 40), well-controlled DM/HTN, mild lung disease	Asymptomatic congenital cardiac disease, well-controlled dysrhythmias, asthma without exacerbation, well-controlled epilepsy, non-insulin dependent diabetes mellitus, abnormal BMI percentile for age, mild/moderate OSA, oncologic state in remission, autism with mild limitations	Normal pregnancy*, well-controlled gestational HTN, controlled preeclampsia without severe features, diet-controlled gestational DM	0.27–0.40
ASA III	A patient with a severe systemic disease	Substantive functional limitations; one or more moderate to severe diseases. Poorly controlled DM or HTN, COPD, morbid obesity (BMI ≥40), active hepatitis, alcohol dependence or abuse, implanted pacemaker, moderate reduction of ejection fraction, ESRD undergoing regularly scheduled dialysis, history (>3 months) of MI, CVA, TIA, or CAD/stents	Uncorrected stable congenital cardiac abnormality, asthma with exacerbation, poorly controlled epilepsy, insulin dependent diabetes mellitus, morbid obesity, malnutrition, severe OSA, oncologic state, renal failure, muscular dystrophy, cystic fibrosis, history of organ transplantation, brain/spinal cord malformation, symptomatic hydrocephalus, premature infant PCA <60 weeks, autism with severe limitations, metabolic disease, difficult airway, long-term parenteral nutrition. Full term infants <6 weeks of age	Preeclampsia with severe features, gestational DM with complications or high insulin requirements, a thrombophilic disease requiring anticoagulation	1.82–4.30
ASA IV	A patient with a severe systemic disease that is a constant threat to life	Recent (<3 months) MI, CVA, TIA or CAD/stents, ongoing cardiac ischemia or severe valve dysfunction, severe reduction of ejection fraction, shock, sepsis, DIC, ARD or ESRD not undergoing regularly scheduled dialysis	Symptomatic congenital cardiac abnormality, congestive heart failure, active sequelae of prematurity, acute hypoxic-ischemic encephalopathy, shock, sepsis, disseminated intravascular coagulation, automatic implantable cardioverter-defibrillator, ventilator dependence, endocrinopathy, severe trauma, severe respiratory distress, advanced oncologic state	Preeclampsia with severe features complicated by HELLP or other adverse event, peripartum cardiomyopathy with EF <40, uncorrected/decompensated heart disease, acquired or congenital	7.80–23.0

ASA V	A moribund patient who is not expected to survive without the operation	Ruptured abdominal/thoracic aneurysm, massive trauma, intracranial bleed with mass effect, ischemic bowel in the face of significant cardiac pathology or multiple organ/system dysfunction	Massive trauma, intracranial hemorrhage with mass effect, patient requiring ECMO, respiratory failure or arrest, malignant hypertension, decompensated congestive heart failure, hepatic encephalopathy, ischemic bowel or multiple organ/system dysfunction	Uterine rupture	9.40–50.7
ASA VI	A declared brain-dead patient whose organs are being removed for donor purposes				

Retrieved from https://www.asahq.org/standards-and-guidelines/asa-physical-status-classification-system#:~:text=The%20%EE%80%80ASA%20Physical%20Status%20Classification%20System%EE%80%81%20has%20been,type%20of%20surgery%2C%20frailty%2C%20level%20of%20deconditioning%20 dead and as a donor whose organs are removed in preparation for transplantation. However, this concept is still not widespread in China.

ASA I and II patients generally have a good tolerance for anesthesia and are less likely to encounter perioperative accidents. ASA III patients' anesthesia has risks and should be adequately prepared for the prevention and treatment of complications, to avoid perioperative accidents. ASA IV patients are at greater risk and should always be prepared for resuscitation. ASA V patients are critically ill, whose anesthetic tolerance is very poor, and face the threat of death at any time. They are exceptionally dangerous for accepting both anesthesia and surgery. Thus the pre-anesthetic preparation becomes even more important. Above all, no matter what classifications patients belong to, they are all at risk of accidents at any time during their perioperative period and it is important to communicate with the surgeons and to inform the family in detail and obtain informed consent prior to surgery.

The ASA classification emphasizes the patient's risk and is based only on the subjective assessment of the anesthetists and surgeons. Besides, it does not take into account the complexity and environmental factors of the procedure. Thus it still requires other criteria, such as the clinical guideline for "Routine Preoperative Tests for Elective Surgery" published by the National Institute for Health and Clinical Excellence on its official website in 2016 [51] which can be a reference.

Medical History

The anesthetists should review and be familiar with the patient's medical history prior to surgery, which enables them to anticipate possible difficult intubations or to avoid serious anesthetic accidents. Preoperative assessment of medical history usually focuses on the function of vital organs such as the heart, lungs, brain, liver and kidneys, with emphasis on a history of anesthesia-related diseases such as cerebrovascular accidents, hypertension, heart disease, myocardial infarction, lung inflammation, asthma, liver and kidney disease, and diabetes. The anesthetists should also inquire the use of hormonal drugs, cardiac drugs, antihypertensive drugs, monoamine oxidase inhibitors, antibiotics, anticoagulants, anticholinesterase drugs and other drugs that may affect anesthesia process, as well as the history of drug allergies. The patient's history of previous surgery (if performed), allergies, blood transfusions and infectious diseases also need to be known.

Assessment of Physical Examination

The assessment of the physical examination includes the patient's gender, age, height, weight, body temperature, respiration, heart rate, pulse, blood pressure, state of consciousness, posture and gait. Particular attention should be paid to patients whose weight exceeds the standard weight by more than 30%, because they are prone to co-morbid chronic respiratory diseases and the incidence of postoperative respiratory complications can be increased by twofold. In addition, changes in cardiovascular, respiratory and metabolic aspects should be noticed as well.

Preoperative Tests

Preoperative tests can be used to provide additional diagnostic and prognostic information to complement the medical history, facilitating the assessment of anesthetic and surgical risks. Refinement of the preoperative tests guides preoperative interventions which aims to reduce perioperative risks and provide baseline results to improve perioperative management strategies. Abnormal test results suggest the possibility of postponing surgery or changes in anesthesia, surgical approach and prognosis; thus avoiding severe perioperative complications. Occasionally, such results may require consultation with other specialties, or the prescription of new medication, or correction of abnormal physiology such as anemia, severe hypertension, hypokalemia, etc. However, there is currently no strong evidence to support the need for additional routine tests in asymptomatic patients, as it remains debatable whether this work-up provides greater benefit to the patient. Therefore, a rational and cost-effective test strategy is indispensible.

Complications

Evaluation and Optimization of the Cardiovascular System

The cardiovascular system is a key component of the anesthetic assessment and the goal of the cardiovascular assessment is to identify patients at high risk, assign their risk levels and develop strategies to reduce the risk. In most cases, a detailed and accurate inquiry of medical history and a focused physical examination are sufficient to diagnose cardiac disease and associated risk factors. For medium- and high-risk patients, some specialist investigations (e.g. cardiac ultrasound, coronary angiography, etc.) are required to classify risk and develop a preoperative intervention strategy. The use of dispensable tests may lead to delays and increased costs, and may even be harmful to patients.

When surgical patients are at risk of a combination of cardiac problems, they may not only develop heart disease intraoperatively, but may also have accidents during the postoperative recovery period. This is particularly true for patients with a history of known coronary heart disease. Known risk factors for ischemic heart disease (coronary atherosclerotic heart disease) include advanced age, family history of coronary heart disease, smoking, hyperlipidemia, diabetes and hypertension. For coronary atherosclerotic heart disease, there are several indicators for classifying risk levels.

(a) ASA Physical Status Classification System. It is used to assess the patient's general health and to predict perioperative morbidity and mortality.
(b) Cardiac Risk Index (Goldman Criteria). This is a multi-factorial index of cardiac risk in the noncardiac surgical setting. It was developed for preoperative identification of patients at risk from major perioperative cardiovascular complications. Nine independent risk factors are evaluated on a point scale (Table 3.2).

Table 3.2 Cardiac risk index (Goldman criteria)

Risk factors		Score (points)
History	Age >70 years	5
	Myocardial infarction within 6 months	10
Cardiac exam	Signs of CHF: Ventricular gallop or JVD Significant aortic stenosis	11 3
Electrocardiogram	Arrhythmia other than sinus or premature atrial contractions 5 or more PVC's per minute	7 7
General medical conditions	$PO_2 < 60$; $PCO_2 > 50$; $K < 3$; $HCO_3 < 20$; $BUN > 50$; creatinine > 3; elevated SGOT; chronic liver disease; bedridden	3
Operation	Emergency Intraperitoneal, intrathoracic or aortic	4 3

The Cardiac Risk Index results range from 0 to 53, where the higher the score, the greater the risk for complications: ① 0–5 points: Class I, incidence of complications is 1%; ② 6–12 points: Class II, incidence of complications is 7%; ③ 13–25 points: Class III, incidence of complications is 14%; ④26–53 points: Class IV, incidence of complications is 78%. Examples of conditions considered as major cardiac events (MACEs) or complications include myocardial infarction, primary cardiac arrest, ventricular fibrillation, complete heart block, and pulmonary edema.

The spectrum of peri- and postoperative complications does not end with cardiac events, and other complications such as cerebrovascular disease or anemia may present.

(c) Revised Cardiac Risk Index (RCRI). It helps in the evaluation of patients undergoing cardiac surgery. It estimates the likelihood of perioperative cardiac events and therefore can support clinical decision-making by weighing the benefits and risks surgery has over different treatment options that might be available for individual cases.
(d) Detsky Modified Cardiac Risk Index. This is a model aimed at revealing the degree of

cardiovascular risk in the perioperative setting in the case of patients who have relevant cardiac risk factors. The index consists of 9 items, all with differing predictive value: age, prior myocardial infarction, unstable angina in the last 6 months, angina pectoris, alveolar pulmonary edema, suspected critical aortic stenosis, arrhythmia, emergency surgery, and general medical status. In contrast to the original Detsky cardiac risk index, the modified version adds new variables (e.g. angina and pulmonary edema), changes the allocation of points and contains a slightly different interpretation (the three risk groups).

The criteria considered in the RCRI includes high-risk surgery such as intraperitoneal, intrathoracic, suprainguinal vascular, history of ischemic heart disease, history of congestive heart failure, history of cerebrovascular disease, preoperative insulin treatment, and preoperative creatinine more than 2 mg/dL.

(e) ACC/AHA Guideline on Perioperative Cardiovascular Evaluation and Management of Patients Undergoing Noncardiac Surgery. The aim of preoperative assessment is not simply to give medical clearance, but to assess the patient's current medical status comprehensively, including cardiac problems that may be encountered during the perioperative period, and provide management and risk recommendations in response to the findings. In addition, a clinical risk profile needs to be created for the patient; thus, when the primary physician, anesthesiologists, and surgeon have to make treatment decisions that may influence short- and long-term cardiac outcomes, the profile can serve as a reliable reference [52].

For patients with chronic heart failure, the most commonly used method of assessing cardiac function is the New York Heart Association (NYHA) Classification for Heart Failure, which is presented below (Table 3.3).

Class I and II patients have good tolerance to anesthesia, while Class III and IV patients' anesthesia tolerance is poor. Classifying patients according to NYHA classification and treating them accordingly.

Assessment and Optimization of Respiratory System

The assessment of the respiratory system should be comprehensive and detailed, including the patient's ventilation and air exchange function, medical history of respiratory disease, smoking history, and other relevant components. The assessment requires detailed patient's medical history and a thorough physical examination to determine whether the patient is at risk of perioperative pulmonary complications. Common respiratory complications include atelectasis, lung infection, pulmonary infarction, acute respiratory distress syndrome, and respiratory failure. Perioperative management comprises of respiratory disease identification, assessment, and pre-optimization. If patients have risk factors such as smoking, it is important to recommend patients to quit smoking before surgery.

Table 3.3 New York Heart Association (NYHA) classification for heart failure

Class	Patient Symptoms
I	No limitation of physical activity. Ordinary physical activity does not cause undue fatigue, palpitation, dyspnea (shortness of breath)
II	Slight limitation of physical activity. Comfortable at rest. Ordinary physical activity results in fatigue, palpitation, dyspnea (shortness of breath)
III	Marked limitation of physical activity. Comfortable at rest. Less than ordinary activity causes fatigue, palpitation, or dyspnea
IV	Unable to carry on any physical activity without discomfort. Symptoms of heart failure at rest. If any physical activity is undertaken, discomfort increases

Retrieved from https://www.heart.org/en/health-topics/heart-failure/what-is-heart-failure/classes-of-heart-failure

Risk factors associated with postoperative pulmonary complications involve age, smoking, obesity, obstructive sleep apnea syndrome, and asthma and chronic obstructive pulmonary disease (COPD). Old age is an independent risk factor for postoperative pulmonary complications, as elderly patients may easily have failed pulmonary elastic recoil, impaired airway protection reflexes, reduced peak expiratory flow, and airway closing. Obesity may lead to reduced functional residual capacity, lung vein-arterial shunt, and hypoxemia. Patients who smoke up to ten packs per year have a high risk of perioperative pulmonary complications. Particularly those who do not quit smoking before surgery have a significantly higher risk of postoperative pulmonary complications compared to those who quit smoking. Smoking patients should be advised to stop smoking at least 1–2 days prior to surgery to reduce their COHb levels as well as the cardiovascular effects of nicotine. Studies have shown that the lung function would only be improved when the patients give up smoking for 6–8 weeks, but this is often difficult to implement in clinical practice. Obstructive sleep apnea syndrome can also be an independent risk factor, which may lead to a significantly higher morbidity and mortality of postoperative complications in patients. Therefore, anesthetists should diagnose this condition during preoperative assessment and provide early treatment. Asthma is a heterogeneous disease of the airway characterized by chronic inflammation, which is manifested by a high sensitivity of the airways to various allergens, and may cause obstruction of the airways and irreversible restriction of airflow. Therefore, the anesthetists should learn the medical history of asthmatic patients' accurately, including the severity of the asthma, precipitating factors, current medication (including when the last dose was administered, whether hormonal medication is being used and the name of the specific drugs), previous admissions for acute asthma attacks, and any intensive care unit visit history. Due to the hyper-responsive nature of the airway in asthmatic patients, the most common risk during general anesthesia is airway overreaction, which can cause bronchospasm, and thus it adversely affects the patient's perioperative airway management. Preoperative disposition for such patients includes identification of the severity of asthma, preoperative treatment with beta2 agonists or/and steroids and, if necessary, suspension of the procedure.

The measurement of peak expiratory flow rate can be an excellent diagnostic aid in pulmonary function tests, which aims to optimize a patient's individual peak expiratory flow rate prior to elective surgery. COPD is a chronic lung disease characterized by progressive and irreversible airflow restriction, with two common symptoms, namely, chronic bronchitis and emphysema, but these two symptoms often appear at the same time. According to studies, COPD is an independent risk factor for perioperative pulmonary complications. Therefore, the pulmonary function test of COPD patients should be paid attention to during the perioperative process, especially in preoperative assessment. Preoperative optimization includes, for example, treatment of patients with concomitant infection, partial bronchospasm and airflow restriction and non-invasive ventilator oxygen therapy. Patients with hypoxemia and pulmonary hypertension should also be identified during the preoperative assessment and, if necessary, a consultation with the relevant department may be sought to further clarify and treat the disease to improve their lung function and tolerance of surgical anesthesia. COPD patients usually show obstructive ventilation in pulmonary function test, with the ratio of first second exertional volume (FEV1) to forced vital capacity (FVC) being reduced.

A preliminary diagnosis of patients' respiratory function can be acquired through their limitations or endurance in daily activities, which can generally be assessed by the MRC (Medical Research Council) Dyspnea scale (Table 3.4).

We generally consider that patients classified as grade 3 or 4 dyspnea are at high risk of developing postoperative respiratory insufficiency because their lung function have already suffered greater impairment.

Simple testing method of lung function such as bedside test can also be adopted by the anesthetists. Common bedside tests of lung function

Table 3.4 MRC dyspnea scale

Grade	Degree of breathlessness related to activity
1	Not troubled by breathless except on strenuous exercise
2	Short of breath when hurrying on a level or when walking up a slight hill
3	Walks slower than most people on the level, stops after a mile or so, or stops after 15 min walking at own pace
4	Stops for breath after walking 100 yards, or after a few minutes on level ground
5	Too breathless to leave the house, or breathless when dressing/undressing

Used with the permission of the Medical Research Council (https://mrc.ukri.org/research/facilities-and-resources-for-researchers/mrc-scales/mrc-dyspnoea-scale-mrc-breathlessness-scale/)

include stair climbing, breath holding test, and match blowing test. First of all, climbing up three flights of stairs is a relatively relax physical activity for normal people, and there are usually no obvious symptoms of breathlessness after completing it. However, relax physical activity can make it difficult for the patient with impaired cardiopulmonary function to breathe and thus unable to complete the activity. Besides, breath holding test may be helpful to identify patient's lung function. Normal people can hold their breath for over 30 s. According to it, patients whose breath holding time is less than 20 s may be deemed as cardiopulmonary insufficiency. Another useful test is match blowing test which refers to placing a lit match in front of the patient and ask the patient to blow out the match. If the distance blown out is shorter than 15 cm, the FEV1% is estimated to be below 60%, FEV1 is below 1.6 L and the maximal voluntary ventilation is below 50 L/min; if the distance is shorter than 7.5 cm, the estimated maximal voluntary ventilation is less than 40 L/min.

For patients with impaired lung function, the anesthetists should prepare adequately, especially those with abnormal pulmonary function findings and high incidence of complications. Consultation and treatment by the relevant departments (respiratory medicine or thoracic surgery) may be required to reduce or prevent postoperative pulmonary complications. Modification of anesthesia, surgical approach, and prognosis should also be considered once abnormal pulmonary function results are detected. Specific preoperative preparations are as follow.

(a) Patients with acute respiratory infections, who are prone to get postoperative atelectasis and lung infection, may choose to postpone surgery, and elective surgery must be performed 1 to 2 weeks after the lung infection being cured.
(b) Providing education on giving up smoking and advising patients to quit smoking as early as possible, preferably 1 to 2 weeks before surgery.
(c) Patients with pneumocardial disease should be improved preoperatively with medication to keep cardiopulmonary function at optimum state and avoid perioperative cardiopulmonary complications.
(d) Patients with asthma can be treated preoperatively with bronchodilators and hormones to improve their conditions and avoid intraoperative airway spasm.
(e) Pre-anesthetic dosing of some interacting drugs should be reduced or even stopped.
(f) High-risk patients are prone to postoperative respiratory failure, which should be explained to their families preoperatively, and require postoperative mechanical ventilation.

Assessment of Nervous System

The assessment of the nervous system involves the assessment of 12 pairs of cranial nerves, motor nerves, sensory nerves, nerve reflexes, and autonomic nerves. The assessment of the cerebral nerves includes 12 pairs of cerebral nerve reflexes which can be divided into superficial, deep and pathological reflexes, and the different reflex results embrace different meanings, which will not be discussed in this section due to space limitations.

The Glasgow Coma Scale (GCS) is used to assess the severity of patients' coma when there is a problem with patients' consciousness, such as stroke, neurosurgery, and other reasons. Whereas, this scale is not used in awake patients. Besides, it has limitations such as it does not involve brainstem reflexes, is not suitable for patients who are intoxicated and who are taking sleeping or sedative medication (Table 3.5).

The higher the GSC score is, the less severe the condition is. On the contrary, the lower the score, the more severe the condition. When the score is below 8, the patient is in relatively severe coma.

Other Diseases

In addition to respiratory and cardiovascular diseases, liver, kidney, endocrine, and coagulation function should be examined in the preoperative assessment as well. Surgical trauma and the effects of anesthetic drugs may further aggravate the impairment of liver function. Patients with severe renal and endocrine dysfunction may not be eligible for elective surgery and require preoperative systemic treatment to adjust their general condition to a relatively ideal state before surgery. If patients have abnormalities in coagulation, which may lead to uncontrollable hemorrhage during or after surgery, the cause should be clarified and addressed before elective surgery is performed.

Table 3.5 Glasgow coma scale

Behavior	Response	Score
Eye opening response	Spontaneously	4
	To speech	3
	To pain	2
	No response	1
Best verbal response	Oriented to time, place, and person	5
	Confused	4
	Inappropriate words	3
	Incomprehensible sounds	2
	No response	1
Best motor response	Obeys commands	6
	Moves to localized pain	5
	Flexion withdrawal from pain	4
	Abnormal flexion (decorticate)	3
	Abnormal extension (decerebrate)	2
	No response	1
Total score:	**Best response**	**15**
	Comatose client	**8 or less**
	Totally unresponsive	**3**

Adapted from https://www.glasgowcomascale.org/what-is-gcs/

Evaluation of Mental Status

The preoperative assessment also requires an assessment of the patient's mental status, as surgery and anesthesia is an unfamiliar and unknown process that out of their control. They are likely to experience fear, anxiety and unease in the preoperative period. Despite the fact that anesthetists are experienced in the perioperative anesthesia management, predicting the possible adverse psychological state of the patients remains a difficult task in light of previous reports.

Anxiety (worrying about what might happen) has long been recognized as a kind of important emotion. Excessive anxiety may be an obstacle to the clinical treatment, which is why patients' psychological state also needs to be evaluated before surgery [53]. Some studies have shown that preoperative assessment and appropriate interventions (including psychotherapy, medication, etc.) can be effective in mitigating patients' anxiety and thus improve their prognosis.

Paranesthesia Examinations and Tests

1. Electrocardiography (ECG)

   ECG can measure patients' heart rate and rhythm and detect cardiac abnormalities such as myocardial ischemia by using different leads. Many cardiac conditions can be initially screened for by ECG in a non-invasive way. Currently, ECG is a routine preoperative test in China. Preoperative ECG is particularly important in high-risk groups, such as men aged over 40 or women aged over 50. The abnormal ECG results, together with the patient's medical history and physical examination results, determine whether further investigations (e.g. echocardiography) are required and, if necessary, a cardiology consultation can be requested to further clarify the diagnosis and management.

2. Echocardiography

   Echocardiography allows observation of the anatomical or pathological structures of the heart and can provide diagnostic evidence for various cardiac diseases (hypertrophic cardiomyopathy, constrictive pericarditis, pericardial effusion, atrial/ventricular defects, valvular heart disease, pulmonary hypertension, etc.).

3. Medical Imaging Study

   Chest X-ray is a routine or necessary preoperative examination. A clear chest X-ray provides a diagnostic basis for most chest, lung, and cardiac diseases and facilitates the preoperative assessment and optimization of the patient. In addition, for different departments such as orthopedics, oral and maxillofacial surgery, urology and general surgery, X-rays of different areas are performed to provide different diagnostic evidence.

   In addition, computed tomography (CT) and magnetic resonance imaging (MRI) techniques are also important components of imaging study. Chest CT provides clearer image information than chest X-ray. Therefore, it better reflects anatomical and pathological structures at all tomographic levels. MRI is a type of tomographic imaging that shows different anatomical structures and pathological tomographic images through different shades of gray [54].

4. Visual Aid

   Traditional methods of preoperative assessment and difficult airway prediction are complex and have poor accuracy, specificity, and sensitivity. Therefore, in recent years, new assessment modalities have been introduced and applied. Based on imaging techniques, visual aid is one of the new modalities. While assessing and anticipating difficult airway, common indicators involve anatomical structures such as thickness of anterior cervical soft tissue, hyoid bone-chin distance, epiglottis, hyoid bone, and pharyngeal cavity volume. However, the existing visual aids are still subjective and sometimes have poor prediction outcomes.

5. Big Data, Machine Learning, and Artificial Intelligence

   With the development and progress of technology, new technologies such as machine learning, artificial intelligence, and big data are becoming more sophisticated and their integration with healthcare industry is becoming closer. Big data is a field that treats ways to analyze, systematically extract information from, or otherwise deal with data sets that are too large or complex to be dealt with by traditional data-processing application software. It was originally associated with three key concepts: volume, variety, and velocity. Current sources of big data in China come from electronic health record data, genomics data, physiological monitoring data, and healthcare data from local and national databases, but there is currently no systematic organization and categorization of these data. In addition, big data is combined with machine learning. Machine learning is a branch of artificial intelligence (AI) and computer science which focuses on the use of data and algorithms to imitate the way that humans learn, gradually improving its accuracy. There are different models of machine learning, and each have different characteristics. Convolutional neural networks, for example, can be used for deep learning and principal component analysis for dimensionality reduction. Besides, artificial intelligence, which has also grown rapidly in recent years, is the science dedicated to developing systems or machines that approach or even surpass humans in some respect, thus contributing further to the development of science.

   The combination of artificial intelligence and medical care model is a popular research and development trend in recent years, which has a lot to do with the current domestic and international environment and the speed of technological development. At present, the national strategic planning and encouraging support policies for artificial intelligence have been launched, and the country has put forward 15 development requirements for medical artificial intelligence and the development of the industry has kept in pace with the policy and technology. Meanwhile, the market is also eager to medical AI under the promotion of the policies and optimistic about the development of the industry, with rising investment and the whole community committed to training and recruiting excellent AI talents. In addition, the "internet + medical care" model provides a large amount of data for learning and verification, and AI can provide new and powerful support and evidence for the clinical medical field after learning and exploring big data, thus forming a beneficial circle.

Intelligent healthcare can be used in a number of areas such as electronic assistance (electronic medical records, medication recommendations, etc.), medical imaging, assisted diagnosis and treatment, disease risk prediction, drug mining, and health management. Moreover, early detection of complications is the next area in which AI can play a role, and closely related to anesthesia. Currently, in reactive management system, harmful reactions are not managed until they occur or present. Such a passive system should be gotten rid of. Instead, cutting-edge technologies like artificial intelligence should be adopted to build active systems, thus radically avoiding harmful processes. To put this more concretely, it is about appropriate patient-specific treatment and prevention of disease in early diagnosis. The words "we tend to overestimate the effect of a technology in the short run and underestimate the effect in the long run," coined by Roy Amara are also suit to the field of intelligent healthcare. For example, the recently propagated algorithms are constrained to predicting in-hospital mortality, hypotension and EEG dual frequency indices, and therefore aroused little attention. To improve the surgery outcomes, we need to explore answers of questions such as which patients will benefit from surgery, when surgery should be performed, which anesthetic technique should be used and which perioperative pathway is most suitable for specific patients. The dynamic information sources need to be retrieved from different data sources, for example, electronic health records, surveillance devices, population health records, and among others, and then combining the above information with evidence-based clinical basis to aid and refine clinical decisions. However, we have not yet achieved this goal. Collecting and analyzing complete and real-time information on patients from different data sources remains a challenge. Professionals of healthcare organizations, including data scientists, both within and outside the health care organization, need to work together to integrate and analyze the data. In other words, perioperative artificial intelligence needs to be achieved through collaborations across the industry [55, 56].

Anesthesiology was one of the first disciplines in the medical field that dabbled in artificial intelligence by being the first to establish the pharmacokinetic-pharmacodynamic concept and model of clinical drugs (PK/PD model), which was the prototype for automated and robotic anesthesia. It will keep to the technological trend in the future with the anesthesia assessment and optimization of the patient being one of its key areas.

References

1. Twigg SR, Wilkie AO. New insights into craniofacial malformations. Hum Mol Genet. 2015;24:R50–9. https://doi.org/10.1093/hmg/ddv228.
2. Nugent N, McGillivary A, Earley MJ. 22q11 chromosome abnormalities and the cleft service. J Plast Reconstr Aesthet Surg. 2010;63:598–602. https://doi.org/10.1016/j.bjps.2009.01.021.
3. Heerva E, Peltonen S, Pirttiniemi P, Happonen RP, Visnapuu V, Peltonen J. Short mandible, maxilla and cranial base are common in patients with neurofibromatosis 1. Eur J Oral Sci. 2011;119:121–7. https://doi.org/10.1111/j.1600-0722.2011.00811.x.
4. Cung W, Freedman LA, Khan NE, Romberg E, Gardner PJ, Bassim CW, et al. Cephalometry in adults and children with neurofibromatosis type 1: implica-

tions for the pathogenesis of sphenoid wing dysplasia and the "NF1 facies". Eur J Med Genet. 2015;58:584–90. https://doi.org/10.1016/j.ejmg.2015.09.001.
5. Visnapuu V, Peltonen S, Tammisalo T, Peltonen J, Happonen RP. Radiographic findings in the jaws of patients with neurofibromatosis 1. J Oral Maxillofac Surg. 2012;70:1351–7. https://doi.org/10.1016/j.joms.2011.06.204.
6. Javed F, Ramalingam S, Ahmed HB, Gupta B, Sundar C, Qadri T, et al. Oral manifestations in patients with neurofibromatosis type-1: a comprehensive literature review. Crit Rev Oncol Hematol. 2014;91:123–9. https://doi.org/10.1016/j.critrevonc.2014.02.007.
7. Alfi D, Lam D, Gateno J. Branchial arch syndromes. Atlas Oral Maxillofac. Surg Clin North Am. 2014;22:167–73. https://doi.org/10.1016/j.cxom.2014.04.003.
8. Akram A, McKnight MM, Bellardie H, Beale V, Evans RD. Craniofacial malformations and the orthodontist. Br Dent J. 2015;218:129–41. https://doi.org/10.1038/sj.bdj.2015.48.
9. Beleza-Meireles A, Hart R, Clayton-Smith J, Oliveira R, Reis CF, Venancio M, et al. Oculo-auriculo-vertebral spectrum: clinical and molecular analysis of 51 patients. Eur J Med Genet. 2015;58:455–65. https://doi.org/10.1016/j.ejmg.2015.07.003.
10. Choi J, Park SW, Kwon GY, Kim SH, Hur JA, Baek SH, et al. Influence of congenital facial nerve palsy on craniofacial growth in craniofacial microsomia. J Plast Reconstr Aesthet Surg. 2014;67:1488–95. https://doi.org/10.1016/j.bjps.2014.07.020.
11. Shibazaki-Yorozuya R, Yamada A, Nagata S, Ueda K, Miller AJ, Maki K. Three-dimensional longitudinal changes in craniofacial growth in untreated hemifacial microsomia patients with cone-beam computed tomography. Am J Orthod Dentofac Orthop. 2014;145:579–94. https://doi.org/10.1016/j.ajodo.2013.09.015.
12. Brandstetter KA, Patel KG. Craniofacial Microsomia. Facial Plast Surg Clin North Am. 2016;24:495–515. https://doi.org/10.1016/j.fsc.2016.06.006.
13. Heike CL, Wallace E, Speltz ML, Siebold B, Werler MM, Hing AV, et al. Characterizing facial features in individuals with craniofacial microsomia: a systematic approach for clinical research. Birth Defects Res Part A Clin Mol Teratol. 2016;106:915–26. https://doi.org/10.1002/bdra.23560.
14. Seow WK, Urban S, Vafaie N, Shusterman S. Morphometric analysis of the primary and permanent dentitions in hemifacial microsomia: a controlled study. J Dent Res. 1998;77:27–38. https://doi.org/10.1177/00220345980770010201.
15. Ongkosuwito EM, van Neck JW, Wattel E, van Adrichem LN, Kuijpers-Jagtman AM. Craniofacial morphology in unilateral hemifacial microsomia. Br J Oral Maxillofac Surg. 2013a;51:902–7. https://doi.org/10.1016/j.bjoms.2012.10.011.
16. Ahiko N, Baba Y, Tsuji M, Suzuki S, Kaneko T, Kindaichi J, et al. Investigation of maxillofacial morphology and dental development in hemifacial microsomia. Cleft Palate Craniofac J. 2015;52:203–9. https://doi.org/10.1597/13-179.
17. Ongkosuwito EM, van Vooren J, van Neck JW, Wattel E, Wolvius EB, van Adrichem LN, et al. Changes of mandibular ramal height, during growth in unilateral hemifacial microsomia patients and unaffected controls. J Craniomaxillofac Surg. 2013b;41:92–7. https://doi.org/10.1016/j.jcms.2012.05.006.
18. Maruko E, Hayes C, Evans CA, Padwa B, Mulliken JB. Hypodontia in hemifacial microsomia. Cleft Palate Craniofac J. 2001;38:15–9. https://doi.org/10.1597/1545-1569(2001)038<0015:HIHM>2.0.CO;2.
19. Ongkosuwito EM, de Gijt P, Wattel E, Carels CE, Kuijpers-Jagtman AM. Dental development in hemifacial microsomia. J Dent Res. 2010;89:1368–72. https://doi.org/10.1177/0022034510378425.
20. Chen EH, Reid RR, Chike-Obi C, Minugh-Purvis N, Whitaker LA, Puchala J, et al. Tongue dysmorphology in craniofacial microsomia. Plast Reconstr Surg. 2009;124:583–9. https://doi.org/10.1097/PRS.0b013e3181addba9.
21. Ye XQ, Jin HX, Shi LS, Fan MW, Song GT, Fan HL, et al. Identification of novel mutations of IRF6 gene in Chinese families with Van der Woude syndrome. Int J Mol Med. 2005;16:851–6. https://doi.org/10.3892/ijmm.16.5.851.
22. Szpalski C, Vandegrift M, Patel PA, Appelboom G, Fisher M, Marcus J, et al. Unilateral craniofacial microsomia: unrecognized cause of pediatric obstructive sleep apnea. J Craniofac Surg. 2015;26:1277–82. https://doi.org/10.1097/SCS.0000000000001551.
23. Dixon J, Trainor P, Dixon MJ. Treacher Collins syndrome. Orthod Craniofac Res. 2007;10:88–95. https://doi.org/10.1111/j.1601-6343.2007.00388.x.
24. Vincent M, Genevieve D, Ostertag A, Marlin S, Lacombe D, Martin-Coignard D, et al. Treacher Collins syndrome: a clinical and molecular study based on a large series of patients. Genet Med. 2016;18:49–56. https://doi.org/10.1038/gim.2015.29.
25. Posnick JC, Ruiz RL. Treacher Collins syndrome: current evaluation, treatment, and future directions. Cleft Palate Craniofac J. 2000;37:434. https://doi.org/10.1597/1545-1569(2000)037<0434:TCSCET>2.0.CO;2.
26. Poswillo D. The pathogenesis of the Treacher Collins syndrome (mandibulofacial dysostosis). Br J Oral Surg. 1975;13:1–26. https://doi.org/10.1016/0007-117X(75)90019-0.
27. Martelli-Junior H, Coletta RD, Miranda RT, Barros LM, Swerts MS, Bonan PR. Orofacial features of Treacher Collins syndrome. Med Oral Patol Oral Cir Bucal. 2009;14:E344–8.
28. da Silva Dalben G, Costa B, Gomide MR. Prevalence of dental anomalies, ectopic eruption and associated oral malformations in subjects with Treacher Collins syndrome. Oral surg. Oral med. Oral Pathol Oral Radiol Endod. 2006;101:588–92. https://doi.org/10.1016/j.tripleo.2005.07.016.
29. Akre H, Overland B, Asten P, Skogedal N, Heimdal K. Obstructive sleep apnea in Treacher Collins syndrome. Eur Arch Otorhinolaryngol. 2012;269:331–7. https://doi.org/10.1007/s00405-011-1649-0.

30. Pereira PM, Schneider A, Pannetier S, Heron D, Hanauer A. Coffin-Lowry syndrome. Eur J Hum Genet. 2010;18:627–33. https://doi.org/10.1038/ejhg.2009.189.
31. Touraine RL, Zeniou M, Hanauer A. A syndromic form of X-linked mental retardation: the coffin-Lowry syndrome. Eur J Pediatr. 2002;161:179–87. https://doi.org/10.1007/s00431-001-0904-6.
32. Lopez-Jimenez J, Gimenez-Prats MJ. Coffin-Lowry syndrome: odontologic characteristics. Review of the literature and presentation of a clinical case. Med Oral. 2003;8:51–6.
33. Gilgenkrantz S, Mujica P, Gruet P, Tridon P, Schweitzer F, Nivelon-Chevallier A, et al. Coffin-Lowry syndrome: a multicenter study. Clin Genet. 1988;34:230–45. https://doi.org/10.1111/j.1399-0004.1988.tb02870.x.
34. Koehne T, Jeschke A, Petermann F, Seitz S, Neven M, Peters S, et al. Rsk2, the kinase mutated in coffin-Lowry syndrome, controls cementum formation. J Dent Res. 2016;95:752–60. https://doi.org/10.1177/0022034516634329.
35. Wilson GN, Oliver WJ. Further delineation of the G syndrome: a manageable genetic cause of infantile dysphagia. J Med Genet. 1988;25:157–63. https://doi.org/10.1136/jmg.25.3.157.
36. Meroni G. X-linked Opitz G/BBB syndrome. In: Pagon RA, Adam MP, Ardinger HH, Wallace SE, Amemiya A, Bean LJH, Bird TD, Fong CT, Mefford HC, Smith RJH, Stephens K, editors. GeneReviews(R). Seattle, WA: University of Washington, Seattle University of Washington, Seattle; 1993. Available online at: https://www.ncbi.nlm.nih.gov/books/NBK1327/.
37. Quaderi NA, Schweiger S, Gaudenz K, Franco B, Rugarli EI, Berger W, et al. Opitz G/BBB syndrome, a defect of midline development, is due to mutations in a new RING finger gene on Xp22. Nat Genet. 1997;17:285–91. https://doi.org/10.1038/ng1197-285.
38. Jacobson Z, Glickstein J, Hensle T, Marion RW. Further delineation of the Opitz G/BBB syndrome: report of an infant with complex congenital heart disease and bladder exstrophy, and review of the literature. Am J Med Genet. 1998;78:294–9. https://doi.org/10.1002/(SICI)1096-8628(19980707)78:3<294::AID-AJMG18>3.0.CO;2-A.
39. De Falco F, Cainarca S, Andolfi G, Ferrentino R, Berti C, Rodriguez CG, et al. X-linked Opitz syndrome: novel mutations in the MID1 gene and redefinition of the clinical spectrum. Am J Med Genet A. 2003;120A:222–8. https://doi.org/10.1002/ajmg.a.10265.
40. Parashar SY, Anderson PJ, Cox TC, McLean N, David DJ. Multidisciplinary management of Opitz G BBB syndrome. Ann Plast Surg. 2005;55:402–7. https://doi.org/10.1097/01.sap.0000174355.56130.0a.
41. Aranda-Orgilles B, Trockenbacher A, Winter J, Aigner J, Kohler A, Jastrzebska E, et al. The Opitz syndrome gene product MID1 assembles a microtubule-associated ribonucleoprotein complex. Hum Genet. 2008;123:163–76. https://doi.org/10.1007/s00439-007-0456-6.
42. Hsieh EW, Vargervik K, Slavotinek AM. Clinical and molecular studies of patients with characteristics of Opitz G/BBB syndrome shows a novel MID1 mutation. Am J Med Genet A. 2008;146a:2337–45. https://doi.org/10.1002/ajmg.a.32368.
43. Bhoj EJ, Li D, Harr MH, Tian L, Wang T, Zhao Y, et al. Expanding the SPECC1L mutation phenotypic spectrum to include Teebi hypertelorism syndrome. Am J Med Genet A. 2015;167a:2497–502. https://doi.org/10.1002/ajmg.a.37217.
44. Antoniades K, Peonidis A, Pehlivanidis C, Kavadia S, Panagiotidis P. Craniofacial manifestations of Smith-Lemli-Opitz syndrome: case report. Int J Oral Maxillofac Surg. 1994;23:363–5. https://doi.org/10.1016/S0901-5027(05)80056-6.
45. Muzzin KB, Harper LF. Smith-Lemli-Opitz syndrome: a review, case report and dental implications. Spec Care Dentist. 2003;23:22–7. https://doi.org/10.1111/j.1754-4505.2003.tb00285.x.
46. Pizzo G, Piscopo MR, Pizzo I, Giuliana G. Oral manifestations of Smith-Lemli-Opitz syndrome: a paediatric case report. Eur J Paediatr Dent. 2008;9:19–22.
47. Cunniff C, Kratz LE, Moser A, Natowicz MR, Kelley RI. Clinical and biochemical spectrum of patients with RSH/Smith-Lemli-Opitz syndrome and abnormal cholesterol metabolism. Am J Med Genet. 1997;68:263–9. https://doi.org/10.1002/(SICI)1096-8628(19970131)68:3<263::AID-AJMG4>3.0.CO;2-N.
48. Porter FD. Cholesterol precursors and facial clefting. J Clin Invest. 2006;116:2322–5. https://doi.org/10.1172/JCI29872.
49. Rajpopat S, Moss C, Mellerio J, Vahlquist A, Ganemo A, Hellstrom-Pigg M, et al. Harlequin ichthyosis: a review of clinical and molecular findings in 45 cases. Arch Dermatol. 2011;147:681–6. https://doi.org/10.1001/archdermatol.2011.9.
50. Liming W, Zhihua C, Mei Z, et al. Study on the prevalence and burden of chronic diseases in the elderly population in China. Chin. J. Endem. 2019;40(3):277–83.
51. Routine preoperative tests for elective surgery. National Institute for health and clinical excellence. Retrieved from https://www.nice.org.uk/guidance/ng45. Accessible date: July 15 2022.
52. Balint M, Bapat S. Preoperative evaluation of neurosurgical patients. Anaesth Intensive Care Med. 2020;21(1):20–5.
53. Davidson S, et al. Preassessment clinic interview and patient anxiety. Saudi J Aneasth. 2016;10(4):402–8.
54. Du X-H, et al. Artificial intelligence (AI) assisted CT/MRI image fusion technique in preoperative evaluation of a pelvic bone osteosarcoma. Front Oncol. 2020;10:1209.
55. Ramkumar PN, et al. Artificial intelligence and arthroplasty at a single institution: real-world applications of machine learning to big data, value-based care, mobile health, and remote patient monitoring. J Arthroplast. 2019;34(10):2204–9.
56. Maheshwari K, et al. Perioperative intelligence: applications of artificial intelligence in perioperative medicine. J Clin Monit Comput. 2020;34:625–8.

Medical Risk Management of Anesthesia for Oral and Maxillofacial Surgery

4

Ming Xia

4.1 Introduction

Risks to patients, staff, and organizations are prevalent in healthcare. Thus, it is necessary for an organization to have qualified personnel responsible for medical risk management to assess, develop, implement, and monitor risk management plans with the goal of minimizing exposure. There are many priorities to a healthcare organization, such as finance, safety, and most importantly, patient care, among which safety is one that cannot be overlooked, and medical risk management is a critical factor in achieving safety in health care.

4.2 Defining "Medical Malpractice"

To discuss medical risk management, it is a priority to be clear about the term "medical malpractice." Medical malpractice is defined as any adverse event that occurs through medical treatment [1]. Medical malpractice is considered to occur even if there are situations where the medical staff is not responsible, these include situations where the medical staff is the victim, or where a patient falls somewhere in the hospital. In the event of a medical incident, the hospital or clinic administrator must immediately report the date, time, place, and circumstances of the medical incident to related organizations. As mentioned above, the term "medical malpractice" is different from the general public's perception of the concept and requires attention.

Medical malpractice is specifically defined as medical negligence where there is negligence in the course of medical treatment and a causal relationship between the adverse event and the negligence. Medical negligence is predominantly found in cases of misdiagnosis, delayed diagnosis, injection accidents, blood transfusion accidents, drug abuse, and nursing errors. In order to determine whether medical negligence was caused by medical negligence, the level of medical care and the circumstances of the medical act at the time should be examined. If the outcome of a judicial decision is that the accident was caused by the negligence of a doctor or medical practitioner, he or she should be held liable under criminal, civil, and administrative law.

The rights of patients are stipulated in the medical malpractice law and the medical law. Medical malpractice is one of the main concerns of medical law and relates to the liability of medical professionals for "negligence in the diagnosis or treatment of a patient which results in injury or death." Negligence is the primary cause

M. Xia (✉)
Department of Anesthesiology, Shanghai Ninth People's Hospital Affiliated to Shanghai Jiao Tong University School of Medicine, Shanghai, China
e-mail: xiaming1980@xzhmu.edu.cn

H. Jiang, M. Xia (eds.), *Anesthesia for Oral and Maxillofacial Surgery*,
https://doi.org/10.1007/978-981-19-7287-4_4

of complaint in allegations of medical malpractice and therefore such action belongs to the category of Tort Law. A treatment agreement is established between the doctor and the patient when they begin conversation and treatment. Possible violations involve failure to comply with the duty to inform the patient or medical malpractice during treatment. Doctors, as professionals, have the duty of care to patients who come to them for medical assistance. If medical malpractice is suspected, a qualified lawyer should be contacted immediately to protect the patient's legal rights. Claims based on liability for medical malpractice may also arise during treatment in hospitals and nursing homes.

4.3 Characteristics of Oral and Maxillofacial Surgery

Oral and maxillofacial surgery involves a narrow field of operation—the mouth—and the close proximity of the mouth to the upper airway, which means that there is a risk of accidents. During treatment, there is a risk of accidental injury from local anesthesia and aggravation of systemic medical conditions due to the use of many fine sharp instruments or inlays and the use of local anesthetics containing vasoconstrictors, which can cause choking and aspiration. In a hyper-aging society, where more patients need to be monitored and managed for systemic conditions, and where there is an active promotion of visiting dental services for patients who find it difficult to come to hospital, there is a potential risk if there is a lapse in response.

In anesthesia, there is an increasing use of various drugs and medical equipment during general anesthesia. Infusion pumps and ventilators account for most of the causes of medical errors and near misses. Oral and maxillofacial surgery for inpatients and bedridden patients has been actively promoted in recent years and patients on ventilators require close attention. In addition, nasal infections caused by the use of suction devices during dental treatment have been reported from dental departments to hospitals and long-term care facilities, so it is essential that a rigorous safety management system incorporating infection control measures is in place and that the entire healthcare team is committed to safety management.

4.4 Characteristics of Medical Malpractice in Oral and Maxillofacial Surgery

According to the data in a report during the year 2013–2014, the number of incident reports for dentistry, orthodontics, pediatric dentistry, and oral surgery is relatively low, but it is generally believed that the actual number is much higher when incident reports for general oral and maxillofacial clinics are included [2]. In terms of the number of medical proceedings (District Court) that have been filed by medical subject, the number of incident reports arising from oral and maxillofacial surgery ranks fourth after medicine, surgery, and plastic surgery.

The incidence of medical malpractice arising from self-funded oral and maxillofacial clinics is relatively high, and patients have high expectations of improved cosmetic results and oral function. Therefore, it is important to always sign an informed consent form. This needs to be carefully explained especially for extractions and occlusion adjustments, as the procedures are irreversible. There have been many cases of medical litigation, such as wrong extraction sites, mistaken baby and permanent teeth, expensive implant surgery, and sensory disturbances after wisdom tooth extraction. In addition, medical negligence involving local or general anesthesia can lead to death, as a result, competence, skill, and knowledge in dealing with the unexpected, as well as the ability to anticipate and avoid danger, are necessary.

4.5 Accidents and Medical Malpractice

In academic classification, medical malpractices are divided into two main categories: accidents and errors caused by force majeure, drug side effects, and blood transfusions, while errors are usually divided into three categories: errors that cause medical errors, errors that by fluke did not cause an accident, and errors that could have been detected and corrected earlier. Medical errors caused by force majeure and error are considered to be the so-called medical malpractices, while cases that did not result in an accident by fluke and cases that could have been detected and corrected are considered to be cases that could have been medical malpractices. The former is referred to as accidents or incidents and are generally understood to be unintended events that occur during the course of medical treatment and cause harm to patients. The latter, also referred to as an incident or near miss, refers to an error that occurred or almost occurred but did not result in a medical error and did not cause harm to the patient. In the USA, all of these are referred to as incidents.

It is generally accepted that "behind every 1 major incident or disaster there are 29 minor incidents or disasters, and behind every minor incident or disaster there are 300 anomalies." "Heinrich's Law" sums up the occurrence of accidents in the form of a pyramid, i.e. behind one accident lies many near misses [3].

Furthermore, even if there is a potential danger, accidents can be avoided through protective measures such as knowledge, technical measures, and organizational safety initiatives, however, in reality, as the Swiss cheese model shows, accidents do not occur in isolation but as a sequence of events and it is difficult to create a perfect barrier, and accidents are likely to break down several layers.

In order to carry out daily medical activities safely, it is effective for an organization to conduct an internal evaluation of its own activities. For an objective internal evaluation, a medical safety management department should be established separately from other departments. In addition to the active reporting of near misses and incidents, it is necessary to consider improvement measures for cases arising from systemic problems in multiple departments and departments, as well as for cases that are difficult to analyze in each department, and to ensure that these measures are thoroughly implemented in the relevant departments. In addition, it is important to continue to check the status of medical and nursing records, the maintenance of consultation manuals and other documentation, compliance with guidelines and procedures, and to carry out daily near-miss reporting.

4.6 Causes and Their Analysis

When a serious incident or accident occurs, people tend to focus on "people" and assume that it is a human error. However, people's behavior is influenced by the environment and the environment is influenced by people, so when a problem occurs, it must be analyzed in terms of both "people" and "environment." In particular, the environment surrounding healthcare is complex, with multiple people involved and a variety of items, medical equipment, and facilities to deal with, so when an adverse event occurs, it is important to focus not only on human error, but also to analyze other factors from different perspectives in order to develop more effective measures to prevent recurrence.

4.6.1 Root Cause Analysis (RCA)

This is a method of planning accident prevention measures based on the root causes obtained by asking "why" to investigate the background factors of a medical accident, but it is not always possible to analyze the incident from all angles [4].

As a popular and widely used technique, RCA assists people to figure out why the problem occurred in the first place. It uses a specific set of steps, with associated tools to trace where a problem comes out and what are the primary causes of the problem, after which, you are able to identify what happened, why it happened and how to prevent it.

Essentially, RCA assumes that systems and events are interrelated. In other words, an action in one area may trigger and be triggered by an action in another area, and another area, and so on. By tracing back one action after another, the original and radical problem will be discovered and at the same time, the process how it progresses into the symptom patients are now facing will also be revealed.

4.6.2 SHEL Model, SHELL Model, and P-mSHELL Model

SHEL model is an accident analysis model proposed by Edwards (1972) and Hawkins (1975), who was an aircraft captain, as a method of analysis that takes into account the complexity of the environment surrounding the people involved [5].

In the SHEL model, the environment (E) includes the people involved (liveware, L), the software (S) (e.g. procedures, manuals, and rules), and the hardware (H) (e.g., the structure, equipment, and facilities of the facility).

The SHELL model revealed that the liveware (L) was at the center, surrounded by the associated software (S), hardware (H), environment (E), and even people other than the liveware (L).

In addition, in healthcare, a healthcare safety analysis model specifically for medical practices was used (P-mSHELL model), adding elements of management (m) and patients (P), such as safety management, to the SHELL model, to be analyzed from different perspectives.

4.6.3 4M4E

4M4E is a method used by NASA to investigate the causes of incidents and organize countermeasures. The specific causes of incidents and accidents are divided into 4 M's: Man, Machine, Media, and Management; and the countermeasures for each cause are the 4 E's: Education, Engineering, Enforcement, and Example. This allows the countermeasures for each cause of accident to be organized. It is a multifaceted method providing analysis on the causes that induce human making mistakes. It refers to the concept of accident investigation adopted by the National Transportation Safety Board (NTSB). Instead of merely launching guidelines on procedures, it provides ideas on how accidents should be evaluated and what lessons should be drawn from accidents. Accordingly, the method has been widely accepted by various industries and is used to review measures related to human error.

References

1. Patel K, Eltorai AS. Medical malpractice cases involving anesthesia awareness. J Clin Anesth. 2021;71:110225. https://doi.org/10.1016/j.jclinane.2021.110225. Epub 2021 Mar 4
2. Blau I, Levin L. Medical malpractice: an introduction for the dental practitioner. Quintessence Int. 2017;48(10):835–40. https://doi.org/10.3290/j.qi.a39106.
3. Maeda S, Kamishiraki E, Starkey J, Ehara K. Patient safety education at Japanese nursing schools: results of a nationwide survey. BMC Res Notes. 2011;17(4):416. https://doi.org/10.1186/1756-0500-4-416.
4. Rayan AA, Hemdan SE, Shetaia AM. Root Cause Analysis of Blunders in Anesthesia. Anesth Essays Res. 2019;13(2):193–8. https://doi.org/10.4103/aer.AER_47_19.
5. Tsuchiya H, Kurosaki H, Hiramoto S, Seki M, Moriuchi K, Kawauchi S, Kurita I. Analysis of medical accidents using the "Why Why Why Analysis" (questions): comparison with conventional analytical techniques. Nihon Hoshasen Gijutsu Gakkai Zasshi. 2005;61(12):1638–44. https://doi.org/10.6009/jjrt.kj00004022975.

Recognition and Management of the Difficult Airway

5

Hong Jiang

5.1 Introduction

Ventilation failure due to difficult airway is the most important cause of anesthesia-related death and disability, and about 30% of anesthesia deaths are related to improper airway management [1]. Difficult airway management is closely related to the safety and quality of anesthesia and is one of the world's most pressing problems in the field of anesthesiology. Oral maxillofacial head and neck surgery involves cranial, maxillary, facial, oral, nasal, orbital, head and neck, and even thoracic cavities, and is an emerging interdisciplinary specialty [2]. In contrast to other surgical patients, there are specificities in the way difficult airways are evaluated, causes of occurrence and management measures (including the choice of airway establishment route, choice of airway establishment equipment, methods of establishing emergency airway and postoperative airway management, etc.) in this type of surgical patients [1].

This chapter will describe the normal anatomy of the airway, the causes and prediction of the occurrence of a difficult airway, and the basic principles and techniques of airway management in oral and maxillofacial head and neck surgery.

H. Jiang (✉)
Department of Anesthesiology, Shanghai Ninth People's Hospital Affiliated to Shanghai Jiao Tong University School of Medicine, Shanghai, China

5.2 Normal Anatomy of the Airway

5.2.1 Nasal Cavity

The nasal cavity is mainly made up of bone and cartilage covered with mucous membrane and is connected to the outside world through the nasal aperture and to the pharyngeal cavity through the postnasal aperture. The bottom wall of the nasal cavity is the roof of the oral cavity, which is composed of bone and palate; the parietal wall is composed of nasal bone, frontal bone, ethmoid bone, and pterygoid bone, etc. Trauma-induced fracture of the skull base here can injure the meninges and produce cerebrospinal fluid nasal leakage; the medial wall is the nasal septum, which is mostly to the left, and there is a bleeding-prone area in the lower part of its anterior part with rich vascular plexus, where about 90% of epistaxis occurs; the lateral wall is divided into upper, middle, and lower nasal passages by the upper, middle, and lower turbinates, and there are openings for each paranasal sinus in the upper and middle nasal passages and the sphenoethmoidal recess.

5.2.2 Larynx

The larynx is connected upward to the pharyngeal cavity via the laryngeal opening and

H. Jiang, M. Xia (eds.), *Anesthesia for Oral and Maxillofacial Surgery*,
https://doi.org/10.1007/978-981-19-7287-4_5

downward to the lower edge of the cricoid cartilage to the trachea, which is surrounded by a cartilaginous scaffold to form a cavity containing joints and muscles and lined with mucosa. In adults, the larynx is located between the upper boundary pair C_4 to C_5 and the lower boundary flat C_6 lower edge. The position of the larynx in pediatric patients is higher than that of adults and decreases gradually with age.

The cartilage of the larynx includes the thyroid cartilage, cricoid cartilage, epiglottis cartilage, and arytenoid cartilages. The thyroid cartilage forms the anterior and lateral walls of the larynx, and the superior anterior angle protrudes forward to form the laryngeal node. The cricoid cartilage is the lower border of the larynx, posterior to the flat C_6, and it is the only complete cartilage ring in the respiratory tract. The cricothyroid membrane between the lower edge of the thyroid cartilage and the upper edge of the cricoid cartilage arch is superficially located and marked on the body surface, so it is often punctured here clinically for surface anesthesia of the vocal cords and endotracheal mucosa, and when laryngeal obstruction occurs, the cricothyroid membrane can be cut here for emergency artificial ventilation. The triangular fissure between the vocal folds is known as the rima glottidis. In adults and children over 10 years of age, the rima glottidis is the narrowest part of the laryngeal cavity, while in children under 10 years of age, the narrowest part is located in the cricoid cartilage below the rima glottidis.

The laryngeal muscles include the posterior cricoarytenoid, lateral cricoarytenoid, cricothyroid, and single cricoarytenoid intercalary muscles, a total of nine muscles. The main function of these muscles is to tense or relax the vocal cords. Laryngospasm can occur when the cricoarytenoid muscle is excited by extreme contraction. The laryngeal sensory and motor nerves are the bilateral superior laryngeal nerve and the recurrent laryngeal nerve. Both the superior laryngeal nerve and the recurrent laryngeal nerve originate from the cervical branch of the vagus nerve. The external branch of the superior laryngeal nerve innervates the cricothyroid muscle, and the internal branch innervates the sensation of the epiglottis, the root of the tongue, and the laryngeal mucosa above the rima glottidis. The recurrent laryngeal nerve innervates all laryngeal muscles except the cricothyroid muscle and the sensation of the laryngeal mucosa below the rima glottidis.

5.2.3 Trachea and Bronchi

The trachea and bronchi are connected between the larynx and the lungs by a "C"-shaped cartilage scaffold containing smooth muscle and connective tissue, lined with mucosa. The trachea starts from the lower edge of the cricoid cartilage and ends at the carina (the plane of the sternal angle, which corresponds to the plane between C_4 and C_5), and divides downward into the left and right main bronchi. The adult trachea is composed of 16–20 cartilages, with a total length of about 10–14 cm and an inner diameter of about 1.5–2 cm. The right common bronchus is about 2–3 cm long, short and straight, forming an angle of 25–30 degrees with the longitudinal axis of the trachea, and can be regarded as a direct continuation of the trachea, and it is often easy to enter the right main bronchus when the tube is inserted too deeply. The left main bronchus is about 4–5 cm long, slender, and forms an angle of 40–50 degrees with the longitudinal axis of the trachea. The length and internal diameter of the trachea and bronchi are not equal at different ages.

The cervical and thoracic vagus nerve branches and the postganglionic fibers from the sympathetic trunk ganglion and stellate ganglion in the upper thorax (T_1–T_5) together form a plexus, which is distributed in the trachea and bronchi and innervates their sensation, mucosal secretion, and smooth muscle contraction and diastole.

5.3 Knowing About Difficult Airway

5.3.1 Definition of Difficult Airway

According to the 2017 edition of the Difficult Airway Management Guidelines drafted and formulated by Chinese Medical Association Chinese Society of Anesthesiology, the definitions are as follows.

1. Difficult airway: a clinical situation in which a professionally trained anesthesiologist with more than 5 years of clinical anesthesia experience experiences difficulty with mask ventilation or intubation, or both [1].
2. Difficult mask ventilation (DMV): experienced anesthesiologists are unable to obtain effective mask ventilation after several attempts or more than 1 min without the help of others. Mask ventilation is divided into four levels according to the difficulty of ventilation, level 1 to 2 can obtain good ventilation, level 3 to 4 is DMV.
3. Difficult laryngoscopy exposure: direct laryngoscopy cannot visualize any part of the vocal cords after more than three efforts.
4. Difficult intubation (DI): regardless of the presence or absence of airway pathology, tracheal intubation by experienced anesthesiologists requires more than three attempts.
5. Difficult supraglottic airway device (SAD) insertion and ventilation: regardless of the presence or absence of airway pathology, SAD insertion by experienced anesthesiologists requires more than three attempts; or after insertion, ventilation is not possible.
6. Difficult invasive airway establishment: difficult positioning or difficult anterior cervical invasive airway establishment, including incisional techniques and puncture techniques.
7. Difficult airways are subdivided into non-emergency and emergency airways according to the presence or absence of difficult mask ventilation.
   (a) Non-emergency airway: only difficult tracheal intubation without difficult mask ventilation. The patient can maintain satisfactory ventilation and oxygenation, allowing sufficient time to consider other methods of airway establishment.
   (b) Emergency airway: An emergency airway is present whenever difficult mask ventilation is present, whether or not it is combined with difficult tracheal intubation. Patients are vulnerable to hypoxia and an emergency airway must be established. A few of these patients are "Cannot Intubate, cannot oxygenate (CICO)," which can lead to serious consequences such as tracheotomy, brain damage, and death.

5.3.2 Characteristics of Difficult Airways in Oral and Maxillofacial Head and Neck Surgery

Firstly, oral, maxillofacial, head, and neck surgical disorders inherently cause anatomical abnormalities in the airway and adjacent structures, so the incidence of difficult airways in patients undergoing this type of surgery is the highest of all surgical procedures and much higher than in patients undergoing general surgery. In a 6-year prospective study in Germany, the incidence of difficult airway was "5.8%" in 102,305 general anesthesia cases, with the incidence of 8.9% and 7.4% in maxillofacial surgery and ENT patients, respectively. The statistics of this discipline for more than 30 years show that the incidence is as high as 15–21%, which is much higher than the general surgery population (1–5%).

Secondly, the causes and manifestations of difficult airways in patients undergoing oral maxillofacial head and neck surgery have significant disease characteristics and therefore special features in terms of airway assessment and management response, which are also significantly different from other surgical patients.

1. Oral maxillofacial head and neck tumors. Tumors may occupy airway space or deform the airway through external compression to the point that airflow in and out is compromised, resulting in complete or incomplete

airway obstruction. The specific location of tumor growth adds to the difficulty of airway operations such as mask ventilation, laryngeal mask ventilation, endotracheal intubation, and extubation. Postoperative delayed removal of tracheal tube or tracheotomy is often required to prevent airway obstruction.

2. Temporomandibular joint disease. Temporomandibular joint disorders are common among oral diseases. Many temporomandibular joint disorders can lead to temporomandibular joint ankylosis, causing difficulty in opening the mouth. Bilateral ankylosis can result in a specific small jaw deformity. Such patients are often associated with difficulty in tracheal intubation or mask ventilation, which greatly increases the difficulty of management.
3. Craniomaxillofacial deformities or syndromes. Many craniomaxillofacial deformities or syndromes are clinically associated with difficult airway. Examples include Apert syndrome, Pierre Robin syndrome, and Treacher Collin syndrome. These syndromes tend to manifest primarily in cranial, orbital, and jaw deformities. Exposure of the airway during tracheal intubation is very difficult under normal circumstances due to the small mandible with a small jaw deformity.
4. Obstructive sleep apnea syndrome (OSAS). These patients tend to have short jaws or hypertrophy of the tonsillar and adenoid hyperplasia, and in severe cases may have respiratory and circulatory comorbidities. Improper management can easily lead to an airway crisis.
5. Oral and maxillofacial head and neck trauma. Due to the direct relationship between the oral cavity and the respiratory and digestive tracts, an alveolar fracture may affect the respiratory tract patency due to tissue swelling, displacement, glossoptosis, foreign body obstruction, etc., and asphyxia may occur in severe cases. External force acting on the middle of the face leads to a fracture of the base of the skull, accompanied by cerebrospinal fluid rhinorrhea. Head and neck injuries can lead to subcutaneous emphysema and hematoma, and dysphagia. It should be noted that one disease often causes multiple manifestations, such as craniomaxillofacial syndromes are often accompanied by OSAS, oral and maxillofacial head and neck tumors or trauma are often accompanied by temporomandibular joint disease or even OSAS, which are also more special for oral and maxillofacial head and neck surgery patients.

Thirdly, oral maxillofacial head and neck surgery patients have the highest degree of difficult airway complexity among all surgical procedures, and therefore the most difficult to manage. The oral maxillofacial head and neck can be divided into three zones, each of which has tumors, malformations, or trauma that can lead to serious airway problems. From top to bottom, they are Zone III: mandibular angle to skull base (complex airway situation and difficult to manage); Zone II: thyroid cartilage to mandibular angle (rapid progression of airway problems, prone to emergency airway); Zone I: clavicle to thyroid cartilage (area where large blood vessels, lungs, and trachea are located, high-risk area for airway problems and high lethality). Moreover, the tissue structure of the oral and maxillofacial head and neck itself is characterized by multiple potential cavities and sinus tracts, which also adds to the complexity of a difficult airway. At the same time, the site of the surgeon's surgery often involves the upper respiratory tract or adjacent tissues, which more or less causes interference to the anesthesia operation, all of which exacerbate the difficulty of difficult airway management.

Fourthly, difficult airway in oral and maxillofacial head and neck surgery can occur at all stages of induction, maintenance, extubation, awakening, and postoperative period of anesthesia, in other words, throughout the perioperative period. In particular, the long duration of postoperative airway management (sometimes up to several weeks) and the high incidence of airway crises during this period are a challenge for anesthesiologists, surgeons, and intensivists alike.

5.3.3 Difficult Airway Assessment

Pre-anesthetic airway assessment is important to help select the appropriate method of induction of anesthesia and tracheal intubation technique to minimize the risk of airway difficulties [3]. There are several methods for predicting airway difficulties, but even the most rigorous and thorough prediction cannot fully detect every case of difficulty [4].

5.3.3.1 Difficult Mask Ventilation

Mask ventilation requires tight coverage of the mouth and nose and opening of the airway. Factors associated with mask ventilation difficulties are: age >55 years; body mass index (BMI) >26 kg/m^2; history of snoring; beard; dental defects; (sensitivity and specificity >70% if two or more of these are met).

5.3.3.2 Difficult Tracheal Intubation

Medical History

All the following conditions should be paid attention to: congenital causes of difficult airway such as Pierre Robin, Klippe Feil, Down syndrome; acquired difficult airway such as rheumatoid arthritis, Still's disease, ankylosing spondylitis, acromegaly, pregnancy, diabetes mellitus, etc.; medical causes such as temporomandibular joint surgery, neck fusion, tracheal surgery, and oral pharyngeal radiotherapy and surgery.

Visiting the patient and reading the history before surgery is very important and is the best way to estimate potentially difficult tracheal intubation early and to avoid serious accidents. During the preoperative visit, it is important to focus on whether the patient has had any previous difficult tracheal intubation, etc. If the patient has a history of difficult tracheal intubation, special attention should be paid to the following four important issues when reviewing the medical record and history to clarify the nature, extent, and management of difficult tracheal intubation: the degree of difficulty of tracheal intubation and the solution used; the patient's position during direct laryngoscopy; the device used for tracheal intubation; and whether the operator is familiar with the patient's previous method of tracheal intubation.

Patients who have had jaw, oral, and pharyngeal surgery should be treated as difficult tracheal intubation at the next procedure, which is a particular emphasis for difficult airway management in oral anesthesia. In such patients, the best approach is to perform awake direct laryngoscopy after appropriate preparation prior to induction of anesthesia to determine if the patient has difficulty with laryngoscopic visualization. If the epiglottis and vocal cords are visible with direct laryngoscopy in the awake state, it is essentially certain that direct laryngoscopic visualization and tracheal intubation are not difficult after induction of anesthesia and muscle relaxation. If the epiglottis and vocal cords are not visible with direct laryngoscopy in the awake state, then the patient should be managed as if a difficult airway had been predicted, preferably with the usual awake tracheal intubation.

General Physical Examination

Anatomic features that lead to difficult tracheal intubation include small mouth, receding jaw, enlarged tongue, stiff head and neck, morbid obesity, and breast enlargement. Burns, tumors, abscesses, radiation therapy injuries, and restrictive scars of the head, face, and neck are also noted. Mechanical restrictions such as decreased mouth opening, jaw advancement, and limited cervical spine movement. Poor dental conditions such as cavities, missing teeth, and buck teeth. Certain orthopedic, neurosurgical, and orthognathic devices such as retractors, external fixation braces, and braces. Nasotracheal intubation needs checking nasal patency. Sometimes a beard can mask certain anatomical features of a difficult airway and requires attention.

Special Examination

(a) Interincisor gap: Interincisor gap refers to the distance between the upper and lower incisors at the maximum mouth opening. The normal value should be greater than or equal to 3 cm (2 fingers); if it is less than 3 cm, then there is a possibility of difficult intubation; less than 2.5 cm, it is difficult to place the laryngeal mask.

(b) Thyromental distance: Thyromental distance refers to the distance between the nail cartilage notch and the mandibular chin prominence when the patient's head is tilted back to the maximum. If the thyromental distance is greater than or equal to 7.0 cm, there is no difficulty in intubation; between 6 cm and 6.5 cm, there is difficulty in intubation, but intubation can be done with laryngoscopic exposure; less than 6 cm (3 fingers), 75% cannot be intubated with the laryngoscope. When the thyromental distance is too short, the patient's larynx is positioned higher and the mandibular gap is relatively small, so the tongue is easy to obscure the view under direct laryngoscopy and cause difficulty in exposing the vocal folds.

(c) Neck mobility: It can be measured through neck flexion and extension and neck joint extension. Neck flexion and extension refer to the range of motion of the patient from maximum neck flexion to neck extension. Normal values are greater than 90° and up to 35° from neutral to maximum posterior elevation; less than 80° makes intubation difficult. Cervical joint extension can be measured by taking lateral radiographs, CT, and MRI. With reduced neck mobility, greater force is required to lift the tongue under direct laryngoscopic exposure to expose the vocal folds, which can make intubation difficult.

(d) Mallampati test: This is a widely used clinical method of airway assessment today. The patient is seated in front of the anesthesiologist and the tongue is stretched to the maximum (without articulation) and the patient is graded according to the pharyngeal structures that can be seen. The higher is the grade, the more difficult is the intubation. Grade III or even IV belongs to difficult tracheal intubation. This classification is a composite indicator and its results are influenced by the patient's mouth opening, tongue size and mobility, as well as other intraoral structures such as the palate and craniocervical joint movements [5].

(e) Mandibular anterior extension: Mandibular anterior extension is an indicator of mandibular mobility. If the patient's lower incisors can extend anteriorly beyond the upper incisors, endotracheal intubation is usually easy. If the patient is unable to align the upper and lower incisors when extending the lower jaw forward, intubation may be difficult. The greater the anterior extension of the lower jaw, the easier it is to reveal the larynx, and the smaller the anterior extension of the lower jaw, the more likely it is that an anterior larynx will occur and make tracheal intubation difficult.

(f) Wilson risk score: Weight, neck mobility, mandibular mobility, mandibular recession, and buck teeth are used as five risk factors to assess the airway, each with a score of 0, 1, and 2, with a total score of 0 to 10. A score of ≥2 is associated with a 75% likelihood of difficult intubation, in addition, there is a 12% likelihood of false positives.

(g) Ancillary tests: After taking a history and performing a physical examination, ancillary tests can be used to help diagnose patients suspected of having a difficult airway. Ultrasound, X-ray, CT, and MRI can help identify a subset of congenital or acquired conditions that can lead to a difficult airway, such as tracheal deviation and cervical spine disease. For patients with suspected difficult airway with high-risk factors, visual laryngoscopy or visual intubation with tools such as flexible laryngoscopy and evaluation under conscious sedation and surface anesthesia is recommended to clarify the laryngoscopy exposure classification. Ancillary examinations are not routinely used in the evaluation of normal airways and are recommended only for patients with suspected or established difficult airways.

Difficulty in Backup Program

Difficulty in Laryngeal Mask Placement

The laryngeal mask has become one of the routine backup options after failed intubation. If the mouth opening is less than 2.5 cm, it is difficult to place the mask, and if the mouth opening is less than 2.0 cm, it is impossible to place the mask; oral and pharyngeal masses (such as bilateral tonsillar enlargement) also affect the placement of the mask [6].

Difficulty in Cricothyrotomy and Tracheotomy.
If tracheotomy is considered, the patient's anatomy of the larynx and trachea should be carefully examined. The feasibility of tracheotomy should be determined based on the patient's obesity, the presence of an anterior cervical mass, whether the trachea is deviated, posterior cervical elevation, history of radiation therapy, and the presence of an external fixation stent.

There are various ways to identify a difficult airway, and numerous scholars have conducted numerous studies over the years, but the results have been unsatisfactory. Due to the complexity of the factors that cause a difficult airway, involving congenital, postnatal developmental, and anatomical malformations due to specific diseases or trauma, it is difficult to obtain a predictive assessment system with high sensitivity and specificity that integrates all factors. Considering the specificity of oral and maxillofacial head and neck surgery and the high incidence of difficult airways, the possibility of unanticipated difficult airways throughout the unoperated period should be prepared as a backup plan [4].

5.4 The Establishment of Difficult Airway

5.4.1 Establishment of the Airway Without Intubation

5.4.1.1 Mask Ventilation

The principle of "ventilation first" should be kept in mind at all times. Regardless of the airway conditions, supply 100% oxygen to each patient with a face mask and ask for help from a superior physician. Keep the patient's head and neck in the "sniffing position." Two-person mask ventilation (one person holds the patient's jaw and presses down on the mask while the other person squeezes the respirator). It is recommended that the oropharyngeal or nasopharyngeal airway be used gently to avoid bleeding. The most important reason for the failure of mask ventilation is the inability to open the upper airway, at which point an oropharyngeal or nasopharyngeal airway can be considered.

5.4.1.2 Supraglottic Airway Device (SAD)

This includes laryngeal mask, intubating laryngeal mask, laryngeal tube, and others. Due to the limitations of head, neck, and maxillofacial surgery, they are generally used for emergency ventilation, or to guide tracheal intubation.

Laryngeal Mask Airway (LMA)

LMA, including the first generation laryngeal mask and two-point laryngeal mask, the first generation laryngeal mask (LMA Classic), has been used less and less in the clinical application because of its poor sealing and high-risk of reflux and aspiration. The second-generation mask is a gastroesophageal drainage tube type mask (double tube mask). ProSeal mask (LMA-ProSeal), Supreme mask (LMA-Supreme), and i-gel mask are the most widely used second-generation masks. They are characterized by a high placement success rate and can improve ventilation as well as replace tracheal intubation to maintain the airway [6, 7].

Intubating Laryngeal Mask

The commonly used ones are LMA-Fastrach, Cookgas Air-Q, Ambu Aura-i, and Block Buster intubating mask. The advantage of the intubation mask is that it can solve both difficult ventilation and difficult tracheal intubation, and has a high success rate of intubation, but is limited by the patient's mouth opening.

Laryngeal Tube (LT)

The laryngeal tube can be used to close the opening between the pharyngeal cavity and the esophagus, which is easy to put in and has less damage.

Others

SLIPA and other supraglottic tools, non-inflatable type, with a high success rate of insertion.

5.4.2 Difficult Airway Intubation

5.4.2.1 Route of Intubation and Endotracheal Tube

The route of intubation is often determined according to the surgical needs, and in principle should avoid obstructing the surgical operation if there is no special contraindication. Orotracheal intubation is appropriate for skull base, orbital, nasal, maxillary, and maxillary sinus surgery, and transnasal intubation is appropriate for intraoral, parotid glands, mandibular, and cervical surgery.

In addition, there are various types of tracheal tubes to meet the needs of different surgeries: RAE catheters are often used in cranial, oral, and maxillofacial head and neck surgeries, with the proximal end of the exposed oral tube bent downward and the proximal end of the exposed nasal cannula bent upward to maximize the exposure of the surgical field; nylon or wire thread catheters are not deformed after bending and are used in surgeries where the head position often needs to be changed to avoid folding and occlusion of the tube The length and capsule size of the special laryngeal microsurgery catheter are the same as the standard 8 mm ID catheter, but it is only available in 4 mm ID, 5 mm ID, and 6 mm ID models, which can be used in laryngeal microsurgery to reduce the catheter in the common access to obstruct the surgical operation. The laryngectomy catheter is inserted directly into the trachea through the tracheostomy opening, and the exposed proximal end is bent downward so that the proximal end of the catheter can be placed in the surgical field during the operation of laryngectomy; the tracheotomy catheter is shorter in length and is inserted directly into the trachea through the tracheostomy opening, and its distal opening is rounded, which can reduce the damage to the tracheal mucosa.

5.4.2.2 Intubation Methods

Surgical Versus Non-surgical

In general, non-surgical intubation has the advantages of high success rate, low risk, and ease of operation, and is often the preferred method for establishing airway management. However, in some cases such as upper airway abscess, laryngeal trauma, severe oropharyngeal deformity due to disease or trauma, and the presence of an acute airway, surgical options such as tracheotomy or cricothyrotomy may be considered.

Awake Versus Non-Awake

Awake intubation should be considered when a difficult airway is anticipated. For uncooperative patients or those with intracranial hypertension, coronary artery disease, or asthma, the risks of difficult intubation should be weighed against the risks of conscious intubation and given full consideration. The awake intubation method can be used in any intubation technique such as direct laryngoscopy, blind nasotracheal intubation, fiberoptic intubation, etc. It has the following advantages: ① preserves spontaneous breathing and maintains effective gas exchange in the lungs; ② airway reflexes are not suppressed, reducing the risk of asphyxia from false suctioning; ③ maintains muscle tension and keeps the airway anatomy in its original position, which is more conducive to tracheal intubation operations; ④ does not require the use of inhaled anesthetics and muscle relaxants, which can avoid the adverse reactions caused by these drugs in certain high-risk patients. There are no absolute contraindications to awake intubation unless the patient is uncooperative (e.g., children, mentally retarded, intoxicated, and aggressive patients) or the patient has a history of allergy to all local anesthetics [8, 9].

There is no denying that at this stage awake intubation is still one of the most effective means of managing a difficult airway, and it is also a technique that troubles many anesthesiologists. There are a lot of anesthesiologists who take a chance and hope to intubate under general anesthesia relaxation but fail to do so. Why blindly put the patient in the dangerous situation of "cannot intubate, cannot ventilate" when there are many awake intubation devices and equipment to choose from? Therefore, as a qualified anesthesiologist, especially in oral and maxillofacial head and neck surgery, one must be proficient in this technique. I am often asked by young anesthesiologists, "Which surface anesthetics and sedative drugs do you recommend most when performing awake intubation?" The difference between the drugs is minimal, and it is perfect surface anesthesia, the right level of sedation, and proficiency that are the keys to successful awake intubation. In a sense, awake intubation is an art that requires a lot of time and practice in order to achieve the best possible results.

Pre-Anesthesia Visits

Whenever possible, be sure to review previous anesthesia records; they have the potential to provide a lot of useful information. Most important is the status of tracheal intubation, especially the most recent one. Others, such as mask ventilation and drug tolerance, are also valuable. The reactions to local anesthetics and apnea due to small doses of anesthetics should be taken into account. Previous surgical procedures, especially oral and maxillofacial head and neck surgery, should also be reviewed whenever possible.

When we determine to perform awake intubation, we should use a calm and unhurried approach to explain to the patient the difference between conventional and awake intubation. The focus of the conversation should be on telling the patient that although the former is a simple and time-saving procedure, the latter is a safe approach that we make based on a comprehensive consideration of the patient's general condition. We must communicate with the patient and confidently recommend the awake intubation method to the patient. Patients should be informed of the complications of awake intubation, including local anesthetic intoxication, possible discomfort caused by the operation, and the unpleasant experience of the time. If the patient refuses awake intubation, the anesthesiologist should promptly communicate with the surgeon and work together to convince the patient.

When the patient is ready for awake intubation, preoperative medications are usually used to relieve the patient's nervousness and to keep the airway dry.

Pre-Anesthetic Medication

Benzodiazepines

Benzodiazepines have excellent anxiety relief, amnesia, sedation, and hypnotic effects. Midazolam is the most commonly used drug because of its easy dose adjustment.

Midazolam has a rapid onset of action and a short duration of action. In addition to sedation and anxiety relief, this drug has good amnesic effects. The oral dose is generally 15 mg before anesthesia, but intramuscular injection is more commonly used, the dose is 0.07–0.1 mg/kg, and intravenous injection is mostly used for induction of anesthesia, the dose is generally 0.2–0.3 mg/kg, and the dosage is mildly reduced for elderly people. This drug has an obvious paracrine amnesia effect, such as combined with fentanyl can be used during awake tracheal intubation by using fentanyl 0.1 mg intravenously before intubation and then injecting midazolam 0.05–0.1 mg/kg to reduce the discomfort and stress caused by intubation and to forget the intubation process after the operation. However, the blood pressure and respiratory status should be closely monitored after the drug is administered to prevent accidental events.

Opioids

These drugs have a good sedative effect and good cough suppressing effect when reaching certain plasma concentrations, which can inhibit the gag reflex and help prevent coughing and dry heaving during airway operation. Fentanyl takes effect 2–3 min after intravenous injection of 1–2 μg/kg and lasts for 0.5–1 h, and is the most commonly used drug for difficult intubation. Remifentanil is an ultra-short-acting anesthetic, metabolized by plasma and tissue esterases, with a half-life of 9 min. It has an onset of action of 1 min in the range of 0.05 μg/(kg min) to 0.5 μg/(kg min) and a duration of action of 5–10 min. Due to the risk of respiratory depression and muscle stiffness, this drug is not recommended for single injections.

Anticholinergics

The purpose of using anticholinergics is to reduce secretions. Excessive secretions can lead to two problems: the field of vision may be blurred whether using direct laryngoscopy or fiberoptic bronchoscopy; the presence of a layer of secretions during airway surface anesthesia will also prevent local anesthetics from reaching the appropriate site, affecting the effectiveness of local anesthetics.

Clinical atropine and long tonic are more commonly used. Routine intravenous or intramuscular injection of 0.4–0.6 mg atropine is used as pre-anesthetic medication, but atropine can cause dry mouth and discomfort, and in patients with chronic obstructive pulmonary disease, it makes sputum dry and thick, which is not easy to discharge, and can lead to tachycardia. The regular adult dosage of 0.5–1 mg of long tonic does not cause tachycardia and has gradually replaced atropine. Since anticholinergics can block the release of secretions, but cannot clear the secretions that have accumulated, it is best to administer the drug 30 min before anesthesia.

Vasoconstrictors of Nasal Mucosa

The nasopharynx and nasal mucosa are richly vascularized. When a patient requires transnasal intubation, adequate surface anesthesia of the nasopharynx and vasoconstriction of the corresponding area are necessary. Commonly used drugs are 4% cocaine or 2% lidocaine mixed with 1% phenylephrine, which produce good local anesthesia and vasoconstriction when applied to the nasopharynx. Furosemide nasal drops can also be used to constrict the nasal mucosal vessels.

Personnel and Equipment

Personnel

Before preparing to start induction, verbal communication with the patient is done to help overcome his or her fears. At least one professional is needed who can immediately participate as an assistant in difficult airway management. For high-risk patients, it is recommended that a physician familiar with surgical airway establishment be present to perform a tracheotomy or cricothyrotomy in a timely manner when the patient is in an emergency situation.

Monitoring Equipment

The ECG, noninvasive blood pressure, pulse oximetry, and end-breath carbon dioxide waveforms should be routinely monitored during induction of anesthesia. The electrocardiogram provides a continuous display of the patient's cardiac activity (e.g., heart rate and rhythm changes, heart block, and myocardial ischemia). Pulse oximetry monitoring allows early detection of blood oxygen deficiency. The presence of five consecutive waveforms on the carbon dioxide waveform graph confirms that the tracheal tube is in the trachea. Invasive monitoring should be prepared if the surgery is more complex or if the patient is in poor general condition.

Difficult Airway Cart

Each anesthesia department should have a difficult airway equipment cart. The difficult airway equipment cart is a mobile unit equipped with specialized equipment for difficult airway management. It includes various intubation tools such as visual laryngoscopes, fiberoptic bronchoscopes and light wands, various types and classifications of tracheal tubes, various emergency ventilation devices, cricothyroid or tracheotomy kits, and simple ventilators. Various types of syringes, sterile dressing kits, disinfectants, adhesive tape, etc. should also be available. The equipment cart should be manned, regularly inspected and replenished, and replaced with equipment so that all kinds of apparatus are in spare condition and clearly marked.

Airway Surface Anesthesia

1. Nasopharyngeal and Oropharyngeal Area Anesthesia.
   (a) Spray Technique.
   Local anesthetic is added to a nebulizer and connected to an oxygen source (flow rate 8–10 L/min). A nebulizer with a long nozzle can spray local anesthetic into the pharynx and vocal fold area. Each spraying operation lasts no more than 10 s, with an interval of 20 s before the next spray, alternating for about 20 min. The remaining drug in the oral cavity must also be aspirated to avoid absorption by the gastrointestinal tract leading to toxicity. In addition, Mucosal Atomization Device (MAD) is a cheap and simple emulsification device with a suitable injection device containing a certain amount of local anesthetic that can be quickly turned into a mist and sprayed into the oropharynx. 7% lidocaine spray is also commonly used and clinically effective as follows: ① ask the patient to open his/her mouth; ② insert a laryngoscope blade, gently lift the root of the tongue, and use the nebulizer to spray the larynx when the patient inhales deeply to administer anesthesia to the epiglottis and vocal fold; ③ in blind nasal intubation, a fine catheter can be inserted through the tracheal tube and sprayed when the patient inhales deeply to perform anesthesia of the pharynx, glottis, and tracheal mucosa [8].
   (b) Nebulization Technique.
   The ultrasonic nebulizer is filled with 5 mL of 4% lidocaine connected to oxygen (6–8 L/min). The size of the spray depends on the oxygen flow rate and the type of nebulizer. The advantages of ultrasonic spraying are ease of handling and safety of use, especially in patients with increased intracranial pressure, eye injuries, and severe coronary artery disease.
   If no special equipment is available, the following method can also be used: the patient is kept in a sitting position and a gauze strip infiltrated with 2 mL of 5% cocaine is filled into both nostrils using Tilley forceps. Then 4 mL to 6 mL of colloid of 2% lidocaine is dripped into the floor of the mouth, and the patient is instructed to swish the solution back in the oropharynx. After approximately 1 min, a suction catheter is gently placed into the posterior pharyngeal wall for the suction of the excess colloid and simultaneously evaluate whether the vomiting reflex is diminished. If needed, an additional 2–4 mL of colloid can be dripped.
2. Transglottic Injection Anesthesia (Cricothyroid Puncture).
   The ideal position for transglottic injection anesthesia is the supine position with the neck hyperextended. In this position, it is easy to expose the lateral cervical strap muscle so that the cricothyroid cartilage and the results above and below it can be easily palpated. The cricothyroid membrane is first located and, after aseptic preparation, the skin and subcutaneous tissue are infiltrated with 1% lidocaine. A 22-gauge trocar needle (posteriorly attached 5 mL syringe containing 4 mL of 2–4% lidocaine) is held and pierced into the cricothyroid membrane. Push posteriorly, in a caudal direction, and verify that the puncture needle position has entered the trachea with an air aspiration test. Once it is confirmed that the anterior end of the puncture needle is located in the trachea, the outer casing is then pushed forward while the puncture needle and syringe are removed. The syringe is reconnected to the outer cuff for an air aspiration test to determine the correct position of the outer cuff. The patient is asked to inhale deeply and 4 mL of 2–4% lidocaine is injected at the end of the inspiration, followed by asking the patient to cough sufficiently to help the

local anesthetic to spread. The complications and contraindications of transglottic injection anesthesia are similar to those of retrograde intubation. Potential complications are bleeding (subcutaneous and endotracheal), infection, subcutaneous emphysema, mediastinal emphysema, pneumothorax, vocal cord injury, and esophageal perforation. Contraindications include increased intracranial and intraocular pressure, concomitant severe cardiac disease, and unfixed cervical fractures.

5.4.3 Commonly Used Difficult Tracheal Intubation Methods

There are dozens of devices used for difficult tracheal intubation, which can be broadly divided into three categories according to the principle of intubation: tracheal tube guidance devices, supraglottic airway devices, and video laryngoscopes.

5.4.3.1 Tracheal Tube Guidance Device

Elastic Bougie
Gum elastic bougie (GEB) has become the preferred device for intubation assistance in the United Kingdom and is also very popular in the USA. When the patient's pharyngeal inlet is not fully exposed, the GEB can help with intubation. The probe is kept forward and reaches near the midline to avoid entering the esophagus or pyriform fossa. When the probe enters the trachea and slides along the cartilaginous ring of the trachea, it is smooth; when the bougie enters until it encounters resistance, it means that the front end of the bougie reaches the rongeur or common bronchus, and the scale is about 20–40 cm. Finally, the tracheal tube is inserted under the guidance of the bougie, and rotating the tracheal tube 90 degrees counterclockwise helps the successful intubation. The final diagnosis is confirmed and the flexible probe is withdrawn. The Frova probe is a newly designed hollow catheter guidance device that can be used not only for intubation but also for changing tracheal tubes. It has an angled end with two lateral holes. The Aintree Airway Switching Catheter is a hollow ventilation/exchange probe that allows for the direct insertion of a fiberoptic bronchoscope. The bougie has an inner diameter of 4.7 mm, is 56 cm long, and has a 3 cm tip that allows the fiberoptic bronchoscope to be exposed for easy positioning and guidance.

Fiber Optic Laryngoscopes
The Shikani Optical Stylet laryngoscope has the advantages of an ordinary fiberoptic bronchoscope, and at the same time has a certain degree of rigidity and plasticity, and is easy to operate, especially for physicians who are not familiar with tracheal intubation. The Flexible Airway Scope Tool is a fiber optic system similar to the Shikani Optical Stylet, with greater flexibility to make nasotracheal intubation possible. Bonfils fiberscope uses a 5 mm fiberscope that is inserted into the patient's laryngeal cavity through the posterior molar route. The Bonfils fiberscope is suitable for patients with cervical spondylosis and limited mouth opening [10]. SensaScope is a hybrid steerable semirigid S-shaped video stylet that can facilitate the management of difficult airway situations in anaesthetized patients [11].

Fiberoptic Bronchoscope
The fiberoptic bronchoscope is thin and soft and can be bent at will, with little irritation to the surrounding tissues and a high success rate of intubation, making it one of the most feasible methods for difficult tracheal intubation. The detailed implementation procedures and precautions are as follows.

Nasotracheal Intubation Using Fiberoptic Bronchoscope
Place the bronchoscope in the nose, determine the position of the inferior turbinate, and feed the front end of the fiberoptic bronchoscope downward along the base of the nose. Push in the fiberoptic bronchoscope and keep the front end in the center of the visual field space. When exiting the posterior nostril into the oropharynx, the patient is asked to breathe deeply or extend the tongue to open the visual field. The anterior end of the fiberoptic bronchoscope is brought as close to the epiglottis as possible, at which point the assistant

sprays lidocaine from the epidural catheter. Make sure that the negative pressure suction access is closed while the local anesthetic is being injected, and do not turn on the suction line until at least 30 s after the injection. Once the sprayed local anesthetic reaches the mucosa, it causes the patient to choke and cough, at which point the visual field is temporarily affected. The front end of the fiberoptic bronchoscope is entered along the lower part of the epiglottis, and the vocal cords can be seen for approximately 30 s. The local anesthetic is sprayed again, at which point lidocaine may be injected directly into the vocal folds, which may take two to three times until vocal cord motion is reduced. The fiberoptic bronchoscope is pushed into the vocal hilum, ideally during the inspiratory phase if controlled access is possible. After seeing the tracheal ring, continue to advance the fiberoptic bronchoscope in the direction of the tracheal bulge, be careful not to touch the tracheal wall as this may interfere with the view. Local anesthetic is re-injected to anesthetize the tracheal wall and the tracheal ridge. This completes the placement of the fiberoptic bronchoscope via the nasal cavity. The guided insertion of the tracheal tube is the most uncomfortable part of the entire fiberoptic bronchoscopy procedure, so additional sedative medication is administered prior to the start of intubation. Apply lubricating gel to the interface between the catheter and the nose; do not apply the entire catheter to avoid too much slippage to interfere with the procedure. It is usually important to inform the patient of the possible discomfort during catheter entry. Gently push the tracheal tube from the nasopharynx along the fiberoptic bronchoscope stem. Rotating the tube 90 degrees counterclockwise before entering the vocal cords will prevent the tip of the tube from resting on the vocal cords or arytenoid cartilage.

Orotracheal Intubation Using Fiberoptic Bronchoscope

A special airway for tracheal intubation (such as Ovassapian airway) needs to be applied or an assistant can use a direct laryngoscope to push away the tongue root and place the mirror stem in the median line, which can significantly shorten the intubation operation time and improve the safety of the patient. A 5% lidocaine ointment is applied to the surface of the ventilator and the ventilator is slowly placed on the floor of the mouth. Gentle suctioning is performed prior to initiation. The fiberoptic bronchoscope is then advanced through the airway. The tip of the fiberoptic bronchoscope enters the mouth when it is beyond the airway. The epiglottis is seen and the fiberoptic bronchoscope is continued until the anterior end passes through the vocal cords and into the trachea. If the surface anesthesia of the airway is inadequate, surface anesthesia can be completed with a gradual spray of lidocaine. Gently insert the tracheal tube through the airway, rotating the tube with your fingers as you advance (do not lubricate the periphery of the tube or your fingers or rotation will be difficult) and push the tube along the stem of the scope until it enters the airway through the larynx. When the tip of the catheter reaches 2 cm to 3 cm above the bulge, exit the fiberoptic bronchoscope and the special airway.

The fiberoptic bronchoscope is used to visualize the tracheal ring and the tracheal ridge, and the position of the catheter can usually be determined at the same time as exiting the fiberoptic bronchoscope.

Light Wand and Blind Intubation Devices

The use of fluoroscopy for tracheal intubation has been reported since the 1950s. The Trachlight™ consists of a handle, a light wand, and a guide core. The Light Wand is a bendable catheter with a light bulb at the front. The operator holds the handle, places the tracheal tube over the light bar, and places it in the patient's larynx, where a bright light spot can be seen moving down the anterior neck of the patient, providing a visual indicator for blind intubation and thus effectively increasing the success rate of difficult intubation. The use of Trachlight™ is limited in patients with significant structural abnormalities of the larynx, excessive obesity, and neck scars. The Trachlight™ technique is still a blind technique, but is particularly useful and simple to perform when fiberoptic bronchoscopy is not available (e.g., in emergency rooms, ambulances, or when there is a large number of secretions and blood in the airway) [12].

The blind tracheal intubation device is a new intubation guidance device developed by the

Department of Anesthesiology of the Ninth People's Hospital of Shanghai Affiliated to Shanghai Jiaotong University School of Medicine to solve the problem of difficult tracheal intubation, consisting of three parts: esophageal tracheal guidance tube, optical fiber, and power box. The distal end of the esophageal tracheal guide tube is a round closed blind end, and there is an elliptical opening in the wall of the tube 6 cm from the apex, and there is a silicone rubber bevel in the lumen under the elliptical opening, and the top of the bevel coincides with the distal end of the elliptical hole. The head end of the optical cable is slightly upturned and the other end can be connected to an external DC power supply. During operation, the patient is lying supine. The esophageal airway is inserted into his or her esophagus so that the oval opening in the wall of the tube is aligned with the vocal cords, at which point clear tubular breath sounds can be heard outside the mouth of the tube. The optical fiber was inserted into the esophageal airway, and as the optical fiber entered the trachea through the elliptical opening, a bright light spot could be seen moving down outside the anterior neck of the patient, and the insertion was stopped when it moved to the superior sternal recess. The esophageal airway is removed and the light cord is used to guide the insertion of the desired tracheal tube. This method addresses the characteristic that tracheal catheters tend to slip into the esophagus in patients with difficult intubation, and changes the previous method of intubation by guiding from the esophagus into the trachea to complete intubation. A blind probe tracheal intubation device was developed for nasotracheal intubation, which is especially suitable for oral and maxillofacial head and neck surgery and plastic surgery. The success rate of intubation is about 95% and does not cause significant fluctuation of hemodynamics during intubation [12].

Intubating Laryngeal Mask

The laryngeal mask has been widely used clinically as a common ventilation tool in patients with airway difficulties in both emergency and non-emergency situations. The mask forms a closed circle around the patient's laryngeal opening and is effective in overcoming upper airway obstruction and maintaining voluntary or positive pressure ventilation. The LMA-Fastrach™ laryngeal mask is designed for blind intubation or fiberoptic bronchoscopy-guided intubation and is a modification of the LMA Classic. The LMA-Fastrach™ has a 95–97% success rate of guided endotracheal intubation via the mouth. The video intubating laryngeal mask, trade name LMA-Ctrach™, has a removable LCD display and operates in a similar manner to the LMA-Fastrach™, which has been reported to significantly increase intubation success rates.

5.4.3.2 Video Laryngoscope

Video laryngoscope is a modification of the traditional direct laryngoscope with an integrated video system. The rigid video laryngoscope is another major invention of the last few decades as it requires non-line-of-sight of the glottis and is effective in overcoming current difficult airway problems such as restricted mouth opening, chin-thoracic adhesions, microstomia, and ankylosing spondylitis. Rigid video laryngoscopes can be divided into two categories according to the presence or absence of tracheal tube guided access [10].

Without Tracheal Tube Guided Access

The GlideScope® is a video laryngoscope manufactured by Saturn Biomedical System, Inc. The GlideScope® lens is only 1.8 cm thick and has an angled front end of 60°, which facilitates the visualization of the voice box and makes tracheal intubation easier with the guidance of the monitor image.

With Tracheal Tube Guided Access

Pantax Airway Scope® AWS-S100 is a newly developed portable rigid video laryngoscope. It integrates an LCD screen and a single-use curved lens. The main feature is that the curved lens has a tracheal tube guidance channel on one side. During operation, the tracheal tube is fed into the trachea through the channel according to the image of the glottis displayed on the LCD screen. The Pantax Airway Scope® significantly improves the success rate of conventional direct laryngoscopic intubation above Cormack-Lehane class III.

Retrograde Guided Intubation

This method has been used successfully in the clinic for many years and is particularly useful in patients with severe maxillofacial trauma, temporomandibular joint ankylosis, and upper airway masses who have difficulty intubating. Cook has designed a set of retrograde guided intubation devices that can be used for tracheal tubes with an internal diameter of 5 mm or more.

5.4.4 Establishment of Surgical Airway

5.4.4.1 Cricothyroid Puncture and Incisional Ventilation

In cases where CICO takes place, this will result in progressive oxygen desaturation. At this point, the patient's airway must be opened urgently. Cricothyroid membrane puncture ventilation: The catheter is 4 mm in diameter (e.g. Quicktrach set) and is punctured through the cricoid membrane, allowing direct mechanical or manual control ventilation. The cricothyroid membrane is first located and the puncture kit is held in the right hand and punctured into the trachea from the cricothyroid membrane in an oblique posterior and inferior direction. Fix the puncture needle core, push the outer cuff forward, pull out the needle core, inflate the cuff and then connect to the anesthesia machine for manual or mechanical ventilation. Cricothyroidotomy ventilation: Firstly, the external laryngeal maneuver is performed to confirm the position of the cricothyroid membrane, the blade is directed toward the operator, a transverse incision is made in the cricothyroid membrane, the cricothyroid membrane is cut, the blade is rotated clockwise so that the blade is directed caudally, the probe is placed against the lower edge of the blade to dive into the trachea, the tracheal tube (ID5.0 mm) is introduced into the trachea along the probe, ventilation is performed, the capsule is inflated, the position of the tube is confirmed by the capnography, and the tube is fixed. A longitudinal incision is recommended in obese or anatomically variant patients.

5.4.4.2 Percutaneous Dilatation Tracheotomy

At present, according to the different methods and instruments of dilation, they can be divided into single-step percutaneous rotary dilatation tracheotomy, modified single-step dilatation technique, and guidewire dilatation clamp technique, among which the most commonly used is the guidewire dilatation clamp method. The guidewire dilating forceps method tracheotomy kit mainly includes a tracheotomy scalpel, a tracheal puncture needle (like the size of a 14-gauge intravenous cannula needle), a steel wire, a hollow dilator, a special dilating forceps with a groove inside to hold the wire, and slide on the wire, and a tracheotomy catheter with a tube inside the core to pass the wire. Usually, the second to third or third to fourth tracheal cartilage ring is chosen as the incision. The skin is cut with a knife, a puncture needle is inserted deep into the trachea at the incision, the wire is inserted into the trachea through the puncture needle, the needle is withdrawn and the wire is left in place, then the dilator is inserted via the wire for initial expansion between the cartilage rings of the trachea so that the special dilating forceps can be inserted with the wire for further lateral expansion, and finally, the tracheotomy catheter is inserted via the wire guide.

5.4.5 Difficult Airway Establishment Process

5.4.5.1 Anticipated Difficult Airway

When the patient is judged to have a difficult airway through pre-anesthetic evaluation, the nature of the difficult airway is analyzed and the appropriate technique is selected, which should be dealt with: ① informing the patient of this particular risk so that the patient and his or her family fully understand and cooperate and sign the informed consent form; ② determining the preferred option for tracheal intubation and at least one alternative option before anesthesia, and rapidly adopting the alternative option when the preferred option fails; ③ administering oxygen by mask under mild sedation, analgesia and adequate surface anesthesia (including cricothyroid puncture endotracheal surface anesthesia), mask administration of oxygen, and attempt laryngoscopic visualization; ④ if the glottis can be seen, direct intubation or fast induction intubation can be performed; ⑤ if the visualization is poor, try to use techniques and airway devices that the operator is familiar with, and prefer minimally invasive methods of awake tracheal intubation; ⑥ during the whole process of difficult airway management, ensure ventilation and oxygenation, closely monitor the change of pulse oximetry of the patient, when it drops to 90%, promptly administer oxygen ventilation with the aid of a mask to ensure the safety of the patient's life as the primary goal; ⑦ if the intubation is not successful for more than three attempts, it is necessary to postpone or abandon anesthesia and surgery to ensure the safety of the patient, and deal with it again after summing up experience and adequate preparation.

5.4.5.2 Unanticipated Difficult Airway

It should be dealt with as follows: ① for ventilation difficulties encountered after induction of general anesthesia, seek help immediately; ② at the same time, efforts should be made to solve ventilation problems in the shortest possible time, such as mask positive pressure ventilation (using oropharyngeal or nasopharyngeal airway), placing supraglottic airway devices such as laryngeal mask to improve ventilation; ③ if ventilation and oxygenation are good, special devices such as visual laryngoscope, intubation mask, and other devices can be tried to assist intubation; ④ if intubation fails, do not attempt repeatedly and consider waking up the patient and choosing awake tracheal intubation; ⑤ if the ventilation and oxygenation situation deteriorates, immediately surgically establish an airway to ensure the patient's life safety.

5.5 Tracheal Tube Fixation

The tube should be securely fastened after recording the scale of the tube from the incisor to prevent accidental slippage. Using tape to attach the tube to the skin at the maxilla is the most common method. Because there is little movement in this area, and there will not be significant displacement of the tube within the airway, and the tube fits snugly against the upper jaw with less interference from the tongue. Wrapping the ends of the tape around the neck for one week reinforces the catheter, but there is a risk of interfering with venous return. Another reliable method is to secure the tube to the incisor by wrapping tape around it or to the corners of the mouth with surgical sutures. The fixation of a nasotracheal tube is similar to that of an orotracheal tube. Alternatively, the tube can be wrapped with sutures and tied to the nasal septum.

Accidental extubation during oral maxillofacial head and neck surgery is a real danger of the procedure. The anesthesiologist should be fully aware of this possibility and maintain constant communication with the surgeon to jointly avoid accidental extubation.

5.6 Management of Postanesthesia Recovery

5.6.1 Extubation

Extubation is smooth in most cases, but in some specific patients, it is even more challenging than intubation. Postoperative edema, changes in facial structures, and postoperative bandaging make mask ventilation impossible. Ventilation tracts may also be unusable due to concerns about disrupting the anatomy of the post-repair oropharynx and nasopharynx.

To ensure safe extubation, the anesthesiologist should consider the following two questions. First, is there an air leak around the tube after the cuff is deflated? Second, if the patient develops airway obstruction during extubation, is emergency ventilation, including surgical airway establishment, feasible? If the answer to both questions is yes, extubation may be attempted.

Adequate oxygenation and suctioning of the patient's airway secretions and gastric contents are needed. If necessary, a small amount of tracheal dilator and a short-acting β1 blocker such as esmolol can help improve the patient's breathing and circulation. Intravenous dexamethasone and elevation of the patient's head prior to extubation may relieve airway edema. Confirm that the patient is fully awake and free of residual inotropic effects, that tidal volume and ventilation per minute are essentially normal, and that SpO_2 is maintained above 95%. As long as there are no contraindications, the patient may be placed semi-recumbent at extubation, which maximizes functional residual air volume and minimizes airway obstruction. If there is a possibility of tongue drop after extubation, the tongue should be withdrawn and fixed with sutures. A ventilation-guided tube, such as a jet ventilation tube (Cook Airway Exchange Catheter) or fiberoptic bronchoscope, should be used for extubation. In this way, the tube retained after extubation can also ensure oxygenation and can be reintroduced at any time. The use of nasogastric tubes or optical fibers as guiding tubes can also have a corresponding effect. The extubation should be gentle. First, try to retreat the tracheal tube to the voice box and observe whether there is tracheal stenosis or collapse, and then slowly remove the tracheal tube. If there are no special circumstances, then the ventilation guide tube will be removed last. An oropharyngeal airway, nasopharyngeal airway, or laryngeal mask may be attempted if a posterior tongue drop is present. A small number of patients may develop laryngeal edema or laryngospasm, and symptoms are usually relieved by treatment with pressurized oxygen and nebulized epinephrine inhalation. If the symptoms continue to worsen or even dyspnea occurs, reintubation or tracheotomy should be considered.

5.6.2 Prophylactic Tracheotomy

Surgery on the floor of the mouth and posterior pharyngeal wall causes local edema with the risk of airway obstruction. If the surgery is extensive and causes significant changes in airway anatomy, and if airway patency cannot be ensured in the short term, prophylactic tracheotomy is the best option. Inhale 100% oxygen before performing an open tracheotomy to avoid hypoxemia by avoiding having sufficient oxygen reserves. Avoid direct electrocautery during tracheotomy to prevent airway burns. Once the trachea is entered and the surgeon can see the trachea the anesthesiologist should gradually push the catheter outward so that the distal end of the catheter is above the tracheotomy opening. Communication with the surgeon during this procedure is important to avoid unexpected situations.

References

1. Jiang H, Zhu YS, Zhang ZY. Identification and Management of Difficult Airway in perioperative period. Shanghai J Stomatol. 2003;12(2):147–9.
2. Zhu YS. Modern anesthesia in Oral and maxillofacial and neck surgery. Jinan: Shandong Science & Technology Press; 2001.
3. Mayhew JF. Airway management for oral and maxillofacial surgery. Int Anesthesiol Clin. 2003;41:57–65.
4. Rincon DA. Predicting difficult intubation. Anesthesiology. 2006;104:618–9.
5. Lee A, Fan LT, Gin T, et al. A systematic review(meta-analysis) of the accuracy of the mallampati tests to predict the difficult airway. Anesth Analg. 2006;102:1867–78.
6. Kurola J, Pere P, Niemi-Murola L, et al. Comparison of airway management with the intubating laryngeal mask, laryngeal tube and CobraPLA by paramedical students in anaesthetized patients. Acta Anaesthesiol Scand. 2006;50:40–4.
7. van Zundert A, Al-Shaikh B, Brimacombe J, et al. Comparison of three disposable extraglottic airway devices in spontaneously breathing adults: theLMA-Unique, the Soft Seal laryngeal mask, and the Cobra perilaryngeal airway. Anesthesiology. 2006;104:1165–9.
8. Sun Y, Jiang H, Zhu Y, et al. Blind intubation device for nasotracheal intubation in 100 oral and maxillofacial surgery patients with anticipated difficult airways: a prospective evaluation. Eur J Anaesthesiol. 2009;26:746–51.
9. Heinrich S, Birkholz T, Irouschek A, Ackermann A, Schmidt J. Incidences and predictors of difficult laryngoscopy in adult patients undergoing general anesthesia: a single-center analysis of 102,305 cases. J Anesth. 2013;27(6):815–21.
10. Leung YY, Hung CT, Tan ST. Evaluation of the new viewmax laryngoscope in a simulated difficult airway. Acta Anaesthesiol Scand. 2006;50:562–7.
11. Biro P, Battig U, Henderson J, et al. First clinical experience of tracheal intubation with the SensaScope, a novel steerable semirigid video stylet. Br J Anaesth. 2006;97:255–61.
12. Sun Y, Liu JX, Jiang H, et al. Cardiovascular responses and airway complications following awake nasal intubation with blind intubation device and fibreoptic bronchoscope: a randomized controlled study. Eur J Anaesthesiol. 2010;27:461–7.

General Anesthetic Techniques in Oral and Maxillofacial Surgery

6

Ming Xia

6.1 Concepts and Methods of General Anesthesia

6.1.1 The Concept of General Anesthesia

When ether and chloroform were used as general anesthetics more than 70 years ago, the main goal of general anesthesia was to lose consciousness. This was because it was believed that if the patient was unconscious, he or she would not feel anxious about the procedure and would not remember any intraoperative pain. However, it has recently become clear that even if the patient is unconscious during anesthesia, nociceptive receptors sense the stimulus of tissue damage and release painful and inflammatory substances such as prostaglandins.

Therefore, the importance of eliminating painful stimuli induced by surgical invasion has been proposed, referring to the loss of consciousness and analgesia as the two elemental components of general anesthesia. In recent years it has also been proposed that the most important thing in providing anesthesia is for the patient to be pain-free during the procedure and that loss of consciousness is not an absolute requirement, depending on the content of the procedure.

On the other hand, in general anesthesia, it is necessary to create an environment in which the procedure can be performed safely and smoothly and to prevent the adverse mental and physical effects of surgical intrusion. For this reason, it has been pointed out that elements of anesthesia, such as amnesia, loss of consciousness, analgesia, suppression of pain reflexes (postural immobilization), and suppression of noxious reflexes, are very necessary. In other words, in general anesthesia, analgesia eliminates nociceptive stimuli caused by the surgical invasion, amnesia, and loss of consciousness prevents adverse psychological effects by eliminating memories of the operation, and a fixed position allows the surgeon to perform the operation smoothly. In addition, it inhibits excessive reflexes of the autonomic nervous system to painful stimuli associated with surgical operations, preventing the elicitation of adverse physical reactions.

Various components of general anesthesia have been proposed, but they can be broadly summarized as: amnesia, loss of consciousness, analgesia, postural immobilization, suppression of nociceptive stress responses, and noxious autonomic reflexes.

In the past, general anesthesia was achieved by adjusting the depth of anesthesia of a single anesthetic to produce a state that satisfied all elements of general anesthesia. However, this

M. Xia (✉)
Department of Anesthesiology, Shanghai Ninth People's Hospital Affiliated to Shanghai Jiao Tong University School of Medicine, Shanghai, China
e-mail: xiaming1980@xzhmu.edu.cn

H. Jiang, M. Xia (eds.), *Anesthesia for Oral and Maxillofacial Surgery*,
https://doi.org/10.1007/978-981-19-7287-4_6

approach required the use of high concentrations (doses) of anesthetic drugs and caused high levels of side effects such as respiratory and circulatory depression. Nowadays, we use small doses of several drugs with different effects in combination to create a state that satisfies all elements of general anesthesia and minimizes the side effects of the anesthetic overdose. In this case, a judicious application of various drug combinations, including inhaled and intravenous anesthetics for amnesia and unconsciousness, as well as opioids and muscle relaxants for analgesia and postural immobilization, can bring the various constituent elements of anesthesia into balance.

Therefore, in addition to the standard monitoring of circulation and respiration, such as blood pressure, pulse, electrocardiogram, and pulse oximetry, it is also necessary to evaluate the monitoring of the components of general anesthesia, such as electroencephalography and muscle relaxation monitoring, in order to be able to achieve the appropriate dosing that meets the various components of general anesthesia.

6.1.2 What Is Ideal General Anesthesia?

6.1.2.1 Reduced Surgical Stimulation

When surgery is performed under general anesthesia, the patient will be stimulated not only by the general anesthesia but also by the surgery. Therefore, the ideal general anesthesia should minimize these stimuli as much as possible.

In general anesthesia, sedative drugs, analgesics, and muscle relaxants are used to reduce consciousness and pain and to suppress noxious reflexes, but the use of these drugs is inherently invasive and can interfere with the body's homeostasis, including breathing and circulation. In addition, operations associated with general anesthesia, such as maintaining intravenous access, tracheal intubation, and intraoperative mechanical ventilation, can also be invasive and disrupt the body's homeostasis. Therefore, it is necessary to choose a method of anesthesia that minimizes these stimuli while maintaining the general anesthetic component and appropriate anesthetic management [1].

Surgical stimuli include tissue damage, such as incisions and exposed tissue, and associated bleeding, pain, and inflammatory responses. In addition, psychological distress, such as anxiety and fear of surgery, is another stimulus. In the days when surgery was performed without anesthetics, many patients died due to surgical irritation, but later, with the widespread use of anesthetic methods in surgery, surgical invasiveness can be reduced by anesthetic administration. To reduce the invasiveness of surgery, it is necessary to appropriately manage memory, consciousness, pain, body fluids, metabolism, and body temperature. It is believed that the postoperative recovery of patients can be facilitated by reducing psychological stress and inhibiting inflammatory cytokine production and protein breakdown.

6.1.2.2 Safety

In the management of general anesthesia, human errors such as "wrong response to the patient" and "wrong medication" often occur. In order to prevent such human errors, it is necessary for all operating room staff to monitor and share information during the perioperative period through the use of the WHO Surgical Safety Checklist and the Incident Report.

In addition, many guidelines have been developed in recent years to promote safe medical care. Guidelines related to general anesthesia include the "Guidelines for Initial Examination of the Anesthesia Machine" and the "Guidelines for Management of the Difficult Airway" [2]. Adapting the necessary guidelines to each case and using them as an adjunct to medical treatment can help improve the safety of general anesthesia.

Although the safety of general anesthesia has improved significantly over the past few decades, continuous efforts are needed to improve safety in order to provide safe general anesthesia.

6.1.3 Indications for Dental General Anesthesia

In the 1940s, since the introduction of lidocaine, the most widely used local anesthetic, most oral and maxillofacial surgical procedures have been performed under local anesthesia. However, in recent years, general anesthesia has been used in many cases because local anesthesia often does not provide adequate intraoperative analgesia and safety due to the increasing complexity of oral and maxillofacial surgical procedures and the gradual expansion of the operative field. General anesthesia is also indicated in cases where dental procedures and minor surgeries cannot be performed while awake. General anesthesia is indicated in the following situations.

6.1.3.1 When Local Anesthetics Do Not Provide Adequate Analgesia and Safety

When performing long surgical procedures with a wide surgical range, such as tumor removal plus lymph node dissection in the head or orthognathic surgery, it is impossible to obtain reliable analgesia by local anesthesia for such procedures. In addition, extensive surgery performed while awake may cause prolonged psychological stress to the patient, making it necessary to minimize the intrusion by choosing general anesthesia.

In patients with extensive tumors or cellulitis, it is difficult to obtain results even with high doses of local anesthetics. In addition, if the inflammation has spread to the airway and may cause airway obstruction, airway management via tracheal intubation and general anesthesia is necessary.

6.1.3.2 Pediatric, Disabled, and Dentophobic Patients Who Cannot Undergo Dental Procedures or Treatments Under Conscious Control

Children and patients with cognitive disabilities may not be able to safely perform dental treatment because they are not cooperative enough to open their mouths or hold certain positions during dental procedures. In addition, in patients suffering from a dentophobia, the autonomic nervous system may be overstimulated by excessive stress and the body's homeostasis may be greatly disturbed. In such patients, treatment should be carried out under general anesthesia, with the main aim of rendering them unconscious and immobilized [3].

6.1.3.3 When Local Anesthetics Cannot Be Used

Patients may have special needs while receiving surgery. Dental patients with "special needs" can involve a variety of disabling conditions, namely, intellectual disability, dementia, physical limitations, movement disorders, behavioral disorders, and chronic medical conditions [4]. Although it is rare, local anesthetics should not be used for patients who are allergic to local anesthetics. When it is difficult to obtain analgesia and perform dental treatment with methods other than local anesthetics, general anesthesia can be used.

6.2 Pre-operative Evaluation

The first step in the pre-operative evaluation is to inquire the medical history of the patient in detail and review the results of their physical examination. After the assessment, the surgeon and anesthesiologist can plan the surgery based on the results. The decision to perform a pre-operative examination and evaluation has been heatedly debated over the past few years and the content of the pre-operative assessment is constantly evolving as it has not yet been shown to have a significant impact on the choice of anesthetic plan. Some studies have shown that for patients who required routine alveolar surgery, a thorough check of medical history and physical examination of patients, including re-evaluation of critical areas, is a major factor in determining the anesthetic options [5, 6].

For patients undergoing oral and maxillofacial (OMF) surgery, depending on their medical history and anticipated surgery, tests that may be required include a complete blood count, chemistry tests, urinalysis, coagulation tests, liver function tests, chest X-ray, and ECG. In general, healthy patients undergoing OMF surgery with an expected blood loss within a certain range only require simple pre-operative examination. In patients requiring tooth extractions, hemostasis needs to be considered as there is difficulty in controlling bleeding from bony extraction sites by primary closure. However, the recommendation to routinely assess coagulation status remains controversial, with some suggesting that coagulation testing should be limited to patients with a history of coagulopathy [6].

The importance of the airway to general anesthesia cannot be overstated and therefore a thorough airway assessment of patients undergoing OMF surgery is essential. If a patient has an underlying airway abnormality, their surgical anesthesia can turn into a tough challenge to the anesthetist. Potential airway anomalies may include congenital anomalies such as Gottenhal syndrome, Crouzon's syndrome, Pierre Robin, Treacher Collins, Down syndrome, and ontogenesis imperfect; or they may be other conditions such as altered airway anatomy due to previous surgical procedures, such as patients who have undergone cervical fusion, head and neck tumor resection with or without radiotherapy, or temporomandibular joint surgery. Patients who have undergone surgical treatment of traumatic head and neck injuries, such as burns, gunshot wounds or mandibular fractures, should be carefully assessed for an airway. Certain medical conditions, such as rheumatoid arthritis, TMJ disease, and infectious processes such as Ludwig's angina, may have a tremendous impact on the airway. OMF procedures may also result in difficult airway conditions, such as mandibular osteotomy with intermaxillary fixation [6].

6.3 Induction

6.3.1 Rapid Induction

An intravenous needle is used to fix a vessel in the dorsum of the hand or forearm. Fixation of lower extremity veins is not usually performed, as this may lead to thrombosis. The patient's mouth should be opened and the condition of the mouth should be checked again (e.g., for unstable teeth or difficulty opening the mouth). After a few minutes of inhalation of 100% oxygen (pre-oxygenation), intravenous anesthesia, such as propofol (1–2.5 mg/kg) or ultra-short-acting barbiturates (3–5 mg/kg), is administered. After the loss of consciousness is confirmed, the airway is opened and secured by hand and artificial respiration with 100% oxygen is started with a mask. Muscle relaxants such as rocuronium (0.6 mg/kg) and vecuronium (0.1 mg/kg) are then given. Because of the intense stimulation associated with the tracheal tube, sevoflurane or desflurane may be inhaled, usually in combination with remifentanil or fentanyl. Once a sufficient degree of muscle relaxation is achieved, intubation can be performed.

Intravenous rapid induction is currently the most commonly used induction method, and almost all inductions of anesthesia in adults without difficulties with endotracheal intubation can be performed using intravenous rapid induction. First of all, the patient is given oxygen denitrogenization through the facemask, intravenous general anesthetics, and pain medications are used to make the patient unconscious and free of pain, and if the airway is confirmed, muscle relaxants are used to keep the airway patent by face mask ventilation, and the patient is given endotracheal intubation after respiratory arrest, which is characterized by a short induction time, can provide perfect muscle relaxation, facilitates laryngoscopic exposure of the vocal cords, and has better intubation conditions, making intubation easy and successful, and there is no concern of laryngospasm and bucking. The biggest shortcoming of rapid induction is the disappearance of spontaneous breathing, and the safety of patients may be affected.

6.3.2 Slow Induction

A low concentration of inhaled anesthetic is administered through a face mask and gradually increased. Typically, induction is initiated with the administration of 4 L/min of nitrous oxide and 2 L/min of oxygen, followed by increasing the concentration of sevoflurane by 0.5% every few breaths. Because anesthesia is transferred to the bloodstream through the lungs, it takes longer than the rapid induction method to render the patient unconscious. This method is indicated for situations where it is difficult to open the airway while awake, such as non-compliant children and mentally retarded patients. In addition, in patients with facial deformities, the mask does not fit adequately and can make manual ventilation after difficulty in rapid induction. Slow induction can be performed slowly while checking the fit of the mask so that if ventilation becomes difficult, induction can be stopped immediately and the patient can be awakened.

Intravenous slow induction is an induction that maintains spontaneous breathing, emphasizing both the achievement of a certain depth of anesthesia and the maintenance of endotracheal intubation under conditions of voluntary breathing. It is mainly used in patients in whom anesthesia assessment of endotracheal intubation may be difficult and is relatively safe because the patient retains spontaneous breathing at all times. Slow induction is characterized by a long induction time, no inotropic agents often supplemented with surface anesthesia, and preservation of spontaneous breathing, which is safer.

6.3.3 Other Induction Methods

VIMA (volatile induction maintenance anesthesia), in which a high concentration of anesthetic is injected into the anesthetic circuit and the patient is made to breathe deeply, can avoid agitation because consciousness is lost in a few breaths. In addition, semi-rapid induction, in which the patient's level of consciousness is reduced with less than the induction dose of intravenous anesthetics and then the patient is completely anesthetized with inhaled anesthetics, has also been devised, and this method combines the advantages of both inhaled and intravenous anesthetics.

The induction of combined intravenous and inhaled anesthesia (CIIA) is also a common induction method in clinical practice. It is possible to first inhale anesthetic gas and then open the vein after sleep and use intravenous anesthetics for induction; it is also possible to first use intravenous anesthetics for anesthesia and then use inhaled anesthetics and intoxicating analgesics and muscle relaxants for induction of anesthesia after the patient has fallen asleep.

Some surgeons choose to administer intramuscular ketamine to an uncooperative child or adult, and the result is often satisfactory. Administration of 2–4 mg/kg of ketamine allows the patient to become cooperative within a few minutes, allowing for successful venipuncture and further titration of the drug. The airway must be carefully assessed according to the patient's response to the drug, but usually ketamine leads to elevated values of cardiovascular and respiratory parameters [7]. The presence of postoperative delirium, particularly if benzodiazepines are not used, can complicate the patient's recovery period.

6.4 Intraoperative Management

6.4.1 Controlled Breathing

This is a method of stopping spontaneous breathing and performing controlled breathing by ventilator or manual method. The main difference between this method and spontaneous breathing is that the airway pressure becomes positive during inspiration. In adults, intermittent positive pressure ventilation (IPPV) is used to deliver gas to the airway at a flow rate of 10 mL/kg and a respiratory rate of 10 breaths/min. Either volume-controlled ventilation (VCV) or pressure-controlled ventilation (PCV) is used.

6.4.1.1 VCV

The single ventilation volume, inspiratory flow (or inspiratory time), and inspiratory flow pattern can be set. The advantage is that the ventilation volume can be maintained. The disadvantage is that the airway pressure can rise abnormally when spontaneous breathing occurs.

6.4.1.2 PVC

The advantage is that it prevents pressure damage to the lungs, but the disadvantage is that ventilation is not guaranteed.

6.4.2 Special Airway Management Methods

6.4.2.1 Positive End-Expiratory Pressure (PEEP)

Positive end-expiratory pressure (PEEP) is a ventilation technique that allows the application of positive pressure of 5–10 cmH_2O at the end of expiration. It is effective in patients with increased pulmonary shunts, such as those with combined pulmonary atelectasis. The combination with controlled breathing is called continuous positive pressure ventilation (CPPV), while PEEP under spontaneous breathing is called continuous positive airway pressure (CPAP).

6.4.2.2 High-Frequency Ventilation (HFV)

High-frequency ventilation (HFV) is a method of artificial ventilation at a rate of 60 breaths per minute or higher, which allows a very small amount of ventilation per breath. This method is used to prevent an increase in airway pressure or to ensure adequate intra-airway ventilation.

6.4.2.3 Pulmonary Protection Ventilation

To prevent postoperative pulmonary complications in patients with lung lesions or in highly invasive procedures, PEEP and pulmonary resuscitation are used to limit ventilation, maintain airway pressures below 30 cmH_2O, tolerate the resulting hypercapnia, and provide adequate airway pressure for a given period. Ventilation using these techniques is referred to as a lung-protective ventilation strategy.

6.4.3 Humidification and Removal of Bacteria

The gas used in anesthesia has a 0% humidity level. When these gases are administered under tracheal intubation, the peripheral airway is exposed to dry gas passing through the tracheal tube, causing sputum to clot and become difficult to remove, and vaporization deprives the body of heat, resulting in a drop in body temperature. In addition, the breathing circuit in anesthesia machines is not completely sterile and the possibility of cross-contamination cannot be denied. For these reasons, artificial noses with decontamination filters are used. This filter prevents bacteria from entering the respiratory tract and can add moisture from the exhaled air to the inhaled air.

6.4.4 Circulatory System Management

The goal of circulatory system management is to maintain the oxygen supply to the tissues. In particular, the prevention of cerebral hypoxia is the most important goal in anesthesia management. Oxygen supply depends on blood flow, which is determined by cardiac output and vascular resistance, but these are not easily measured. Therefore, blood flow is predicted from blood pressure and the oxygen supply to the tissues is estimated. In the brain, blood flow is constant on average between 60 and 150 mmHg, and blood pressure should be adjusted intraoperatively to maintain this range. Usually, it is measured by noninvasive methods such as auscultation or electronic oscillometry. Hemodynamic methods, in which internal pressure is measured directly through a catheter inserted into an artery, are used in high-risk patients with an ASA (American Society of Anesthesiologists) classification of III or higher, in patients in whom significant bleeding is expected, and in patients who require frequent blood sampling. If blood pressure is high, the burden on the circulatory system increases and blood loss increases. Conversely, low blood pressure can lead to organ ischemia. Therefore, it is generally recommended that intraoperative blood pressure be maintained at approximately ±20% of the pre-operative value.

When blood pressure decreases, the dose of anesthetics should be reduced, also, fluids, blood transfusions and blood pressure-raising drugs should be carefully administered. Conversely, when blood pressure rises, the dose of anesthetics should be increased to provide adequate sedation and analgesia, and antihypertensive medications should be administered if necessary. Cardiac function should be estimated from ECG measurements using the second lead or CS5 lead. In these leads, the underlying waveform is easily identified and ST-segment changes are easily confirmed. Heart rate can also be calculated from the ECG waveforms.

6.4.5 Other Management

6.4.5.1 Body Temperature

Patients receiving general anesthesia are naked and receive dry gas inhalation and cold infusion for a long time. In addition, anesthetic drugs suppress metabolism and reduce heat production. As a result, body temperature tends to drop during anesthesia. Therefore, deep body temperatures, such as rectal and bladder temperatures, should be monitored and maintained at 35–37 °C with a heating blanket. The difference between surface temperature measured in the axilla or forehead and deep body temperature can become significant if the peripheral vasculature is constricted due to insufficient circulating blood [8].

6.4.5.2 Urine Output

Generally, a catheter is inserted into the bladder if the procedure takes longer than 1 h. If the preoperative function is normal, urine output is influenced by circulating blood volume and blood pressure, and these volumes should be adjusted to maintain 0.5–1.0 mL/kg/h or higher.

6.4.5.3 Acid-Base Balance

Although H^+ is continuously produced in the body due to metabolism, the pH of the blood is maintained within a certain range through the action of the buffer system and regulation by the lungs and kidneys. When the body's balance is disturbed by massive bleeding or elevated body temperature, blood gas analysis should be performed and electrolytes and respiratory rate should be adjusted to maintain $pH = 7.4 \pm 0.05$ [9].

6.4.6 Special Management Methods

6.4.6.1 Controlled Hypotension

This is a method of anesthesia that artificially lowers blood pressure during surgery to reduce blood loss. Excessive lowering of blood pressure can cause ischemia in vital organs, so care should be taken not to exceed the lower limit of automatic control capacity. In particular, hypertensive patients should not be lowered to the same level as healthy patients because the control range is shifted upward. Vasodilators such as nitrates and prostaglandin E1 are commonly used, but even with these drugs, patients should be administered slowly to target levels and blood pressure should be restored after confirmation of hemostasis. If circulating blood volume is inadequate, organ ischemia can easily occur due to vasodilation, so adequate rehydration should be provided.

6.4.6.2 Low-Flow Anesthesia

Since the oxygen intake of a healthy person at rest is about 250 mL/min, the flow rate can be reduced to a few hundred mL/min by measuring the amount of oxygen consumed by the body and the amount of anesthetic entering the body and supplying the appropriate amount of gas accurately. This type of anesthesia is called low-flow anesthesia. In practice, a gas flow rate of 1–1.5 L/min is often used, with some of the gas being expelled out of the circuit.

6.5 Post-anesthesia Awakening

The process of suspending the anesthetic state and regaining consciousness after surgery is called post-anesthesia awakening. As with induction of anesthesia, complications are likely to occur because the patient's general condition changes significantly within a short period of time.

6.5.1 Discontinuation of Anesthetic Drugs

Discontinue the use of anesthetics and ventilate with 100% oxygen. If anesthesia is maintained with inhaled anesthetics, it will be expelled through exhalation. In intravenous anesthetics, the metabolic rate and excretion rate are inherent properties of the drug, so the time to regain consciousness depends on the time after cessation of drug administration.

6.5.2 Intraoral and Intraairway Suctioning and Monitoring of Awakening Status

The anesthesiologist can determine the state of awakening from the patient's response to commands, the recovery of inotropic drugs, and vital signs. Sufficient intra-tracheal and intra-oral suctioning are performed to prevent aspiration after removal of the tracheal tube (extubation).

6.5.3 Extubation

If vital signs are normal and consciousness, reflexes, and muscle strength are restored, the patient can be extubated. After extubation, the patient should be monitored in the recovery room for postoperative bleeding, posterior tongue drop, and airway edema.

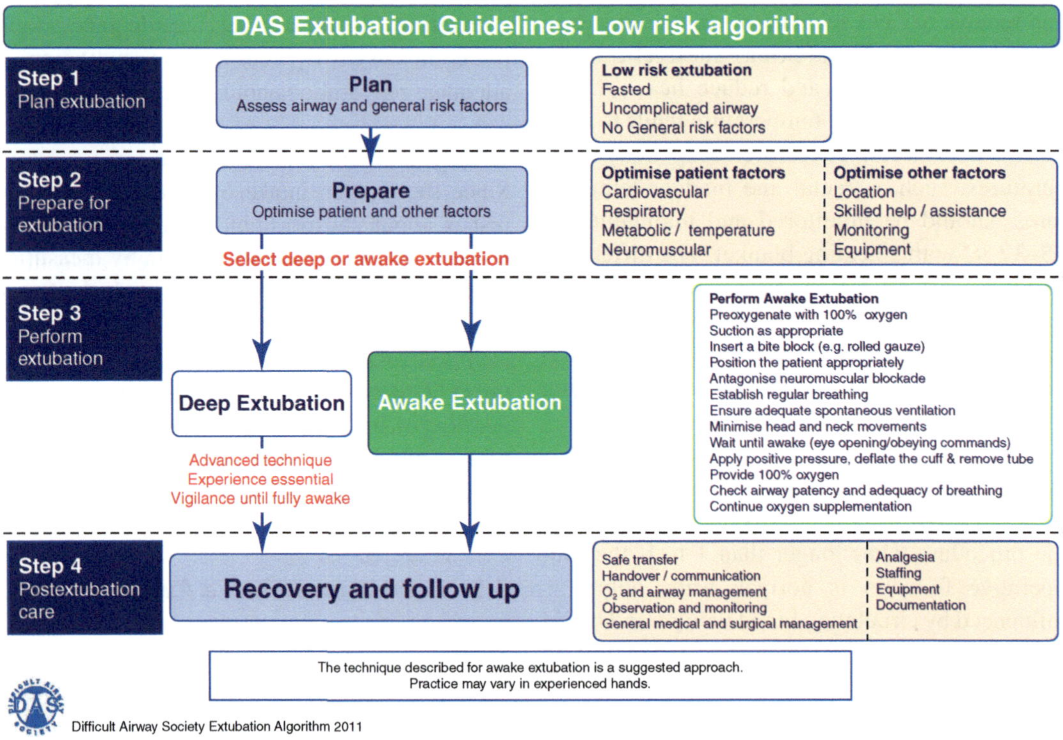

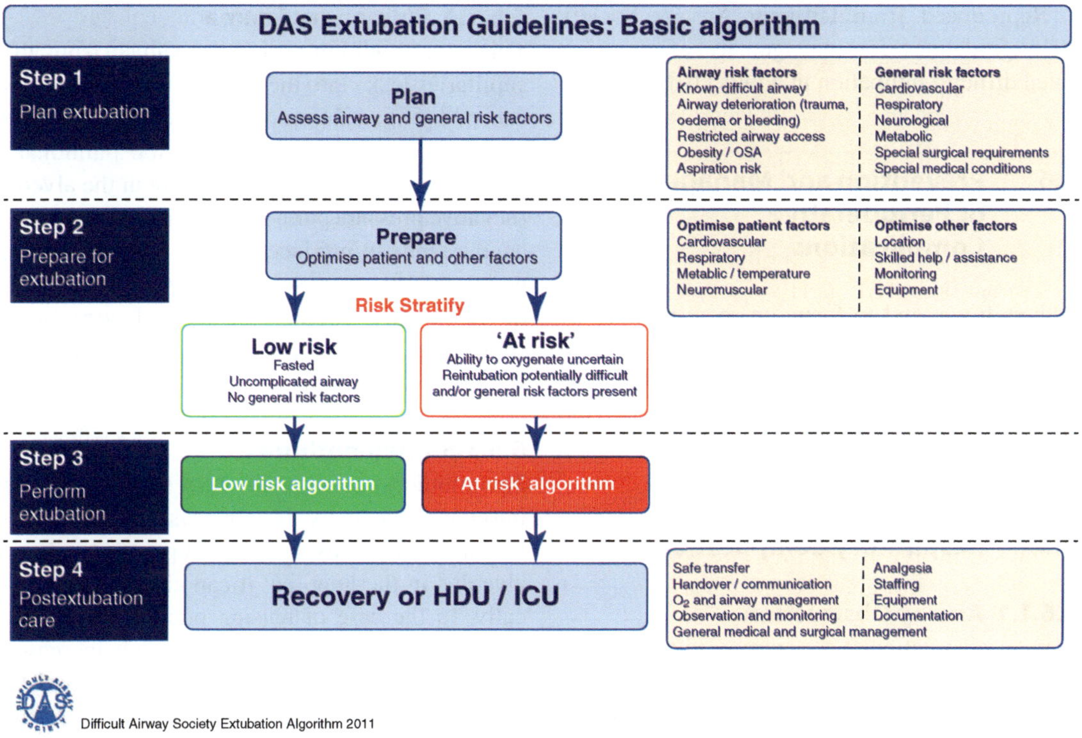
DAS Extubation Guidelines: Basic algorithm
Step 1
Plan extubation
Plan
Assess airway and general risk factors
Airway risk factors
Known difficult airway
Airway deterioration (trauma, oedema or bleeding)
Restricted airway access
Obesity / OSA
Aspiration risk
General risk factors
Cardiovascular
Respiratory
Neurological
Metabolic
Special surgical requirements
Special medical conditions
Step 2
Prepare for extubation
Prepare
Optimise patient and other factors
Optimise patient factors
Cardiovascular
Respiratory
Metabolic / temperature
Neuromuscular
Optimise other factors
Location
Skilled help / assistance
Monitoring
Equipment
Risk Stratify
Low risk
Fasted
Uncomplicated airway
No general risk factors
'At risk'
Ability to oxygenate uncertain
Reintubation potentially difficult
and/or general risk factors present
Step 3
Perform extubation
Low risk algorithm
'At risk' algorithm
Step 4
Postextubation care
Recovery or HDU / ICU
Safe transfer
Handover / communication
O_2 and airway management
Observation and monitoring
General medical and surgical management
Analgesia
Staffing
Equipment
Documentation
Difficult Airway Society Extubation Algorithm 2011

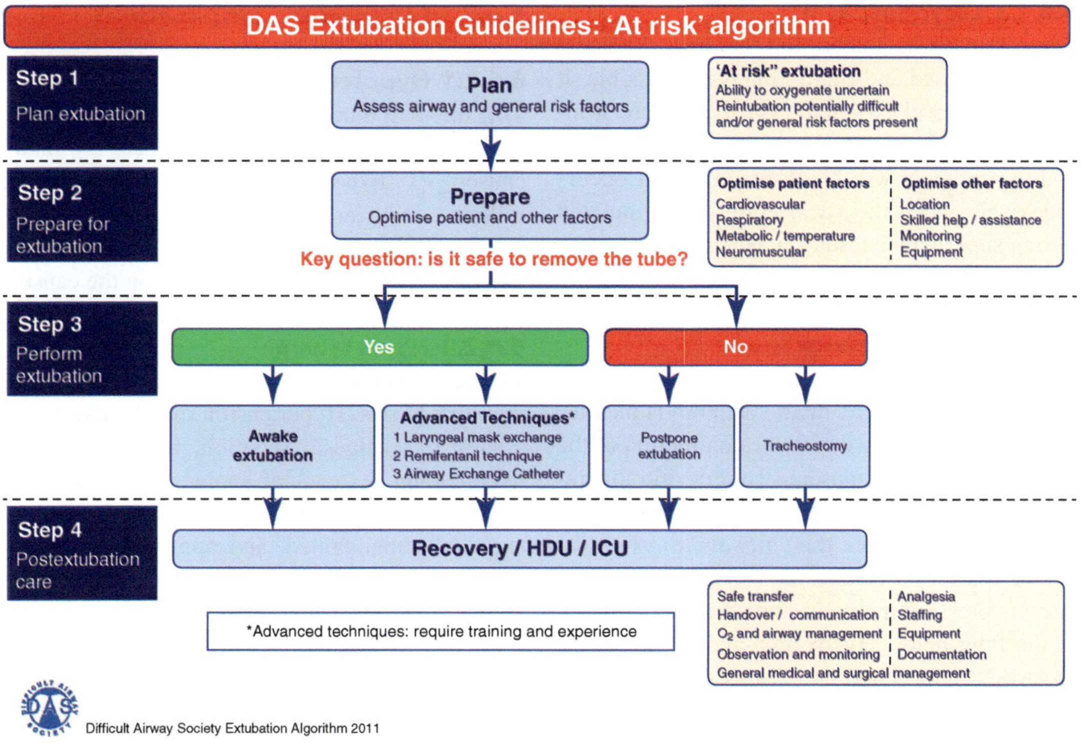
DAS Extubation Guidelines: 'At risk' algorithm
Step 1
Plan extubation
Plan
Assess airway and general risk factors
'At risk" extubation
Ability to oxygenate uncertain
Reintubation potentially difficult
and/or general risk factors present
Step 2
Prepare for extubation
Prepare
Optimise patient and other factors
Optimise patient factors
Cardiovascular
Respiratory
Metabolic / temperature
Neuromuscular
Optimise other factors
Location
Skilled help / assistance
Monitoring
Equipment
Key question: is it safe to remove the tube?
Step 3
Perform extubation
Yes
No
Awake extubation
Advanced Techniques*
1 Laryngeal mask exchange
2 Remifentanil technique
3 Airway Exchange Catheter
Postpone extubation
Tracheostomy
Step 4
Postextubation care
Recovery / HDU / ICU
*Advanced techniques: require training and experience
Safe transfer
Handover / communication
O_2 and airway management
Observation and monitoring
General medical and surgical management
Analgesia
Staffing
Equipment
Documentation
Difficult Airway Society Extubation Algorithm 2011

Reproduced from Difficult Airway Society 2015 guidelines for management of unanticipated difficult intubation in adults [10].

6.6 Prevention and Management of Perioperative Complications

Although we tend to focus on securing intravenous access and tracheal intubation, many complications can occur during surgery. Here, we describe the most frequently encountered complications.

6.6.1 Respiratory Complications

6.6.1.1 Airway Obstruction

Airway obstruction is a common intraoperative complication. Hypoxemia and hypercarbia may occur even under tracheal intubation and should be investigated and improved for the cause.

6.6.1.2 Laryngospasm

Laryngospasm is a condition in which the vocal cords are closed and ventilation is not possible. It occurs reflexively when the vocal cords are stimulated during superficial anesthesia. Hypoxemia and hypercapnia will be observed, and it occurs reflexively when the vocal cords are stimulated during superficial anesthesia. Narcotics and muscle relaxants should be used.

6.6.1.3 Bronchospasm

This presents as an asthmatic attack during general anesthesia, and its main symptom is the narrowing of the airway due to the contraction of the bronchial smooth muscle. Except intraoperatively, these attacks are caused by strong mechanical stimulation of the airway or by the administration of histamine-releasing drugs. Airway pressure increases and wheezing is heard in the lung fields. Hypoxemia and hyperoxemia are present. Bronchodilator drugs such as inhaled anesthetics and beta2 stimulant (agonist) drugs may be given for relief.

6.6.1.4 Pulmonary Edema

This is a condition in which exudate from the capillaries leaks into the alveoli of the lungs. It is caused by heart failure, stroke, reopening of the lungs after atelectasis (re-expansion pulmonary edema), or strong negative pressure in the alveoli (negative pressure pulmonary edema). Pulmonary edema tends to produce impaired gas exchange, which leads to hypoxemia. After the occurrence of pulmonary edema, mechanical ventilation should be performed with PEEP and diuretics should be applied.

6.6.1.5 Pneumothorax

Pneumothorax is a condition in which air flows into the chest cavity. In most cases, pneumothorax is usually caused by the rupture of a large alveolus in the lung, but it can also occur medically. In the case of tension pneumothorax, the pressure in the chest cavity is extremely increased by the one-way valve mechanism at the site of the leak and a chest drain should be inserted urgently.

6.6.2 Circulatory Complications

6.6.2.1 Hypotension

This refers to blood pressure that is 30% or lower than the resting blood pressure. There are many causes of hypotension, including bleeding, reflexes, and heart failure. Fluids, blood transfusions, or vasoconstrictors and catecholamine should be administered depending on the cause.

6.6.2.2 Hypertension

This refers to blood pressure that is 30% or higher than that at rest. Hypertension may be caused by a lack of analgesic sedation, hypoxemia, and hypercapnia. A level of analgesia and sedation commensurate with the degree of surgical injury should be maintained, and appropriate ventilation should be maintained.

6.6.2.3 Cardiac Arrhythmias

Arrhythmias include tachycardia (more than 100 beats/minute), bradycardia (less than 50 beats/minute), and various other arrhythmias. The major antiarrhythmic drugs classified by Vaughan Williams are listed in Table 5-IX-7.

If this syndrome is suspected, the following measures should be taken:

1. Immediately stop the use of volatile drugs and hyperventilate with 100% oxygen.
2. Dantrolene should be administered at an initial dose of 1–2 mg/kg. If symptoms do not improve, administer additional dantrolene at a rate of 1 mg/kg until the total dose is 7 mg/kg. Dantrolene inhibits calcium release from the sarcoplasmic reticulum and normalizes hypermetabolism.
3. Chills may occur and body temperature may rise if the temperature is below 38 °C.
4. For hyperkalemia caused by muscle tonus, hyperkalemia can be treated by glucose-insulin therapy (using the fact that potassium is accompanied by glucose as it is transferred into the cells by insulin. Infusion of 500 mL of 50% glucose solution with 100 units of lidocaine is given and blood potassium concentration is measured at the same time of administration) or administration of $CaCl_2$-(2–5 mg/kg) to counteract it.
5. Lidocaine should be administered for arrhythmias and sodium bicarbonate to correct acidosis.
6. To prevent renal failure due to myoglobin excretion, maintain urine output (2 mL/kg/h) by providing adequate fluids and diuretics.
7. Muscle biopsy should be performed in patients after the onset of the syndrome or in patients with a family history of the syndrome. If a family member has experienced general anesthesia, be sure to confirm their anesthetic procedure.

It is most important to avoid the use of all volatile anesthetics and succinylcholine in patients suspected of having a predisposition to this syndrome. The following drugs are currently considered for anesthetic management: barbiturates, propofol, benzodiazepines, non-depolarizing muscle relaxants, opioids, nitrous oxide, and local anesthetics.

6.6.2.4 Acidosis

The production of lactic acid and the accumulation of carbon dioxide can lead to a blood pH in the body below 7.0. In addition, ketoacidosis and renal insufficiency due to acute exacerbation of diabetes mellitus, which often occurs with massive blood transfusions, can be observed due to the combination of circulatory collapse and hypothermia during massive bleeding.

Treatment of the cause of hypothermia should be prioritized, but correction with sodium bicarbonate should be considered when the pH is below 7.2. Overcorrection of acidosis shifts the oxygen dissociation curve of hemoglobin to the left, which is detrimental to the oxygenation of peripheral tissues.

6.6.3 Other Complications

6.6.3.1 Anaphylaxis

Anaphylaxis occurs when large amounts of chemical transmitters (e.g., histamine) based or not based on antigen-antibody reactions are released into the bloodstream. All drugs can cause allergy, with a particularly high incidence caused by antibiotics, muscle relaxants, and blood products, and in recent years, there have been many case reports of latex (gloves, catheters, etc.) induced cases. In the presence of anaphylaxis, the administration of epinephrine may be effective in response.

6.6.3.2 Hypothermia

This refers to a state in which the central temperature is below 35 °C. As described in the section on maintenance of anesthesia, patients undergoing surgery are prone to hypothermia because they are naked and receive dry gas inhalation and fluids for a prolonged period. It is recommended that a higher room temperature be maintained to warm the patient.

6.6.3.3 Peripheral Nerve Injury

Peripheral nerve injury is usually caused by prolonged nerve compression. To protect the patient from this complication, an effective approach is to avoid unnatural postures and use cushions at the site of compression.

6.6.3.4 Osteofascial Compartment Syndrome

When pressure increases in a compartment surrounded by bone and muscle, the muscles, blood vessels, and nerves in the compartment are compressed, leading to tissue necrosis and nerve paralysis. This is called "osteofascial compartment syndrome" and is caused by prolonged unnatural positioning during anesthesia. When the internal pressure exceeds 40 mmHg, decompression through fasciotomy is necessary.

6.6.3.5 Intraoperative Awareness

Intraoperative awareness refers to the recovery of consciousness during surgery and the presence of intraoperative memory. It is caused by the lack of sedative drugs or analgesics. It is more likely to occur during total intravenous anesthesia (TIVA), in which the three components of general anesthesia, analgesia, sedation, and muscle relaxation, are controlled independently.

References

1. Munz SM, Murdoch-Kinch CA, DesRosiers DA, Buchanan SF, Stefanac SJ, Fitzgerald M. 5 - Interprofessional treatment planning. In: Stefanac SJ, Nesbit SP, editors. Diagnosis and treatment planning in dentistry. 3rd ed. St. Louis: Mosby; 2017. p. 121–138.e5. https://doi.org/10.1016/B978-0-323-28730-2.00014-5.
2. Apfelbaum JL, Hagberg CA, Connis RT, Abdelmalak BB, Agarkar M, Dutton RP, Fiadjoe JE, Greif R, Klock PA, Mercier D, Myatra SN, O'Sullivan EP, Rosenblatt WH, Sorbello M, Tung A. 2022 American Society of Anesthesiologists Practice Guidelines for Management of the Difficult Airway. Anesthesiology. 2022;136(1):31–81. https://doi.org/10.1097/ALN.0000000000004002.
3. López-Velasco A, Puche-Torres M, Carrera-Hueso FJ, Silvestre FJ. General anesthesia for oral and dental care in paediatric patients with special needs: a systematic review. J Clin Exp Dent. 2021;13(3):e303–12. https://doi.org/10.4317/jced.57852.
4. Dougherty N. The dental patient with special needs: a review of indications for treatment under general anesthesia. Spec Care Dentist. 2009;29(1):17–20. https://doi.org/10.1111/j.1754-4505.2008.00057.x.
5. Haug RH, Reifeis RL. A prospective evaluation of the value of preoperative laboratory testing for office anesthesia and sedation. J Oral Maxillofac Surg. 1999;57:16–20.
6. Krohner RG. Anesthetic considerations and techniques for oral and maxillofacial surgery. Int Anesthesiol Clin. 2003;41(3):67–89. https://doi.org/10.1097/00004311-200341030-00007.
7. Karm MH, Chi SI, Kim J, Kim HJ, Seo KS, Bahk JH, Park CJ. Effects of airway evaluation parameters on the laryngeal view grade in mandibular prognathism and retrognathism patients. J Dent Anesth Pain Med. 2016;16(3):185–91. https://doi.org/10.17245/jdapm.2016.16.3.185; Epub 2016 Sep 30.
8. Parikh BR, Rosenberg H. Chapter 14 - Temperature monitoring. In: Ehrenwerth J, Eisenkraft JB, Berry JM, editors. Anesthesia equipment. 2nd ed. St. Louis: W.B. Saunders; 2013. p. 295–306. https://doi.org/10.1016/B978-0-323-11237-6.00014-5.
9. Hardman JG, Hopkins PM, Struys MM, editors. Oxford textbook of anaesthesia. Oxford: Oxford University Press; 2017. https://oxfordmedicine.com/view/10.1093/med/9780199642045.001.0001/med-9780199642045. Accessed 26 May 2022.
10. Frerk C, Mitchell VS, McNarry AF, Mendonca C, Bhagrath R, Patel A, O'Sullivan EP, Woodall NM, Ahmad I. Difficult Airway Society intubation guidelines working group. Br J Anaesth. 2015;115(6):827–48. https://doi.org/10.1093/bja/aev371.

7 Local Anesthetic Techniques in Oral and Maxillofacial Surgery

Xi Chen and Jian Cao

7.1 Introduction

Local anesthesia refers to the injection or application of local anesthetics to temporarily block the conduction of the corresponding nerve impulses so that the area innervated by these nerves produces a painless effect. It is a kind of anesthesia technique frequently used in oral and maxillofacial surgery due to its great range of advantages, including simple operation, precise analgesic effect, patients' cooperation while keeping consciousness, and few perioperative complications. Particularly, dental treatment such as caries filling, root canal treatment, tooth extraction, local excision of small oral masses, tumor biopsy, abscess excision, and so on can be effectively managed under local anesthesia. Furthermore, it is also the most significant pain management skill in oral and maxillofacial surgery [1].

7.2 Common Local Anesthetics

Local anesthetics are defined as drugs that act on nerve trunks or nerve endings, which can temporarily and reversibly block the occurrence or conduction of the nerve impulse and cause the loss of sensation in the innervated area under the condition that the patient remains conscious.

Local anesthetics are often divided into two categories according to the different molecular structures: amide and ester local anesthetics. Amide local anesthetics are mainly lidocaine, articaine, mepivacaine, bupivacaine, ropivacaine, etc., and ester local anesthetics are mainly cocaine, procaine, tetracaine, etc. Whereas, esters have been no longer as popular as amides in dental treatment considering the allergenicity of the former.

The dissociation constants, lipid solubility, tissue diffusivity, and protein binding percentage of different local anesthetics are different, and their local anesthetic effect and onset of action time are also different. In addition, the volume of local anesthetics used, whether to add vasoconstrictors, etc. also affect the effect of local anesthesia, resulting in different clinical anesthetic effects [2, 3]. Table 7.1 summarizes the physical and chemical properties, onset of action, anesthetic properties, and maximum dosage of several local anesthetics frequently used in the clinical practice:

X. Chen
Department of Anesthesiology, Shanghai Ninth People's Hospital Affiliated to Shanghai Jiao Tong University School of Medicine, Shanghai, China
e-mail: chenx1853@sh9hospital.org.cn

J. Cao (✉)
Department of Oral and Craniomaxillofacial Surgery, Shanghai Ninth People's Hospital Affiliated to Shanghai Jiao Tong University School of Medicine, Shanghai, China

H. Jiang, M. Xia (eds.), *Anesthesia for Oral and Maxillofacial Surgery*,
https://doi.org/10.1007/978-981-19-7287-4_7

Table 7.1 Comparison of common local anesthetics

	Procaine	Tetracaine	Lidocaine	Bupivacaine	Ropivacaine
Physical and chemical properties					
pKa	8.9	8.4	7.8	8.1	8.1
Lipid solubility	Low	High	Medium	High	High
Plasma protein binding (%)	5.8	76	64	95	94
Anesthetic properties					
Relative effectiveness	1	8	2	8	8
Diffusivity	Weak	Weak	Strong	Medium	Medium
Toxicity	Weak	Strong	Medium	Medium	Medium
Onset of action					
Topical anesthesia	/	Slow	Medium	/	/
Local infiltration	Fast	/	Fast	Fast	Fast
Nerve block	Slow	Slow	Fast	Medium	Medium
Duration of action (h)	0.75–1	2–3	1–2	5–6	4–6
Maximum dosage of one time[a] (mg)	1000	40(topical anesthesia) 80(nerve block)	100(topical anesthesia) 400(nerve block)	150	150

[a]The maximum dosage here refers to adult doses and should also be determined by the general condition of the patient and the site

Among kinds of local anesthetics, lidocaine is often used as the gold standard to evaluate other anesthesia drugs in terms of safety and effectiveness.

7.2.1 Adverse Reactions of Local Anesthetics

The common clinical adverse reactions to local anesthetics include toxic reactions and allergic reactions.

Toxic reactions to local anesthetics can occur when the amount of local anesthetics is overdosed, accidentally injected into the blood vessels, absorbed too quickly and too much, or when the patient is weak and with poor tolerance, and in severe cases, the patient may experience numbness of the tongue, dizziness, irritability or drowsiness, disorientation, convulsions, loss of consciousness, or even coma and other neurological symptoms, as well as symptoms of the cardiovascular system such as decreased blood pressure, slowed heart rate, or even cardiac arrest. If not treated in time, the patient's life can be endangered. The main therapeutic measures include symptomatic supportive treatment such as oxygen absorption, and if necessary, intravenous injection of 20% fat emulsion at 1.5 mL/kg or continuous intravenous infusion at 0.25 mL/(kg·min). Local anesthetic toxic reactions can be prevented by controlling the amount of drug used, adding an appropriate amount of epinephrine, injecting local anesthetic after no blood in retraction and injecting local anesthetic slowly [4].

Allergic reactions to local anesthetics refer to the use of a small amount of local anesthetics will appear hives, pharyngeal edema, hypotension, angioneurotic edema, and bronchospasm, and other allergic symptoms, in critical cases, they can be even life-threatening, but attention should be paid to differentiate from toxic reactions to local anesthetics, epinephrine reactions, and to make a good differential diagnosis. Once the allergic reaction occurs, the injection of local anesthetics should be stopped immediately, oxygenation and maintenance of the usual airway and circulatory stability should be performed, vasopressors, epinephrine, glucocorticoids, and antihistamines can be used [5].

7.3 Commonly Used Local Anesthesia Methods

The selection of injection methods is another critical factor affecting the success of local anesthesia. Commonly adopted local anesthesia methods in oral and maxillofacial surgery include topical anesthesia, infiltration anesthesia, nerve block anesthesia, etc. Presently, block anesthesia is frequently used in mandibular local anesthesia, and infiltration anesthesia is usually used for maxilla [6].

7.3.1 Topical Anesthesia

The definition of topical anesthesia is to apply or spray a penetrating local anesthetic to the skin or mucosal surface of the operation area so that it penetrates through the mucosa or skin and temporarily blocks the conduction of nerve impulses of nerve endings located below the mucosa or skin to produce anesthesia in the mucosa or skin.

Indications include superficial mucosal or subcutaneous abscess incision and drainage, extraction of loose deciduous teeth, etc.

Commonly used anesthetic: 1–2% bupivacaine.

7.3.2 Infiltration Anesthesia

Infiltration anesthesia is defined as the injection of local anesthetic into the tissue of the oral and maxillofacial surgery area to block the nerve conduction in the area and achieve local anesthesia.

7.3.2.1 Basic Operation

Infiltration anesthesia is performed by first injecting a needle at one end of the surgical incision line into the skin or submucosa to form a mound after the injection of local anesthetic. The needle is then withdrawn, and the needle is inserted at the edge of the previous mound, and a new mound is created by injecting local anesthetics until the entire incision line is covered. When the operative area is small, the needle can be removed without pulling out, and the mound band is formed by continuously advancing along the incision line and injecting drugs while advancing. When the lesion is deeper, local anesthetics can be injected into the subcutaneous or submucosal tissues via the dermal mound to produce anesthesia in the deeper tissues, and then cut the skin or mucosa and subcutaneous or submucosal tissues after the anesthesia takes effect, and local anesthetic can be injected again during the operation if necessary, but the total amount of anesthetics should be controlled.

7.3.2.2 Indications

Indications of infiltration anesthesia include surgical mucocele excision, excision or biopsy of small skin mucosal masses, extraction of deciduous teeth, extraction of adult maxillary teeth, etc.

Local anesthetics commonly used for infiltration anesthesia are 0.5% procaine or 0.25–0.5% lidocaine.

7.3.2.3 Precautions

Infiltration anesthesia requires the injection of a larger volume of local anesthetic solution to create greater tension and facilitate extensive contact between local anesthetic and nerve endings within the tissue to enhance the clinical local anesthetic effect.

Local anesthetics should be appropriately diluted to reduce the concentration, and the total amount of anesthetics should be controlled to avoid overdose toxic reactions.

Each injection of local anesthetic solution should be pumped back before each injection to prevent local anesthetic from accidentally entering the blood vessels resulting in toxic reactions to local anesthetics.

Epinephrine can be added to the local anesthetic solution to slow down the absorption rate of local anesthetics to prolong the local anesthetic time, and the concentration of epinephrine is generally between 1:200,000 and 1:400,000 (i.e., 2.5–5 μg/mL).

7.3.2.4 Maxillary Buccal Infiltration Anesthesia

1. Basic operation: The needle is pierced beneath the buccal mucosa of maxillary alveolar bone, and the local anesthetic is slowly injected

after drawing back no blood. The local anesthetic penetrates the maxillary bone and acts on the dental pulp to achieve anesthesia, and the anesthetic effect is detected after 2 min.
2. Advantages: simple and easy to operate; only the nerve endings are anesthetized, and the nerve stem function is not affected.
3. Disadvantages: limited anesthetic area; need to penetrate through the bone cortex to be effective; risk of spreading infection when an infection exists in the operative area, should be avoided as much as possible.

7.3.2.5 Palatal Infiltration Anesthesia

1. Basic operation: the tip of the needle is pierced into the palatal submucosa, and the local anesthetic solution is slowly injected after confirming that there is no blood in the retraction, and the local anesthetic penetrates the palate, which can anesthetize the palatal mucosa and the palatal side of the periodontal membrane, and the anesthetic effect is detected after 2 min.
2. Advantages: simple operation and more precise effect.
3. Disadvantages: poor compliance of the palatal mucosa, high resistance to drug injection, and strong patient discomfort.

7.3.3 Nerve Block Anesthesia

Nerve block anesthesia is defined as the injection of a local anesthetic solution into the nerve trunk or its branches that innervate the operative area, temporarily blocking its nerve conduction and producing anesthesia. Block anesthesia is commonly used in oral and maxillofacial surgery, such as posterior superior alveolar nerve block, middle superior alveolar nerve block, infraorbital nerve block, anterior palatal nerve block, inferior alveolar nerve block, and long buccal nerve block.

Indications include tooth extraction, periodontal disease treatment, caries filling, root canal treatment, small mass removal, mass excision (resection) biopsy, etc.

Commonly used drugs are 2% lidocaine, 3–4% proparacaine, 4% articaine, 2% mepivacaine, 0.25–0.75% bupivacaine or levobupivacaine, etc. [7].

7.3.3.1 Upper Alveolar Posterior Nerve Block Anesthesia (Tuberosity Injection)

Basic operation: The entry point of posterior maxillary alveolar nerve block anesthesia is the oral vestibule of the distal mid-buccal root of the maxillary second molar, and the needle is inserted into the posterior wall of the maxillary tuberosity at an angle of 45° to the posterior medial side of the maxillary tuberosity for about 2 cm, and then 1–1.5 mL of local anesthetic solution is injected slowly after confirming that there is no blood in the retraction.

Anesthetized area: posterior maxillary alveolar nerve block anesthesia blocks the pulp, periodontium, alveolar process, gingival mucosa, and periosteum of the ipsilateral maxillary molars (except for the buccal side of the first molar near the mesial root).

There is a risk of hematoma, and compression of the pterygoid plexus region for more than 5 min is required.

7.3.3.2 Upper Alveolar Nerve Block Anesthesia

Basic operation: The entry point is the buccal vestibular sulcus of the second premolar, and the tip of the needle reaches the periosteum at the tip of the second premolar root, and then 1.5 mL of local anesthetic solution is injected slowly after confirming that there is no blood in the retraction. Sometimes the infraorbital nerve block can be used instead.

Anesthetized area: ipsilateral maxillary premolar and first molar near the buccal root.

7.3.3.3 Upper Alveolar Anterior Nerve Block Anesthesia

Basic operation: The entry point is the vestibular sulcus of the maxillary cuspid, the needle tip reaches the periosteum of the apical region, and 1.5 mL of local anesthetic solution is injected slowly after confirming that there is no blood in the retraction.

Anesthetized area: ipsilateral maxillary cuspid and upper incisor.

7.3.3.4 Infraorbital Nerve Block Anesthesia

Basic operation: The entry point is at the buccal vestibular sulcus of the maxillary premolar, the needle tip is parallel to the root tip of the premolar and travels upward to the bone surface of the infraorbital foramen, then slightly retreat the needle to the subperiosteum, confirm that there is no blood in the retraction and then slowly inject 1 mL of local anesthetic solution.

Anesthetized area: ipsilateral upper lip and part of the skin of the nose.

7.3.3.5 Palatal Major Nerve Block Anesthesia

Basic operation: The entry point is the palatal foramen at the palatal side of the distal middle of the maxillary second molar, and after entering the needle for several millimeters and with no blood in the retraction, inject 0.2 mL of local anesthetic solution.

Anesthetized area: ipsilateral maxillary cuspid to third molar palatal gingiva, periodontal membrane, alveolar process, and maxillary periosteum.

7.3.3.6 Nasopalatal Nerve Block Anesthesia

Basic operation: The entry point is the incisive papilla on one side, and the needle is inserted about several millimeters, and then 0.2 mL of local anesthetic solution is injected slowly after confirming that there is no blood in the retraction.

Anesthetized area: bilateral maxillary anterior teeth and palatal gingiva, periodontium, alveolar bone, hard palate mucosa, and periosteum.

7.3.3.7 Inferior Alveolar Nerve Block Anesthesia

Definition: Inferior alveolar nerve block is the injection of local anesthetic solution into the pterygomaxillary fissure to block the inferior alveolar nerve, also known as the pterygomaxillary injection method.

Basic operation: The patient opens the mouth widely, and the entry point is the midpoint between the medial oblique ridge and the pterygomandibular ligament. The needle reaches the bone surface (1.5–2.5 cm), back off slightly, and then confirm that there is no blood in the retraction before slowly injecting 1.5–2 mL of local anesthetic solution. The lingual and buccal long nerves are usually also anesthetized during the standard inferior alveolar nerve block [8].

Anesthetized area: ipsilateral mandible, mandibular teeth, gingiva and periodontium, bicuspid to incisal labial gingiva, mucoperiosteum, and lower lip, with lower lip numbness as the main sign of successful inferior alveolar nerve block.

The anesthetized area of lingual nerve block: ipsilateral tongue with burning, swelling, and numbness, with the most obvious symptoms at the tip of the tongue.

Anesthetized area of buccal long nerve block: ipsilateral mandibular second premolar and molar buccal gingiva, periodontium, mucoperiosteum, buccal mucosa, buccal muscle, and skin. Local swelling and numbness may be observed.

When performing the inferior alveolar nerve block, attention should be paid to the morphology of the mandible, and the angle and depth of needle entry should be adjusted according to the changes in the position of the mandibular foramen:

1. The wider the width of the ascending branch of the mandible, the farther the distance from the mandibular foramen to the anterior edge of the ascending branch, the deeper the needle should go.
2. The wider the mandibular arch, the more the needle tip should lean back towards the contralateral molar area as far as possible when entering the needle.
3. The greater the angle of the mandibular angle, the higher the position of the mandibular foramen, and the position of the needle entry point should be appropriately adjusted during needle entry.

7.3.3.8 Chin Nerve Block Anesthesia

Basic operation: The needle entry point is the mucosal turn, the tip of the needle is directed toward the bone tissue between the tips of the premolar teeth, and 1.5 mL of local anesthetic is slowly injected after reaching the bone surface and with no blood in retraction when slightly withdrawing the needle.

Anesthetized area: lower anterior teeth and lower premolar teeth.

7.3.4 Comparing Advantages and Disadvantages of Infiltration Anesthesia and Nerve Block (Table 7.2)

Overall, the success rates of single injection methods are disappointed in achieving the desired goals. In fact, the failure rate of inferior alveolar nerve block is 20–47% [8, 9].

Table 7.2 A comparison between the infiltration anesthesia and nerve block

	Infiltration anesthesia	Nerve block
Advantages	Easy to operate and have a command of	Wide anesthetized area
	The nerve endings are anesthetized, with no influence on nerve trunks	The entry point of the needle is far from the infected area
Disadvantages	Local anesthetics need to penetrate through the bone cortex to take effect	Difficult to operate
	Limited anesthetized area	Endings of other nerve trunks cannot be anesthetized
	Infection can be diffused when the need enters the infected area	Possibility of hematoma
		Possibility of nerve injuries

For decades, the possibility of combining two or more injection methods has been explored. Rogers et al. reported that the anesthetic effect of inferior alveolar nerve block supplemented by a buccal injection of 4% articaine has better performance than inferior alveolar nerve block injection used alone, particularly in terms of anesthesia continuity [10]. Another study reported similar results that the successful anesthesia rate of combing inferior alveolar nerve block with buccal injection, the latter served as a supplement, is 84% [11].

7.4 Conclusion

Oral and maxillofacial surgery plays a critical role in dental treatment and effective local anesthesia not only elevates the treatment outcomes, but also eliminates patients' anxiety. The first use of cocaine in maxillofacial surgery as a local anesthesia method in 1884 revealed the golden age of the development of local anesthesia agents [12]. The new anesthetics have replaced the conventional ones. Procaine, which was widely used in the last century, decayed in dental clinics because of its own allergenicity. Amides, with the first introduction of lidocaine, have gradually overwhelmed in dental local anesthesia. Other amides, including articaine, mepivacaine, and bupivacaine, have come into use. The injection techniques of local anesthetics have also been optimizing till these days. For instance, with the emergence of computer-aided injection system, the success rate of local anesthesia seems to embrace a prospective future.

The update of local anesthesia techniques in oral and maxillofacial surgery should never be hindered by the great satisfaction brought by the achievements we now possess. How to further improve the success rate of anesthesia, how to research and develop efficient and safe local anesthesia agents, and how to provide a more comfort healthcare environment should become the ultimate pursued goal.

References

1. Wang YH, Wang DR, Liu JY, Pan J. Local anesthesia in oral and maxillofacial surgery: a review of current opinion. J Dent Sci. 2021;16(4):1055–65. https://doi.org/10.1016/j.jds.2020.12.003; Epub 2020 Dec 17.
2. Ogle OE, Mahjoubi G. Local anesthesia: agents, techniques, and complications. Dent Clin North Am. 2012;56(1):133–48, ix. https://doi.org/10.1016/j.cden.2011.08.003.
3. Suzuki T, Kosugi K, Suto T, Tobe M, Tabata Y, Yokoo S, Saito S. Sustained~release lidocaine sheet for pain following tooth extraction: a randomized, single~blind, dose~response, controlled, clinical study of efficacy and safety. PLoS One. 2018;13(7):e0200059. https://doi.org/10.1371/journal.pone.0200059.
4. Singaravelu Ramesh A, Boretsky K. Local anesthetic systemic toxicity in children: a review of recent case reports and current literature. Reg Anesth Pain Med. 2021;46(10):909–14. https://doi.org/10.1136/rapm~2021~102529; Epub 2021 Jun 7.
5. Cummings DR, Yamashita DD, McAndrews JP. Complications of local anesthesia used in oral and maxillofacial surgery. Oral Maxillofac Surg Clin North Am. 2011;23(3):369–77. https://doi.org/10.1016/j.coms.2011.04.009.
6. Kanaa MD, Whitworth JM, Corbett IP, Meechan JG. Articaine and lidocaine mandibular buccal infiltration anesthesia: a prospective randomized double-blind cross-over study. J Endod. 2006;32:296–8.
7. Bortoluzzi MC, de Camargo SP, Cecato R, Pochapski MT, Chibinski ACR. Anaesthetic efficacy of 4% articaine compared with 2% mepivacaine: a randomized, double~blind, crossover clinical trial. Int J Oral Maxillofac Surg. 2018;47(7):933–9. https://doi.org/10.1016/j.ijom.2017.11.011; Epub 2017 Dec 2.
8. Crowley C, Drum M, Reader A, Nusstein J, Fowler S, Beck M. Anesthetic efficacy of supine and upright positions for the inferior alveolar nerve block: a prospective, randomized study. J Endod. 2018;44(2):202–5. https://doi.org/10.1016/j.joen.2017.09.014; Epub 2017 Dec 6.
9. Steinkruger G, Nusstein J, Reader A, Beck M, Weaver J. The significance of needle bevel orientation in achieving a successful inferior alveolar nerve block. J Am Dent Assoc. 2006;137:1685–91.
10. Rogers BS, Botero TM, McDonald NJ, Gardner RJ, Peters MC. Efficacy of articaine versus lidocaine as a supplemental buccal infiltration in mandibular molars with irreversible pulpitis: a prospective, randomized, double-blind study. J Endod. 2014;40:753–8.
11. Kanaa MD, Whitworth JM, Meechan JG. A prospective randomized trial of different supplementary local anesthetic techniques after failure of inferior alveolar nerve block in patients with irreversible pulpitis in mandibular teeth. J Endod. 2012;38:421–5.
12. Meechan JG. Practical dental local anaesthesia. 2nd ed. Surrey: Quintessence Publishing Company; 2010.

8 Conscious Sedation and Analgesia

Ming Xia

8.1 The Concept of Sedation

8.1.1 Background

Historically, oral and maxillofacial surgery has been the object of fear, and in recent years, many countries have reported their need and demand for sedation for oral and maxillofacial surgery [1, 2].

In general, oral and maxillofacial diseases are painful and many invasive procedures are also painful unless the patient is anesthetized. Oral and maxillofacial surgery is invasive procedure and is a source of stimulation that causes stress (stress response). The stimulus is called a "stressor" and oral and maxillofacial surgery is a "stressor" that induces physical and mental stress. Since oral and maxillofacial diseases are common, treatment for these diseases is referred to as a familiar "stressor."

Local anesthesia has been widely used for pain control as a stress countermeasure during oral and maxillofacial surgery, and less irritating dental instruments have been developed, and comfort-oriented equipment and facilities have become popular. However, it is generally believed that the anxiety and fear associated with oral and maxillofacial surgery remain latent, and when combined with physical and mental stimulation they may induce systemic complications such as vagal reflexes, hyperventilation syndrome, and acute exacerbation of systemic diseases [3].

Patients with fear and anxiety about oral and maxillofacial surgery may avoid the corresponding procedures. This may not only affect their eating habits due to worsening diseases but may also harm their general health due to severe oral and maxillofacial diseases. In addition, special treatment is necessary for patients with cognitive impairments who refuse oral and maxillofacial surgery due to intense anxiety or fear, or for patients with what is known as the "gag reflex" (i.e., a strong reflex triggered when a foreign body enters the mouth).

Under such circumstances, sedation is introduced into oral and maxillofacial procedures. Sedation is the reduction of irritability or agitation by administration of sedative drugs, generally to facilitate a medical procedure or diagnostic procedure. Due to the unique background of dentistry, a method called psych-sedation (psychological sedation) has been developed in dentistry to effectively manage anxiety and fear of dental treatment. Psych-sedation is a method of managing patients using medications to reduce fear, anxiety, and stress about dental treatment and to perform the treatment comfortably and safely. It is a method of perioperative management using analgesics or sedatives, but it is necessary to

M. Xia (✉)
Department of Anesthesiology, Shanghai Ninth People's Hospital Affiliated to Shanghai Jiao Tong University School of Medicine, Shanghai, China
e-mail: xiaming1980@xzhmu.edu.cn

H. Jiang, M. Xia (eds.), *Anesthesia for Oral and Maxillofacial Surgery*,
https://doi.org/10.1007/978-981-19-7287-4_8

understand its position in anesthesia and to take into account the specificities of dental treatment. It is a term specialized for dental treatment, and later in this chapter, we will still use the term "sedation."

8.1.2 Classification

American Society of Anesthesiologists (ASA) categorizes sedation into minimal sedation, moderate sedation, and deep sedation.

For minimal sedation, it is a drug-induced state during which patients respond normally to verbal commands. Though under such circumstances, patients' cognitive function and physical coordination may be weakened or damaged, their airway reflexes, and ventilatory and cardiovascular functions are unchanged.

To go a step further, moderate sedation, also called conscious sedation, is a drug-induced state during which patients' consciousness is depressed, responding purposefully to verbal commands, either alone or with mild physical stimulation. In this condition, patients can rely on the spontaneous ventilation, requiring no interventions to keep a patent airway, while their cardiovascular function is unaffected [4].

Readers may naturally infer that the next category of sedation after moderate sedation is deep sedation. Surprisingly, there is an intermediate sedation state, called monitored anesthesia care (MAC). MAC denotes a specific anesthesia service performed by a qualified anesthesiologist for a diagnostic or treatment procedure. Indications for MAC embrace the requirement for deeper levels of analgesia and sedation than that provided by moderate sedation, including potential switch to general or regional anesthesia.

The next level is the deep sedation. It is also a drug-induced depression of consciousness during which patients cannot be easily aroused, yet they respond purposefully after repeated or painful stimulation. In this state, patients are unable to maintain spontaneous ventilation. Therefore, they need interventions to keep a patent airway. Their cardiovascular function is still unimpaired.

General anesthesia may sound more familiar to common people compared to other types of sedation, as it has been widely used in various types of surgeries. The drug-induced state deprives of patients' consciousness completely, making them arousable, even following painful stimulation. During general anesthesia, patients cannot independently perform ventilatory function; thus they need positive pressure ventilation and assistance in maintaining a patent airway. Their cardiovascular function is affected.

8.2 Sedation in Oral and Maxillofacial Surgery

8.2.1 The Purpose of Applying Sedation

By applying sedation, the following effects can be obtained: (1) alleviation of anxiety and fear of dental treatment; (2) stabilization of circulatory dynamics; (3) prevention and suppression of hyperventilation; (4) prevention and relief of skeletal muscle tension and involuntary movements; (5) suppression of abnormal neural reflexes (vasovagal reflex, abnormal vomiting reflex, etc.); (6) behavioral modification; and (7) prevention of spastic attacks and amnesia. However, since the effect varies depending on the type of anesthetic or sedative used and the level of sedation, the choice of anesthetic or sedative and the target level of sedation should be determined according to the actual purpose.

8.2.2 Indications

1. Patients who have strong anxiety and fear toward oral and maxillofacial surgery.
2. Patients who have mood swings or loss of consciousness during oral and maxillofacial procedures and are considered to experience strong influence from psychological factors.
3. Patients with abnormal gag reflex.
4. Patients with systemic diseases such as hypertension and heart disease who wish to reduce their stress.
5. Oral and maxillofacial procedures with long duration and large trauma under local anesthesia.

6. Oral and maxillofacial procedures for patients who do not cooperate with treatment.
7. Oral and maxillofacial procedures for patients with central nervous system diseases who have severe involuntary movements.

8.2.3 Characteristics of Sedation in Oral and Maxillofacial Surgery

Characteristics of sedation in oral and maxillofacial surgery: the surgical field and airway overlap; frequent treatment is required; the procedure is mainly for outpatients and is a day case; the procedure is often performed on an outpatient basis. Therefore, special care is needed to ensure safety.

In particular, the surgical area and the airway are in the same area. It is important to keep the patient at a level of sedation that maintains consciousness and upper airway reflexes so that spontaneous breathing can be maintained even if water accumulates in the mouth. In other words, the goal is to achieve a level of sedation, i.e., conscious sedation, that preserves the autonomic reflex function of the airway and can respond appropriately to physical stimuli and verbal commands.

However, in patients with cognitive impairment who strongly resist oral and maxillofacial surgery, deep sedation may be required to control their behaviors. In such cases, deep sedation may be necessary because it is necessary to deliberately deprive the patient of consciousness for some time since the patient often exhibits refusal as long as he or she is conscious. If the central nervous system is depressed until consciousness is lost, the ecological defense reflexes and the mechanisms that maintain upper airway patency may also be compromised.

8.3 Types and Medication of Sedation

8.3.1 Types of Sedation

In sedation, there are several routes of administration of sedatives or anesthetics: inhalation, intravenous, intramuscular, oral, nasal, and transrectal. Intramuscular, oral, nasal, and transrectal administration methods are relatively easy to perform and have been applied to pediatric imaging studies and pre-anesthetic pretreatment. While inhalation and continuous intravenous (IV) administration are dose-controlled, sedation by other routes is less adjustable and may be hazardous due to inadequate or excessive maintenance of sedation levels, depending on the individual patient. Inhalation sedation (IS) and intravenous sedation (IVS) are indicated for safe and effective psychiatric sedation in dental treatment.

8.3.2 Other Methods

Intramuscular, rectal, nasal, or oral sedation may be used when it is difficult to establish vein access, to find a suitable vessel, or to avoid the disadvantages of intravenous methods. However, these methods are less certain of effect, less immediate, and less adjustable than intravenous methods, and their application is limited. There are also methods to achieve sedation through auditory and visual stimulation without the use of a sedative. When selecting a sedation method, it is necessary to consider the advantages and disadvantages of each method, such as the patient's level of stress and cooperation, the degree of invasiveness of dental procedures and sedation methods, and the reliability and adjustability of the sedative.

Oral anxiolytic and sedative drugs are known as oral sedation, and it is the simplest and most non-invasive method of administration. It is slowly absorbed in the digestive system and has a high safety margin. It can be used as a premedication to reduce anxiety before the patient arrives at the hospital or before treatment begins, but it has the disadvantage of being insufficiently effective as a sedative during dental treatment, slow onset of action, and difficulty in adjusting sedation levels after administration. In addition, when adequate sedation is attempted with this method, multiple doses or large amounts of medication are often required, over-sedation thereby causing airway and respiratory complications and increasing the likelihood of delayed recovery and delayed discharge.

8.3.3 Medication

Nitrous oxide (nitrous oxide) is primarily used for inhalation sedation (IS), while benzodiazepines and propofol are primarily used for intravenous sedation (IVS). Opioids and IV analgesics may also be used as adjuncts. In addition, benzodiazepines and opioid antagonists may be used and as needed.

8.4 Inhalation Sedation

Inhalation sedation is used to reduce mental tension and fear of dental treatment by inhaling low concentrations of inhaled anesthetics while maintaining consciousness. This method allows the patient to enter a state where he or she can cooperate with the treatment without stress.

Nitrous oxide inhalation has been used for general anesthesia and was first used by Seldin in the USA in the 1930s for "sedation" of dental patients. In 1972, the American Medical Association changed the name of the method from "nitrous oxide (laughing gas) analgesia," which had been used until then, to "Psych-sedation," In other words, this method can obtain a mild increase in pain threshold, but its purpose is only sedation, and the main principle is to ensure a good analgesic effect in painful dental treatment by local anesthesia.

Although various volatile inhalation anesthetics can be used for inhalation sedation, only nitrous oxide inhalation sedation is described in this article.

8.4.1 Characteristics of Nitrous Oxide and Its Application in Inhalation Sedation

The blood gas partition coefficient and cerebral blood partition coefficient of nitrous oxide are 0.47 and 1.1, respectively, which are small among inhaled anesthetics. The metabolic rate of nitrous oxide in vivo was 0.004%, which was the lowest among inhaled anesthetics. Following inhalation of 30% nitrous oxide, blood concentrations increased rapidly within 3 min after the start of inhalation and decreased rapidly within 3 min after cessation of inhalation. The route of excretion is primarily by exhalation, with a small amount excreted through the skin.

The anesthetic effect of nitrous oxide is significantly weaker than that of other inhaled anesthetics, with a minimum alveolar concentration (MAC, 50% of patients without body movement when the skin is incised) of 105%. Therefore, nitrous oxide is not usually used alone as a general anesthetic.

Nitrous oxide can be administered at low concentrations to achieve good sedation without the patient losing consciousness. Adequate sedation is usually achieved after 10 min of inhalation. Optimal sedation during dental treatment is a state of reduced mental tension and a level of consciousness that ensures adequate communication and cooperation during oral and maxillofacial surgery.

Even in this degree of sedation, a slight analgesic effect can be observed and an amnestic effect, albeit slight, can be expected. In nitrous oxide inhalation sedation, the inhalation concentration of nitrous oxide is usually 20–30%, but there is individual variation in the effect, and effort is required to set the appropriate concentration when examining the patient's signs. If the inhalation concentration is increased too much in anticipation of a decreased level of consciousness, analgesic effect, or amnesic effect, the patient can easily become agitated or unconscious, which not only prevents the patient from cooperating during the dental treatment but also leads to making the procedure less safe, which is originally the most important feature of this method. The concentration of nitrous oxide at which half of the volunteers obtained the amnesic effect was reported to be about 53% (0.5 MAC).

The analgesic effect is stronger compared to other inhaled anesthetics. The currently accepted mechanism of action is to cause the release of endogenous opioid peptides (endorphins, enkephalins, etc.) in the midbrain and to inhibit the transmission of pain information to the central nervous system through the activity of the descending inhibitory system. There are many reports on the reduction of pain by nitrous oxide via the noradrenergic system.

Although the site of action of the nitrous oxide molecule is not yet clear, inhibition of N-Methyl-D-Aspartate (NMDA) receptors and nicotinic acetylcholine receptors are considered as possible mechanisms.

The analgesic effect of nitrous oxide has been demonstrated, with inhalation of 30% nitrous oxide resulting in an increased response threshold to electrical stimulation of the teeth equivalent to a 20% concentration of 15 mg morphine, which is stronger than a 50% concentration of 100 mg intravenous pethidine. In addition, inhalation of 30% nitrous oxide significantly inhibited the increase in plasma norepinephrine during intravenous indwelling needle puncture. In any case, complete painlessness cannot be expected at concentrations of 30% or less used in inhaled sedation, and local anesthesia is essential for painful dental treatment.

8.4.2 Indications and Contraindications

1. Indicated Patients.
   (a) Patients with anxiety or fear of oral and maxillofacial surgery.
   (b) Patients with systemic diseases that are less resistant to invasive treatment.
   (c) Patients who have experienced a systemic accident caused by stress during dental treatment.
   (d) Patients who have a strong vomiting reflex.
2. Indications.
   (a) Oral and maxillofacial surgery with a relatively long duration (e.g., extraction of multiple teeth, or placement of multiple implants).
   (b) Oral and maxillofacial surgery that is relatively invasive (e.g., extraction of implanted wisdom teeth, strong pulling on the corners of the mouth or strong pressure on the jaw).
3. Non-Indicated Patients.
   (a) Patients with nasal congestion and mouth breathing.
   (b) Patients who do not understand the need for the treatment and are completely uncooperative.
   (c) Patients who do not want to wear a nasal mask (they do not like the smell of rubber and have preconceived notions that it will cause breathing difficulties).
4. Contraindications to Nitrous Oxide Inhalation Sedation.
   (a) Patients with closed cavities in the body (elevated middle ear pressure due to otitis media, pneumothorax, pneumopericardium, intestinal obstruction, pneumoperitoneum, etc.).
   (b) Patients who have recently undergone gas tamponade during ophthalmic surgery.
   (c) Patients in the first trimester (within 3 months) of pregnancy.

In addition, patients with epilepsy, hysteria, or hyperventilation syndrome may induce seizures and should be avoided.

8.4.3 Advantages and Disadvantages of Nitrous Oxide Inhalation Sedation

1. Advantages.
   (a) No airway stimulation, smooth induction.
   (b) Highly adjustable for rapid awakening.
   (c) Safe because it does not inhibit organ functions at usual concentrations (respiration, circulation, swallowing, and cough reflexes are not inhibited).
   (d) Has a mild analgesic effect.
   (e) Non-invasive treatment is possible.
   (f) It can supply oxygen at the same time.
2. Disadvantages.
   (a) Expensive inhalation sedation equipment is required.

(b) Unstable sedation effect (affected by mouth breathing and conversation).
(c) Nasal mask must be used (interferes with treatment, not suitable for patients with nasal obstruction or patients with nasal breathing difficulties).
(d) Environmental contamination (indoor and outdoor).

8.5 Intravenous Sedation

Intravenous sedation has been widely used in oral and maxillofacial surgery as a method of sedation. Although it requires maintenance of intravenous access, it has advantages over inhalation sedation because it is more effective and easier to manage systemic emergencies. After all, intravenous access is maintained. However, since intravenous administration has the potential to induce systemic complications in a short period, accurate knowledge and precise skills are required to ensure safety.

8.5.1 Medication

According to a national survey in Japan, benzodiazepines such as midazolam and propofol are commonly used for intravenous sedation in dental treatment, and they may be used alone or in combination. These drugs are used as intravenous anesthetics to induce and maintain general anesthesia, and by adjusting the method and dose of administration, a state suitable for intravenous sedation purposes can be ensured and maintained. In recent years, dexmedetomidine, an alpha2-adrenoceptor agonist, has also come into use.

Drugs with sedative effects used for intravenous sedation are sometimes referred to as sedative drugs (when referring to sedatives below, intravenous anesthetics are also included). In some cases, sedatives and analgesics are used together in intravenous sedation, such as nonsteroidal anti-inflammatory drugs (NSAIDs) flurbiprofen esters and acetaminophen [5]. As mentioned above, a variety of drugs are used in intravenous sedation in dentistry, and the methods of administration are varied. The various drugs and their methods of administration are described below. The pharmacokinetic parameters of the major drugs are shown in Table 8.1.

8.5.1.1 Benzodiazepines

Benzodiazepines refer to compounds that contain a benzodiazepine backbone in their structural formula. Benzodiazepines are the most widely used intravenous sedatives and have hypnotic, sedative, anxiolytic, amnesic, anticonvulsant, and central muscle relaxant effects. These effects are manifested by promoting the action of $GABA_A$ receptors, an inhibitory neurotransmitter in the brain (γ-aminobutyric acid).

Midazolam

Midazolam has a large clearance and short excretion half-life compared with other benzodiaze-

Table 8.1 Pharmacokinetic parameters of the major drugs used in intravenous sedation

	Plasma protein binding rate (%)	Excretion half-life (h)	Clearance (mL/kg/min)	Vdss (L/kg)
Midazolam	96–98[a]	1.7–2.6[b]	6.4–11[b]	1.1–1.7[b]
Diazepam	97.5–98.6[a]	20–50[b]	0.2–0.5[b]	0.7–1.7[b]
Flunitrazepam	77.6–79.6[a]	24[a]	2.27[a]	0.58[a]
Propofol	97–99[a]	4–7[b]	20–30[b]	2–10[b]
Dexmedetomidine	>94[a]	2–3[b]	10–30[b]	2–3[b]
Flumazenil	54–64[a]	0.7–1.3[b]	5–20[b]	0.6–1.6[b]
Ketamine	21.9–46.9[c]	2.5–2.8[b]	12–17[b]	3.1[b]

Vdss volume of distribution by the steady-state method
[a] Inscription of different drugs
[b] Reves JG et al. [6]
[c] Dayton PG et al. [7]

pines and is characterized by rapid metabolism and a short duration of action. Intravenous midazolam is mainly metabolized by cytochrome P-450 (CYP) in the liver, and the main metabolite is α-hydroxymidazolam. Its clinical potency is 20–30% that of midazolam, but it is excreted from the body relatively quickly because its clearance is higher than that of midazolam. Therefore, midazolam is less likely to have a prolonged duration of action due to the effects of metabolites. The same is true for other benzodiazepines; however, metabolism is prolonged by aging, cirrhosis, and other declines in hepatic function, and is affected by concomitant use of drugs that affect CYP. Habitual alcohol consumption may increase the clearance of midazolam.

The usual intravenous dose for general anesthesia is 0.2–0.3 mg/kg, but the appropriate dose for sedation is 0.05–0.075 mg/kg. midazolam (0.07 mg/kg) is slightly more sedating than diazepam (0.2 mg/kg), and recovery of sedation levels and psychomotor function is faster. An infusion rate of 0.015 mg/kg/min is generally considered safe. However, the patient's sedation level, respiratory and circulatory status should still be monitored during dosing, and dosing should be discontinued when optimal sedation levels are achieved. At a dose of 0.075 mg/kg, recovery of mental activity takes approximately 90 min and recovery of motor function takes approximately 120 min.

Diazepam

Diazepam has a small clearance and a long excretion half-life. Diazepam is mainly metabolized by CYP in the liver and excreted after glucuronidation; it is metabolized by CYP3A4, CYP2C19, and CYP2C9 in CYP. The metabolism of CYP2C19 varies depending on the ethnicity of the person, and it is also widely known that it is highly mutated in Asians. The metabolism of diazepam is affected by age (metabolism is delayed in the elderly) and enhanced by smoking. The metabolites nordazepam and oxazepam are both pharmacologically active and have long half-lives. This means that the pharmacological effects of diazepam take longer to fully wear off.

Diazepam has moderate anxiolytic, sedative, hypnotic, anticonvulsant, and muscle relaxant effects and is mainly used for its anxiolytic and anticonvulsant effects. For sedation, 0.2–0.4 mg/kg of diazepam is administered intravenously, with blood levels of 300–400 ng/mL in the sedated state, while anticonvulsant and hypnotic require blood levels over 600 ng/mL.

While observing the patient, 2 mg was infused every 30 s at a dose of 0.2–0.4 mg/kg for approximately 1 h. Due to the long duration of action and the time required for recovery, patients should be monitored for at least 120 min after the administration of 0.2 mg/kg before being allowed to go home. When treating outpatients, it is necessary to pay attention to the recovery of motor function as well as mental function.

Diazepam is often used for its anticonvulsant effects and is the drug of choice for the treatment of seizures and febrile convulsions, as well as for the treatment of convulsions caused by local anesthetic intoxication.

8.5.1.2 Propofol

Propofol is an intravenous anesthetic agent used to induce and maintain general anesthesia. It is also used for sedation during artificial respiration in intensive care units and is frequently used for intravenous sedation in dental practice.

Propofol acts primarily by binding to $GABA_A$ receptor subunits, thereby potentiating the action of $GABA_A$ receptors and inhibiting neural activity. It has an indirect effect on $GABA_A$ receptors through the enhancement of Cl^- channel activity by GABA, and a direct effect on Cl^- channels at high doses. In addition, propofol can inhibit acetylcholine release from the hippocampal and frontal association areas, acting indirectly on α_2-adrenergic receptors, and the CNS effects of propofol are also thought to be associated with inhibition of N-methyl-D-aspartate (NMDA)-type glutamate receptors. In addition, propofol increases dopamine concentrations in the nucleus ambiguus, which increases euphoria.

Propofol is characterized by high clearance and rapid metabolism. The immediate half-time (context-sensitive half-time, the time from administration to 50% drug concentration) of intravenous infusion is shorter than that of other sedatives. Because of the rapid recovery even after prolonged continuous administration, continuous intravenous administration can be performed in small doses in intravenous sedation. Metabolites are excreted in the liver after glucuronidation by glucuronosyltransferase or sulfate conjugation. The metabolites are inactive. Because the clearance of propofol is greater than hepatic blood flow, it is generally believed to be metabolized outside the liver.

Depending on the dose used, propofol can cause amnesia, sedation, and hypnotic effects. The effective dose to cause loss of consciousness at 50% (ED_{50}) is 1.0–1.5 mg/kg in a single intravenous infusion, but amnesia and sedation can occur even below this hypnotic dose. By adjusting the dose, it has been able to be applied for wakeful sedation and deep sedation in intravenous infusion sedation.

There is a way to predict the blood and site of action (brain) concentrations of propofol by using a dedicated syringe pump and automatically controlling the rate of administration to maintain the set target blood concentration. TCI (target-controlled infusion) was developed for general anesthesia, but it has also been used for intravenous sedation in dentistry. In conscious sedation, the target blood concentration corresponding to the optimal level of sedation is 1.0–1.5 μg/mL or 1.2–1.4 μg/mL. However, because the pharmacokinetic parameters included in the syringe pump do not necessarily reflect the pharmacokinetics of individual patients, there may be differences between the set target blood concentration and the actual concentration, and because there are individual differences in drug sensitivity, even in the case of intravenous sedation with TCI, it is necessary to adjust the target blood concentration appropriately, while carefully observing clinical symptoms.

8.5.1.3 Dexmedetomidine

Dexmedetomidine is an α_2 adrenoceptor agonist with pharmacological effects such as sedation, analgesia, anxiolysis, and relief of sympathetic nervous system hyperactivity. Dexmedetomidine is highly selective for α_2 adrenergic receptors and its selectivity for α_2 adrenergic receptors is 1600 times higher than that of α_1 adrenergic receptors.

Dexmedetomidine sedation is characterized by low respiratory depression and the patient's ability to respond quickly to calls.

Dexmedetomidine undergoes extensive metabolism in the liver, undergoing N-glucuronidation, hydroxylation, and N-alkylation, with hydroxylation involving CYP2A6, CYP2E1, CYP2D6, CYP3A4, and CYP2C9 CYPs. Metabolites do not stimulate α_2-adrenergic receptors, and if they do, it is very weak and does not pose a clinical problem.

Unlike intravenous anesthetics, dexmedetomidine has a sedative effect similar to physiological sleep and the patient can easily respond to the stimulus. Dexmedetomidine stimulates α_2 receptors in the nucleus accumbens and produces a sedative effect that is dependent on the dose used. α_2 receptors are of three subtypes, α_2A, α_2B, and α_2C, and dexmedetomidine acts on all of these receptors, but sedation is only associated with α_2A receptors.

The recommended method of dexmedetomidine administration is a continuous intravenous infusion with an initial loading dose of 6 μg/kg/h for 10 min, followed by a maintenance dose of 0.2–0.7 μg/kg/h. This method has been reported to provide an optimal level of sedation equivalent to that of propofol.

8.5.1.4 Antagonists

An antagonist is a substance that binds to a receptor but has no effect on it. Antagonists are used in the treatment of drug overdose or the diagnosis of drug addiction because they antagonize the action of agonists.

In general, antagonists compete with agonists to occupy receptors and produce effects. Thus, the situation varies according to the strength of binding of the agonist to the receptor and the strength of binding of the antagonist to the receptor but is essentially determined by the respective concentrations of agonist and antagonist in the vicinity of the receptor. If blood concentrations are used instead of concentrations near the receptor, the use of an antagonist will not produce sufficient effects when the blood concentration of the agonist is high. In addition, when an antagonist with a short half-life is used to antagonize the effects or side effects of an agonist with a long half-life, the effects or side effects of the agonist will reappear if the blood concentration of the antagonist decreases more rapidly than the blood concentration of the agonist. Therefore, when using an antagonist during rehabilitation, one should fully understand its pharmacokinetics in the blood and be aware of the re-emergence of its action or side effects. In the case of benzodiazepines, it is necessary to be concerned about the reappearance of sedation.

Benzodiazepines have antagonists for their respective receptor agonists and can be used to treat the side effects or overreactions to a benzodiazepine overdose. However, doses of benzodiazepines should be adjusted to eliminate the need for antagonists, and antagonists should be used only as an emergency measure. In addition, the effects of antagonists are not absolute, so their pharmacological characteristics should be fully understood at the time of use.

Flumazenil is an antagonist of benzodiazepine receptors. It is used to alleviate the effects of benzodiazepine-induced respiratory depression and delayed awakening after surgery during general anesthesia and intravenous sedation. It is also used in the treatment of patients with benzodiazepine intoxication and the diagnosis of patients with unexplained coma.

The usual initial dose is 0.2 mg administered slowly intravenously. If the desired wakefulness is not achieved within 4 min of administration, another 0.1 mg should be given, and thereafter, 0.1 mg should be given every 1 min as needed until the total dose is 1 mg. It is important to note that the dose should be adjusted according to the benzodiazepine administration and the patient's condition.

Flumazenil 0.004 mg/kg given within 30 min of midazolam 0.05 mg/kg administration was reported to have a significant antagonistic effect on balance function, clinical findings, and computational tests 10–30 min after administration compared to controls who did not receive flumazenil. However, a decrease in the effect of flumazenil has been observed 40–50 min after flumazenil administration. This reappearance of the antagonized sedation state occurs because flumazenil has a shorter half-life than benzodiazepine. Therefore, when flumazenil is used to antagonize the sedative effects of benzodiazepines, it is necessary to monitor for at least 60 min after flumazenil administration, even if adequate recovery is observed.

8.5.1.5 Other Drugs Used for Intravenous Sedation

Flurbiprofen Axetil

Flurbiprofen axetil is a propionic acid nonsteroidal drug used for intravenous administration. Like propofol, it is dissolved in a fat emulsion consisting of soybean oil, egg yolk lecithin, and glycerin concentrate, and is sold as a white emulsion.

In adult oral surgery, 50 mg administered intravenously during or before the end of the procedure for postoperative analgesia is as effective as 50 mg of diclofenac sodium suppositories. Postoperative pain disappears within 10–70 min (mean 36 min) and analgesia can last for more than 5 h, but there are reports that the drug should be administered early when the pain is mild. On the other hand, it has been reported that in oral surgery, there is no difference in effect between preoperative administration and administration immediately before the end of the surgery, and no prior analgesic effect has been observed, so the appropriate time to administer the drug is before or early after the end of surgery.

Although the same precautions should be taken as for other NSAIDs, it is necessary to be aware of the patient's condition when administering the drug and to administer it as slowly as possible (at least 1 min).

Ketamine

Ketamine is a general anesthetic that suppresses the thalamus and neocortex and activates the limbic system, hence its name as a dissociative anesthetic. Due to its strong analgesic effect, it is sometimes used as an intravenous sedative. Although ketamine can be used alone, it is not used as a primary agent in intravenous sedation for dental treatment but is used in combination with a sedative such as a benzodiazepine as an adjunct to achieve the desired sedative effect. However, the overdose of ketamine or concomitant use with other drugs has the potential to inhibit the body's defensive reflexes and lead to serious complications. Optimal levels of conscious sedation should always be maintained, and it should be ensured that, in the patient's environment, there is a timely switch to general anesthetic management in the event of excessive sedation levels, including securing the airway via tracheal intubation.

8.5.2 Assessment and Monitoring of Sedation Levels

There are two ways to assess sedation levels: (1) using an assessment form depending on the patient's condition; (2) using electroencephalography (EEG) monitor for objective quantitative assessment.

8.5.2.1 Assessment of Sedation Levels with an Assessment Form

Basically, drugs show pharmacological effects in a dose-dependent manner, but even if the doses are the same, the pharmacokinetics vary depending on the patient's systemic background, and even if the blood levels are the same, there are individual differences in the patient's condition and response. In intravenous sedation, the patient's condition and response must be continuously observed and the level of sedation assessed to maintain the desired level of sedation. Items used to subjectively assess the level of sedation include (1) patient's subjective symptoms, (2) response to call, (3) adaptation to instructions, (4) vital signs, (5) facial and limb conditions, and (6) ocular (eyelid) conditions. For example, in the awake sedated state, the patient is free of anxiety and somewhat drowsy but can respond promptly to calls and accept instructions and manipulations without difficulty. In addition, breathing is shallow but within normal limits, pulse and blood pressure are within normal limits, the face and extremities are not tense, and the eyes are open or the upper eyelids are drooping (Verrill's sign). Such a state is the optimal level of sedation, and the dose of sedative should be adjusted to maintain this level.

To ensure and maintain optimal levels of sedation, one approach is to score and assess the patient's condition using an assessment scale. The scoring of sedation levels includes the Ramsay Sedation Scale (Fig. 8.1) [8], the OAA/S score (Observer's Assessment of Alertness/Sedation Scale, Fig. 8.2) [9], RASS (Richmond Agitation-Sedation Scale, Fig. 8.3) [10, 11], VAS (Visual Analogue Scale, Fig. 8.4) [12], and FAS (Facial Anxiety Scale, Fig. 8.5). For conscious sedation for dental treatment or tumor resection, a Ramsay sedation score of 2 to 3, an OAA/S score of 3 to 4, and a RASS score of 0 to 3 are recommended.

1	The patient is anxious and agitated or restless, or both
2	The patient is cooperative, oriented, and tranquil
3	The patient responds to commands only
4	The patient exhibits brisk response to a light glabellar tap or loud auditory stimulus
5	The patient exhibits a sluggish response to a light glabellar tap or loud auditory stimulus
6	The patient exhibits no response

Fig. 8.1 Ramsay Sedation Scale

Score	Sedation level	Responsiveness	Speech	Facial expresssion	Eyes
5	Alert	Responds readily to name	Normal	Normal	Clear, no ptosis
4	Light	Lethargic response to name	Mild slowing	Mild relaxation	Glazed or mild ptosis
3	Moderate	Response only after name is called loudly	Slurring or prominent slowing	Marked relaxation	Glazed and marked ptosis
2	Deep	Response only after mild prodding or shaking	Few recognizable words	–	–
1	Deep sleep	Response only after painful stimulus	–	–	–

Fig. 8.2 OAA/S

Richmond Agitation Sedation Scale (RASS) *

Score	Term	Description	
+4	Combative	Overtly combative violent, immediate danger to staff	
+3	Very agitated	Pulls or removes tube(s) or catheter(s); aggressive	
+2	Agitated	Frequent non-purposeful movement, fights ventilator	
+1	Restless	Anxious but movements not aggressive vigorous	
0	Alert and calm		
-1	Drowsy	Not fully alert, but has sustained awakening (eye-opening/eye contact) to *voice* **(≥10 seconds)**	**Verbal Stimulation**
-2	Light sedation	Briefly awakens with eye contact to *voice* **(<10 seconds)**	**Verbal Stimulation**
-3	Moderate sedation	Movement or eye opening to *voice* **(but no eye contact)**	**Verbal Stimulation**
-4	Deep sedation	No response to voice but movement or eye opening to *physical* stimulation	**Physical Stimulation**
-5	Unarousable	No response to *voice or physical* stimulation	**Physical Stimulation**

Procedure for RASS Assessment

1. Observe patien
   a. Patient is alert restless or agitated. **(score 0 to +4)**
2. If not alert, state patients name and *say* to open eyes and look at speaker.
   b. Patient awakens with sustained eye opening and eye contact. **(score -1)**
   c. Patient awakens with eye opening and eye contact but not sustained. **(score -2)**
   d. Patient has any mo, ement in response to voice but no eye contact. **(score -3)**
3. When no response to verbal stimulation, physically stimulate patient by shaking shoulder and/or rubbing sternum.
   e. Patient has any movement to physical stimulation. **(score -4)**
   f. Patient has no response to any stimulation. **(score-5)**

Fig. 8.3 RASS

Behaviorally modified intravenous sedation of uncooperative patients with disabilities requires higher doses of sedation than normal patients to achieve and maintain a practical level of sedation. As a result, deep sedation is often performed and in most cases, the scores of the usual evalua-

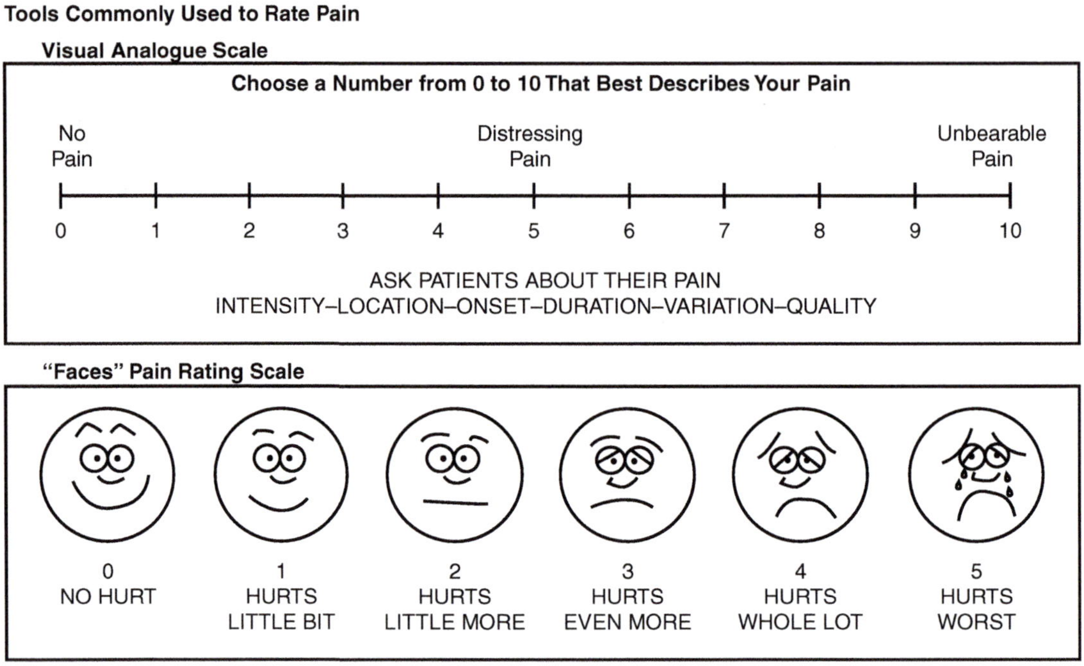

Fig. 8.4 VAS

Anxiety Level	None	Mild	Mild-Moderate	Moderate	Moderate-High	Highest
Faces						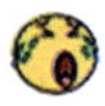

Fig. 8.5 FAS

tion scales do not yield an adequate evaluation. In the case of deep sedation for behavioral modification of dental treatment, valid indicators for evaluating the level of sedation for successful dental treatment include "eye closure," "loss of eyelash reflex," "smooth occlusion," etc.

8.5.2.2 Objective Quantitative Evaluation of Sedation Level

EEG monitoring is used to monitor the depth of anesthesia during general anesthesia and can be applied to monitor the level of sedation. The most commonly used EEG monitor analyzes the EEG and monitors the value of the depth of anesthesia (bispectral index, BIS). BIS values range from 0 to 100, with values close to 100 meaning that the patient is awake. The BIS value for general anesthesia is usually 40–60. The depth of anesthesia for propofol or midazolam, i.e. the level of sedation, correlates well with the BIS value. For intravenous sedation in dentistry, the optimal level of sedation is a BIS value between 70 and 85. However, in behaviorally adjusted deep sedation during dental treatment of patients with disabilities, intraoperative BIS values at clinically optimal sedation levels may be below 70 [13].

The BIS was originally developed for depth of anesthesia in general anesthesia and was then used only as an indicator of the degree of central nervous system activity. Although it is a useful indicator for objectively assessing the level of sedation, it is important to note that in some cases it does not necessarily reflect the actual level of sedation. First, the BIS value does not reflect the optimal level of intravenous sedation in the absence of stimulation, as it decreases to about 30 during natural sleep. In addition, opioids alone do not affect BIS values, but they do reduce the BIS values of sedative drugs. In general, BIS values for intravenous sedation are sensitive to the environment and tend to be unstable, so the patient's symptoms should always be observed and a comprehensive assessment of sedation levels should be made in conjunction with other objective assessments [14].

8.6 Classification and Pathogenesis of Pain

8.6.1 Definition and Classification of Pain

8.6.1.1 Definition of Pain

International Association for Study of Pain (IASP) defines pain as "an unpleasant sensory and emotional experience associated with actual or potential tissue damage or described in terms of such damage." The first half defines pain as pain that can be imagined due to a definite cause, such as tissue damage, while the second part shows that the sensation and emotion of pain can occur even in the absence of such a cause.

It is important to understand that there are many different types of pain, as described below, including pain that is not generally considered to be the cause of pain, such as associated pain or pain caused by a mental or psychological disorder. Pain is considered a very important sensation because it is essentially a way to escape physical harm. However, in the case of chronic pain, which persists even after the tissue damage has healed, or cancer pain at the end of life, does not play an early warning role, but rather a pain itself becomes the subject of the disease, i.e., the main goal of treatment is to relieve pain.

Even in oral and maxillofacial regions, there is a wide variety of pains that have been classified in many ways and are being described in detail. However, there are still some pains that are not yet understood or difficult to treat and for which further cognition is desired. Here, the most common pain classifications and their explanations are introduced.

8.6.1.2 Classification of Pain

Classification According to Etiology

Traditionally, chronic pain associated with cancer has often been seen as a separate category, as this type of pain tends to have a complex etiology and is treated more aggressively. However, there is no evidence to suggest that the neurological mechanisms of cancer pain are any different from other chronic pain. Other contributing factors to pain include acute injuries, underlying diseases or physical conditions, and a history of treatment associated with these injuries or diseases, such as surgery [15].

Classification According to Pathophysiology

Pain can also be categorized according to its pathophysiology as nociceptive pain, neuropathic pain or, in the case of chronic pain, central sensitization, the classification criteria of which depends on the types of injury/damage and the pathophysiological pathway leading to the pain sensation.

Nociceptive pain generally refers to the normal physiological response to tissue damage caused by trauma, non-healing injury or inflammation. Nociceptive pain can be divided into two categories, namely somatic pain and visceral pain. The former refers to injury to the musculoskeletal system and the latter refers to injury to internal organs and is usually felt indirectly.

The Aδ and C fiber endings of peripheral nerves are receptive to nociceptive stimuli and their membranes are known to contain various ion channels that respond to different stimuli. In response to different stimuli, the corresponding channels are opened and cations enter the cell. Subsequently, potential-dependent Na^+ channels open, allowing large amounts of Na^+ to enter the cell, generating action potentials.

The definition of neuropathic pain is the pain induced by a lesion or disease of the somatosensory nervous system, usually due to abnormal nerve activity. Neuropathic pain includes both central or peripheral categories, based mainly on whether the lesion occurred in the peripheral or central nervous system. Moreover, there are two main characters of neuropathic pain: recurrent paroxysmal pain and persistent pain.

Philosophical in nature, the definition of central sensitization, also known as nociplastic pain, refers to pain arising from altered nociception in the absence of clear evidence of actual or threatened tissue damage leading to peripheral neuroreceptor activation, or evidence of disease or lesions of the somatosensory system causing pain [15].

Classification According to Anatomical Location

Classifying pain according to anatomy allows the location of the patient's pain to be identified. When patients seek medical advice for pain, the first thing they confide in the doctor is often the part of the body that feels the pain. Somatic pain is pain specific to the part of the body that is injured, where pain receptors are activated in the bones, muscles, skin, joints, ligaments, tendons and connective tissues. Similarly, visceral pain generally arises in the viscera, but pain associated with visceral injury is difficult to be identified accurately because of the low density of nociceptive receptors in the viscera and the poor representation of afferent fibers in cortical mapping. According to a European survey, the most common sites of chronic pain, irrespective of acute pain conditions, were the back and joints, closely followed by neck and headache-related pain.

8.6.2 Diagnosis of Pain

8.6.2.1 Medical History

General Information

1. Age
2. Gender
3. Job

   Occupational muscle tension, such as using a computer for long periods in an office job or pinning a phone to your shoulder while talking, can cause muscle pain. In addition, when considering medication, great care should be taken when prescribing antispasmodics and antidepressants if the occupation involves driving a car or working at a high altitude.
4. Life style and chewing habits

   Wind instruments may be associated with the development of TMD. Tobacco and coffee can strain the sympathetic nervous system and affect local circulation, and thus patients should also be asked about related habits. The presence of bad habits in mastication or disorders of jaw movement may also be a trigger for TMD and masticatory muscle pain. Habits such as teeth grinding and clenching are also associated with muscle pain.

Main Symptoms

Patients in pain clinics are often unable to express their pain or abnormal sensations in clear language. In addition, they may be unable to speak if talking provokes pain or if the pain is severe. In such cases, infiltration or nerve block anesthesia should be administered to the area where the pain is thought to occur and the patient should be provided with pain relief prior to the interview.

History and Routine Medication

1. History

   A history of general systemic diseases should be obtained from the patient, with special attention to trauma, cerebrovascular disease, psychiatric and neurological disorders, diabetes mellitus, and orthopedic, ophthalmologic, and otorhinolaryngologic disorders. Mental disorders, such as depression and neurosis, may also be associated with symptoms such as pain and discomfort in the mouth and face.
2. Routine Medication

   Many conventional medications have side effects, such as mouth ulcers and taste disorders. In addition, older patients may be taking more than ten different medications, but the patient himself or herself is likely unaware of what medications he or she is taking. In some cases, the patient may already be taking the medication to be prescribed. Therefore, it is necessary to ask the patient's primary care physician about his or her current general condition and the type of medications he or she is taking.

Family History of Diseases

Check for chronic pain, especially intractable pain conditions.

Current Symptoms

Ask the patient about the location, nature, intensity, duration, and frequency of current pain, as well as pain triggers and relief measures. The presence or absence of systemic symptoms should also be noted.

1. Location

   Ask the patient in detail, such as the left, right, upper and lower jaw, teeth, tongue, oral mucosa and facial skin, joint areas, head (temporal, occipital, whole head, etc.), neck and shoulders, etc. It may also be helpful to ask the patient to point out the area of pain. In some cases, the patient may complain of pain throughout the mouth, but be unable to pinpoint the exact location.0000
2. Features

   There are a variety of ways to describe the pain. For example, throbbing pain, stabbing pain, electric shock (shock pain), pressing pain, pain like pricking with a needle, burning pain like hot water poured over the body, etc. Therefore, it is important to record the patient's description of the pain truthfully. In some cases, it is difficult to describe the pain in words, in which case some examples can be given to help the patient describe it.
3. Intensity.

   The VAS (visual analogue scale) is a subjective method of pain assessment in which a 10-cm (100-mm) horizontal line is shown to the patient to indicate: the left end represents 0 (no pain) and the right end represents 10 (unbearable pain); the patient is asked to indicate where the current pain and have the patient indicate where the pain is currently located. There is also a numerical rating scale (NRS) in which the patient is asked to rate the current level of pain on a scale of 0 to 10, with 0 being no pain at all and 10 being the most painful.
4. Frequency.

   Ask the patient about the frequency of pain episodes, in days, weeks, months, years, etc.
5. Duration.

   Ask the patient to describe in detail whether the pain is momentary or constant and whether it lasts for a few seconds, minutes, hours, or a full day.
6. Temporal characteristics and diurnal variation of pain.

   Ask the patient about the time of day when the pain is most severe and understand its temporal characteristics and diurnal variation.
7. Triggers and aggravating factors.

   Know the factors that trigger the pain (e.g., talking, eating, opening doors, coughing, swallowing, washing, drinking, etc.). Also, check whether the pain is spontaneous and whether there are precipitating factors. Ask about aggravating factors, i.e., what makes the pain worse.
8. Relief measures.

   Patients should be asked specifically what they can do to relieve pain when it occurs, and whether they can relieve pain by applying hot and cold compresses, eating and drinking, or taking pain medication.
9. Complications.

   Attention should be paid to the presence of autonomic symptoms (e.g., lacrimation, nasal congestion, increased nasal discharge, abnormal sweating), muscle spasms, headache, dizziness, light-headedness, and pain outside the mouth and face.
10. Whole-Body Condition.

    Ask the patient about his or her daily life and activities. Special attention should be paid to the patient's mental status, i.e., whether the patient is energetic, depressed, anxious, or nervous, as these factors can affect the level of pain. Attention should also be paid to the patient's fever, sleep status, and appetite. Attention should also be paid to any shoulder stiffness, headache or muscle pain, gastrointestinal symptoms such as diarrhea or constipation, blood pressure, and pulse rate.

8.6.2.2 Examination

Systemic Examination

Patients in pain may fidget from the moment they enter the waiting room, they may hold their head in their hands, or their face may display an expression of pain. However, it is important to note that patients in chronic pain do not always exhibit this expression or posture. The patient's gait should be carefully observed to determine if he can walk on his own or needs assistance. If the patient is overweight or underweight, systemic diseases are often present. In addition, the patient's posture should be examined, including the balance of muscle tone from left to right and right to front and back of the body. The extremities should also be checked for paralysis or involuntary movements.

Local Medical Examination (Maxillofacial and Oral Cavity)

1. Eyes.

   The size of the eye fissure and the presence of drooping eyes are examined. The examiner then places a finger approximately 40 cm in front of the subject's eye and asks the subject to look at it and move the finger to check eye movements such as up and down, side to side, and the degree of vergence reflex (convergence of the eyes). The eye movements should be checked for smooth or restricted eye movements, and for double vision. In addition, the pupil should be checked for abnormal pupil size (constriction or clouding) and abnormal pupillary reflexes. In a healthy adult, the pupil is a regular circle with both sides being the same size. The pupil is usually 2.5–4.5 mm in diameter but tends to get smaller with age. In general, pupils smaller than 2 mm are referred to as miosis, and pupils larger than 5 mm are referred to as dilation. Since the light reflex occurs not only in the light-receiving eye but also in the contralateral eye, the bilateral light reflex can be used to some extent to estimate the site of the lesion.

2. Ear.

   A tuning fork is placed close to the examinee's ear and gradually moved away to see if he can hear it (air conduction test). When no sound can be heard, the hearing of the other ear is checked and compared with the subject's hearing. If there is a hearing loss, the tuning fork is then placed in the middle of the forehead and the subject is asked which ear he hears better (Weber test). If the tuning fork resonates on the impaired side of the hearing, the hearing loss is considered conductive; if the tuning fork resonates on the healthy side, the hearing loss is considered sensorineural.

   A tuning fork is placed on the temporal bone mastoid (bone conduction test) to test the difference between bone conduction and air conduction. If air conduction is better, the hearing loss is considered sensorineural, and if bone conduction is better, the hearing loss is considered conductive (Linney test). The Linney test or Weber test may be effective in cases where there is a pain in the trigeminal region, or where there is widespread paresthesia, as this condition may indicate a tumor, especially of the auditory nerve.

3. Maxillofacial, Head, and Neck.

   The color and condition of the skin of the maxillofacial region should be examined visually, as well as for any swelling or deformity. In addition, palpation should be performed at the bony foramina where each branch of the trigeminal nerve comes out, namely the supraorbital foramen (first branch), infraorbital foramen (second branch), and foramen ovale (third branch) areas. Confirm if there are trigger points where even minor stimuli can induce pain.

   In addition, the temporomandibular joint and muscles (temporalis, masseter, sternocleidomastoid, anterior and posterior belly of the trapezius, and trapezius) should be palpated to confirm the presence or absence of pain. The area of tenderness should be examined by applying even pressure to the right and left sides and shifting slightly. The muscles should be checked for pressure pain during palpation, as well as for recurrence or worsening of dental pain. In addition, the jaw should be examined for restricted opening and closing, murmurs or pain, deviation of the jaw, and loss of chewing power with forceful clenching of the teeth. Confirm whether the movement of the head and neck is restricted or whether the pain is triggered by movement. In addition, check for left-right differences in forehead wrinkles, eye closures, and mouth lifts. The movement of the head and shoulders should also be checked. The patient is instructed to rotate the head to the left and place the hand on the left chin, applying resistance to check muscle strength. Also, palpate the contraction of the sternocleidomastoid muscle on the right side. The same manner of examination was performed for the right side. After observing the height of the shoulder, the hands were placed on the patient's shoulders and the patient was instructed to lift the shoulder against resistance to check the strength of the superior trapezius muscle.

4. Oral Cavity and Nose.

   Examines the teeth, periodontal tissue, tongue, and oral mucosa. The mucous membranes are examined for color and texture, and swelling, malformations, defects, abnormal dentures and occlusion, abnormal salivary characteristics, abnormal taste, and dryness of the mouth. The apical area should also be examined for pain due to gingival pressure. Painful occlusion, including lateral movement, should be examined. Diagnosis is often more difficult, especially in cases of fractured teeth with loss of nerve, and should be checked for pain by applying vertical and horizontal occlusal pressure to the split tooth or toothpick. The patient should also be made to open his or her mouth to check for tongue atrophy and to check if the tongue can be extended forward; if it cannot be extended, or is off to the side, sublingual nerve palsy should be suspected.

   Have the patient continuously say vowels such as "aa," repeat single syllables such as "papa, tata, kaka" and repeat three syllables such as "pataka" to check for The presence of dysarthria. Coughing and swallowing can also be used to check for the presence of this disorder. The subject is asked to pronounce the "a" sound and to observe the symmetry of the pharyngeal and palatal movements.

   In cases of unilateral paresis, the posterior wall of the pharynx is pulled toward the healthy side (curtain sign). Sensation in the pharynx and palate should be examined by palpation with a tongue depressor. Contraction of the pharynx and soft palate, i.e. the reflexes of the pharynx and soft palate, should be examined. The sense of smell is then tested by pinching the nose on both sides and asking the patient if he/she can smell coffee powder.

5. Skin and Mucous.

   The skin should be examined for redness, swelling, and warmth. If inflammation is suspected, blood tests and imaging should be considered (see below). If a rash, blisters, or erythema are present, herpes zoster should be suspected. However, in chronic pain, such skin and mucosal abnormalities are often not present.

Function and Disorders of the Cranial Nerves

To assess pain and sensory disturbances in the oral and maxillofacial regions, it is necessary to understand the function and disorders of the cranial nerves. Cranial nerves can be classified as sensory, motor, or a mixture containing both, and some also contain parasympathetic functions.

8.7 Analgesia

8.7.1 Common Analgesics

Including non-steroidal anti-inflammatory drugs (NSAIDs), opioids, and adjuvant analgesics.

8.7.1.1 Non-Steroidal Anti-Inflammatory Drugs (NSAIDs)

Clinical Pharmacology

NSAIDs are one of the analgesic drugs commonly used in clinical work, which have antipyretic, analgesic, anti-inflammatory, and anti-rheumatic effects. NSAIDs can reduce the production of prostaglandins by inhibiting peripheral cyclooxygenase (COX), which leads to antipyretic, analgesic, and anti-inflammatory effects. Relieve joint pain, muscle pain, headache, neuralgia, and bone metastasis pain, especially for mild to moderate chronic dull pain. However, NSAIDs are less effective for acute pain, severe pain due to severe trauma, and smooth muscle colic. The long-term application generally does not produce addiction [16].

In recent years, due to the discovery of the existence of two cyclooxygenases in the human body, namely COX-1, which has the effect of repairing the gastric mucosa, and COX-2, which can cause an inflammatory response and damage the gastric mucosa, traditional NSAIDs such as aspirin, ibuprofen, naproxen, etc., often cause damage to the gastric mucosa and may even lead to bleeding gastric ulcers. Selective COX-2 inhibitors reduce the side effects of the gastrointestinal tract, with better safety and wider applicability.

Commonly Used NSAIDs

1. Ibuprofen.

   It is fast absorbed orally and can be absorbed through the synovial cavity, thus acting on the joints, with strong antipyretic and analgesic effects and less adverse effects than aspirin.
2. Meloxicam.

   The effect on COX-2 is about 20 times that of COX-1, selective inhibition of COX-2, strong effect, slow absorption.
3. Celecoxib.

   It is a specific inhibitor of COX-2. It has a good analgesic effect, almost no gastrointestinal reactions and nephrotoxic reactions, and is well tolerated by patients, and was once widely respected. However, after COX-2 specific inhibitor rofecoxib was forced to withdraw from the market due to acute cardiovascular and cerebrovascular accidents after use, celecoxib was also issued a safety warning by FDA.
4. Flurbiprofen Ester.

   The effect is exerted by using lipid microspheres as the drug carrier and targeting distribution to the site of trauma or tumor to inhibit prostaglandin synthesis. This drug is for intravenous use and is indicated when oral drugs cannot be taken or when oral drugs are less effective.

8.7.1.2 Weak Opioids

Weak opioids are used for mild to moderate pain, with less physical dependence and addiction.

Codeine

The analgesic effect is 1/2 of morphine, the starting dose is 30 mg per dose, orally administered every 4–6 h, the dose can be as high as 130 mg per dose. The main side effect is constipation, which can be reduced by laxatives.

Buprenorphine

It can be administered rectally or sublingually, and the pain relief effect is 60–80 times that of morphine. Side effects are nausea and constipation.

Tramadol

Tramadol is a synthetic opioid analgesic that inhibits the reuptake of norepinephrine and 5hydroxytryptamine at brain synapses. Its affinity for opioid receptors is only 1/1000 of morphine, and it is easily replaced by other strong opioids. The analgesic effect is similar to that of pethidine, and it is effective for moderate or severe pain, and can be given orally, intravenously, intramuscularly, or even epidurally. Commonly used doses have no significant effect on respiration, and the effect on circulation is slight, with few side effects. For adults, 50–100 mg each time, three times daily, total amount not to exceed 400 mg daily.

8.7.1.3 Strong Opioid Drugs

Strong opioids are the main drugs for the treatment of moderate and severe pain, representing morphine.

Clinical Pharmacology of Morphine

The pharmacological effect of morphine is dose-related. The analgesic effect begins to appear at small doses, and the effect of emetic and constipation appears at the same time. When increasing the dose, there may appear drowsiness, in addition, too large a dose will result in respiratory depression. The optimal dose for analgesia is the dose that gives pain relief without drowsiness. Since the optimal dose varies widely among individuals, it is best to start with a small dose and gradually increase it to the optimal dose. Side effects such as nausea and constipation can be prevented with the combination of antiemetics and laxatives.

Continuous administration of analgesic doses of morphine is slow to develop resistance and somatic dependence and does not prevent clinical use. Since morphine has no high limit effect, even if resistance occurs, the pain relief will be maintained again with a slight increase in dose. Patients who have been treated with morphine for a long time will develop somatic dependence and will experience withdrawal syndrome once the drug is suddenly stopped, which is a normal reaction and does not usually occur if the drug is slowly reduced over 2 weeks and morphine is eventually stopped.

Use of Morphine

Currently, morphine extended-release is more commonly used in the form of continuous drug administration.

1. Morphine Sustained-Release Agent.

   Morphine is released slowly after oral administration, and the effect is maintained for 10–12 h, usually taken once every 12 h.
2. Morphine Continuous Intravenous Administration.

   It has the advantage of maintaining stable blood concentration and reducing the side effects of word administration. The disadvantage is the need to maintain continuous intravenous access.
3. Continuous Subcutaneous Injection of Morphine.

   The method of microinjection by the analgesic pump is adopted, and a fine needle is placed directly under the skin connected to the micropump, and the drug is absorbed directly into the peripheral vein under the skin. Compared with continuous intravenous administration, continuous subcutaneous injection reduces the complications such as puncture difficulties, phlebitis, and systemic infections, and is more suitable for patients with regular outpatient follow-up.
4. Other Methods.

   The optional analgesic methods include fentanyl transdermal patch, which slowly penetrates the subcutis and can maintain the analgesic effect for 48–72 h with a single dose.
5. Caution.

   When the pain is reduced, it means that the drug produces a good response, and it can be assumed that further increase of the drug dose will be more effective. If the pain does not disappear after increasing the dose of the drug, the pain medication should be replaced with a more potent one. Pay attention to the equivalence of opioids when replacing drugs, for example, the equivalent analgesic dose of 10 mg of intramuscular morphine, 75 mg of pethidine, 130 mg of codeine, and 0.1 mg of fentanyl.

8.7.1.4 5-Hydroxytryptamines

5-hydroxytryptamine (5-HT) is a monoamine neurotransmitter whose receptors are expressed in neural tissue as well as in blood vessels. In the dorsal horn of the spinal cord, 5-HTergic neurons are part of the inhibition of endogenous pain. Except for 5-HT_3, all other 5-HT receptors belong to G protein-coupled receptors. 5-$HT_{1B/1D}$ agonists (triptans) can be effective in neurovascular headaches (migraine, cluster headache).

Triptans can be administered orally, subcutaneously, or via intranasal drip, and is commonly used in the treatment of migraine. They are contraindicated in patients with risk factors for coronary artery disease, cerebrovascular and peripheral vascular disease, as they can narrow coronary arteries by 20% at clinical doses. Triptans, when combined with monoamine oxidase inhibitors, propranolol, cimetidine, drugs metabolized by hepatic P450, and P-glycoprotein pump inhibitors, have a mutual synergistic effect.

8.7.1.5 Anti-epileptic Drugs

Anti-epileptic drugs are used to treat neuropathic pain caused by peripheral nervous system damage (e.g., diabetes, scarring) or central nervous system damage (e.g., stroke). The pathogenesis includes ectopic activities of regenerative sensitized injurious receptors; reactivation of injurious receptors; or spontaneous neuronal activity; or it may be any combination of these mechanisms. These mechanisms may cause multilevel afferent neuronal sensitization. Anti-epileptic drugs can be divided into four types according to different mechanisms of action: (1) drugs that work by blocking activated voltage-sensitive sodium channels, including carbamazepine, phenytoin sodium, and lamotrigine; (2) drugs that work by blocking voltage-dependent calcium channels, including gabapentin and pregabalin; (3) drugs that work by inhibiting the release of presynaptic excitatory neurotransmitters, including gabapentin and lamotrigine; and (4) drugs that increase GABA receptor activity. Anti-epileptic drugs are indicated for the treatment of neuropathic pain and the prevention of migraine.

Pregabalin (lyrica) is a calcium channel blocker that is used to improve headaches, sleep disorders, etc. Pregabalin is used for the treatment of chronic pain as well as neuropathic pain. Dosage: The starting dose is 150 mg/day, titrated regularly for 5–7 days, and the maximum dose should not be greater than 600 mg/day.

8.7.1.6 Antidepressants

Antidepressants are used to treat neuropathic pain and headaches. According to the mechanism of action, tricyclic antidepressants can be divided into three major categories, which are nonselective norepinephrine/5-HT reuptake inhibitors (amitriptyline, imipramine, clomipramine, venlafaxine), selective norepinephrine reuptake inhibitors (desipramine, nortriptyline), and selective 5-HT reuptake inhibitors (citalopram, paroxetine, fluoxetine). Antidepressants can excite endogenous monoaminergic pain inhibitory neurons in the spinal cord and brain by blocking reuptake effects. In addition, it has the effects of antagonizing NMDA receptors, increasing endogenous opioid levels, blocking sodium channels, and opening potassium channels, thus inhibiting peripheral and central nervous system sensitization.

Adverse effects of antidepressants include sedation, nausea, constipation, dizziness, drowsiness, and blurred vision. To achieve better therapeutic effects as well as to avoid adverse drug reactions, clinical monitoring of blood levels of tricyclic antidepressants is often required. Tricyclic antidepressants block ion channels in the heart can lead to arrhythmias and are contraindicated in patients with recent myocardial infarction, arrhythmia, or cardiac dysfunction.

8.7.1.7 Other Analgesics and Adjuvant Drugs

Local Anesthetics

Local anesthetics can be used for patients with chronic pain syndrome, including topical, oral, intravenous, trigger point injection, regional block. Systemic drugs (such as oral mexiletine) have different effects in various neurological diseases, and mexiletine can be used as a third-line drug for diabetic neuropathy patients. When using local anesthetics, patients need to be closely monitored for adverse reactions.

α_2 Adrenergic Agonists

Such as clonidine and dexmedetomidine, α_2 adrenergic receptors belong to the G protein-coupled receptor family and have similar effects to opioids. They produce inhibitory effects by opening potassium channels, inhibiting presynaptic calcium channels, inhibiting adenylate cyclase activity, reducing neurotransmitter release, and decreasing postsynaptic transmission. In patients with complex regional pain syndrome, neuropathic pain, and cancer pain, the application of clonidine can produce analgesic effects, but adverse drug reactions such as excessive sedation, hypertension, and bradycardia should be alerted.

Baclofen
The drug can activate the presynaptic and postsynaptic $GABA_B$ receptors, resulting in decreased excitability and neurotransmission and enhanced inhibitory neurotransmission. Baclofen is often used for trigeminal neuralgia and central neuropathic pain. The most common side effects are drowsiness, dizziness, and gastrointestinal discomfort.

Antiemetics
Antiemetics are important adjuvant drugs in the treatment of acute pain and cancer pain. They should be used as early as possible and in combination.

8.7.2 Nerve Block Therapy

8.7.2.1 Concept of Nerve Block
Blocking nerve conduction by injecting drugs or giving physical stimulation directly into or near nerve tissue such as nerve trunk endings, plexus, cerebral nerve, spinal nerve root, sympathetic ganglion, etc. is called nerve block. There are two types of blocks, chemical and physical. Chemical nerve blocks mainly use local anesthetic drugs to block nerve conduction function and can be used for intraoperative analgesia and are also commonly used for pain management. Nerve blocks using conventional local anesthetics are generally reversible. As the effects of the drugs wear off, the locally blocked nerve conduction function can be gradually restored. However, nerve blocks with high concentrations of local anesthetics or nerve-destroying drugs for certain therapeutic purposes can block nerve conduction for longer periods or even permanently. In addition, the clinical use of physical means such as heating, pressure and cooling to block nerve conduction is called physical nerve block.

8.7.2.2 Mechanism of Nerve Block

Blocking the Nerve Conduction Pathway of Nociception
Local anesthetics and nerve destruction drugs inhibit the flow of sodium and potassium ions inside and outside the nerve cell, and even cause cell membrane degeneration and necrosis, thus blocking the conduction of nerve impulses in the nerve fiber.

Block the Vicious Circle of Pain
The pain-causing substances produced by the pain can intensify the pain, and this vicious circle makes the pain persist for a long time and gradually worsen. The use of nerve block treatment, acting on the pain site, while blocking the conduction of nociceptive stimuli, can well relieve local muscle tension and vascular spasm, improve local blood circulation, reduce the accumulation of blocking metabolites, which is more conducive to lifting the vicious cycle of pain than analgesic drug treatment so that the internal environment tends to stabilize and pain disappears. As the patient's fear, anxiety, and psychological changes of disease and pain will also stimulate the sympathetic nerve and aggravate the above vicious cycle If we can cooperate with psychological and pharmacological treatment, we can achieve better results.

Improve Blood Circulation
Nerve block treatment can improve local microcirculation, of which sympathetic nerve block plays a very important therapeutic role. For pain caused by peripheral circulation disorder, sympathetic nerve block can make the blood vessels within the innervation area dilate, release vascular spasm and relieve vascular obstruction, thus improving blood circulation and promoting the formation of collateral circulation.

Anti-inflammatory Effect
Nerve block therapy has an anti-inflammatory effect, especially since the sympathetic block is more significant. In recent years, endogenous antibiotics, i.e. natural antibiotics, have been dis-

covered, and he is a tiny protein inside the white blood cells. Endogenous antibiotics are not fully effective when blood circulation is impaired. Sympathetic nerve block can improve blood circulation and promote the full effect of endogenous antibiotics, enhancing the natural healing ability.

8.7.2.3 Characteristics of Nerve Block Therapy

Reliable Analgesic Effect

Nerve block therapy can achieve temporary or permanent analgesia in most pain patients and become the beginning of the treatment with the original disease. Although this does not mean that nerve block therapy can treat all pain, and the most appropriate method should be selected. However, at present, among most pain treatment methods, nerve block therapy is still one of the most dominant treatment tools.

Helping to Diagnose Diseases

It is difficult to make a clear diagnosis quickly for some diseases, and experimental blocking of the associated nerve can be an important tool for diagnosis and differential diagnosis. For example, it is difficult to confirm the diagnosis of glossopharyngeal neuralgia based on clinical manifestations alone, and a glossopharyngeal nerve block can help to make a clear diagnosis. Similarly, the clinical diagnosis of the affected branch of trigeminal neuralgia is often made by nerve block.

Controllable

Unlike systemic drug therapy, nerve block treatment is highly controllable, and by adjusting the type, concentration, dose, and injection site of drugs, the nerve block can be limited to a certain range, and the application of nerve destructive drugs and physical destruction methods can make the analgesic effect long-lasting. The scope of nerve block treatment is not only limited to painful diseases, but is expanding. Recent studies have shown that stellate ganglion block can be used to treat dozens of non-painful diseases such as primary hypertension, sudden deafness, and facial nerve palsy, in addition to herpes zoster on the head and face.

Small Side Effects

The drugs used in nerve blocks have no serious side effects and do not require special equipment and devices.

High Operation Technique Requirement

The effect of nerve block is closely related to the operation technique. If the block is successful, the effect is remarkable; if the block fails, not only is it ineffective, but also irritation symptoms and even serious comorbidities may occur. This is another major feature of this treatment method, and also the disadvantage of this treatment method. Therefore, in addition to having rich anatomical, neurophysiological, and clinical knowledge, the operator must be proficient in the operation techniques of various nerve block techniques, strengthen monitoring as well as the follow-up, and achieve institutionalization and standardization.

8.7.2.4 Indications and Contraindications of Nerve Block

Indications

The indications for nerve block treatment are very broad, and almost all parts of the body and pain of various nature can be treated with nerve block. Its treatment is not only limited to various acute and chronic pain but also can be used for many non-painful symptoms and diseases, such as chronic sinusitis, retinal vascular occlusion, facial nerve palsy, primary hypertension, etc. When selecting indications, attention should be paid to the developmental changes of the disease process, and it should not be used for all patients regardless of the timing. For example, for patients with early trigeminal neuralgia, drug therapy can be tried first, and when drug therapy is not effective or cannot be continued due to side effects of drug therapy, then nerve block therapy can be chosen. For some painful diseases that nerve block therapy has achieved efficacy, attention should also be paid to the combination of drug therapy, physical therapy, to increase and consolidate the efficacy and prevent a recurrence.

Contraindications

1. Uncooperative patients, including patients with schizophrenia and Alzheimer's disease;
2. Patients with infected lesions at the puncture site;
3. Patients with a bleeding tendency or undergoing anticoagulation therapy;
4. Patients who are allergic to local anesthetic drugs.

The pros and cons of implementing nerve block therapy should also be considered comprehensively for patients of advanced age, poor general condition, and serious organic diseases. In addition, delayed treatment due to analgesia masking the disease needs to be avoided.

8.7.2.5 Commonly Used Facial and Cervical Nerve Block Treatments

The sensory nerves in the maxillofacial neck include the cervical nerve, sympathetic nerve, as well as the trigeminal nerve, facial nerve, glossopharyngeal nerve, vagus nerve, and several other pairs of brain nerves. These nerves are involved in sensory transmission in the maxillofacial neck together. The most commonly used maxillofacial and cervical nerve blocks include trigeminal ganglion block, glossopharyngeal nerve block, and stellate ganglion block.

Trigeminal Ganglion Block

Trigeminal neuralgia is one of the common neuropathic pain disorders in clinical practice. The trigeminal ganglion block is often used for treatment. The block route is to enter the needle from below the posterior 1/3 of the zygomatic arch, 2.5 cm above the lateral corner of the mouth directly opposite the maxillary second molar, stab along the inner surface of the mandibular branch to reach the base of the pterygoid process posteriorly and reach the foramen ovale anteriorly, confirm the needle position with X-ray, then retreat the needle and penetrate the foramen ovale posteriorly and superiorly to reach the trigeminal ganglion at the trigeminal nerve pressure trace, carefully retract, after confirming that there is no blood or cerebrospinal fluid reflux, inject the blocking agent.

Because the subarachnoid space extends into the trigeminal nerve cavity, even a small amount of local anesthetic accidentally enters the cerebrospinal fluid and spreads rapidly to the brainstem, causing serious consequences such as loss of consciousness or cardiac arrest, so trigeminal ganglion blocks must be performed with caution. For the sake of safety, trigeminal ganglion block is mostly performed under the guidance of imaging technology in clinical practice.

Linguopharyngeal Nerve Block

The needle can be inserted vertically from below the external orifice of the external auditory canal, slightly in front of the anterior edge of the mastoid process, continue to insert the needle 1.25–2.50 cm past the posterior aspect of the styloid process. The tip of the needle can reach below the jugular foramen, and local anesthetics can be injected to achieve the purpose of blocking the glossopharyngeal nerve. It is worth noting that cerebral nerves X and XI, and the cervical sympathetic trunk can be blocked at the same time when the glossopharyngeal nerve block is performed. In addition, the glossopharyngeal nerve block can also be performed by inserting the needle vertically between the midpoint of the mastoid tip and the mandibular angle, with the tip of the needle passing a little in front of the styloid process, and injecting the local anesthetic into the front of the styloid process.

Stellate Ganglion Block

The paratracheal approach is used commonly in clinical practice, that is, 2.5 cm above the sternoclavicular joint and 1.5 cm lateral intersection of the anterior midline to the base of the transverse process of the 7th cervical vertebrae, using the fingers to push the common carotid artery to the lateral side, the tip of the needle meets the bone, and injects local anesthetic after there is no retraction of blood or cerebrospinal fluid. If the block is effective, Horner's syndrome (miosis of the affected pupil, ptosis of the upper eyelid and entropion of the eye, etc.) may occur. Attention should be paid to prevent complications such as pneumothorax, total spinal anesthesia, and retropharyngeal nerve block in clinical practice.

8.7.3 Treatment of Acute Pain

8.7.3.1 Treatment of Postoperative Pain

There are several options for postoperative pain management, including systemic administration of analgesics and regional (intralesional and peripheral) analgesic techniques. Based on the patient's wishes and active individualized assessment of the pros and cons of each treatment method, the clinician can select the most appropriate postoperative analgesic regimen for each patient. Since postoperative oral and maxillofacial surgery mostly involves head and neck pain, intradural analgesia often fails to meet the analgesic needs [17].

Route of Analgesic Administration

1. Oral Administration.

   The choice of oral analgesic drugs is suitable for patients with high bioavailability and those who are suitable for oral administration after surgery. The disease itself, surgical trauma, and anesthesia can inhibit gastrointestinal motility, and it is generally believed that oral drugs have delayed absorption, slow onset of action, and poor effect. Therefore, the analgesic effect of oral administration is poor in patients with moderate or severe postoperative pain, and it is not recommended.

2. Intramuscular Injection.

   This route is a classical clinical drug delivery method. Commonly used drugs include pethidine, tramadol, buprenorphine hydrochloride, and so on. However, the absorption of the drug depends on the lipid solubility of the drug and the local blood flow of the injection. The concentration of intramuscular injection in blood fluctuates greatly, which leads to incomplete analgesia or complications as well as injection pain. Therefore, the intramuscular injection route is used less and less in clinical practice.

3. Intravenous Injection.

   Intravenous injection is the fastest route to effective analgesia. Continuous intravenous infusion can reduce the fluctuation of drug concentration and has a definite effect on the continuous relief of postoperative pain. Commonly used drugs are morphine, fentanyl, and pethidine. The use of medium and long half-life opioids may result in accumulation, leading to serious complications such as respiratory depression. To improve the analgesic effect and safety of continuous intravenous drug administration, patient-controlled analgesia is mostly used.

4. Skin Mucosa and Regional Routes.

   These routes are also commonly used clinically effective methods.

8.7.3.2 Patient-Controlled Analgesia

PCA is developed by combining the concept of on-demand analgesia proposed in the last two decades with artificial intelligence technology. The PCA device includes a drug injection pump, an automatic control device, an infusion line, and a one-way valve to prevent regurgitation. According to different drug delivery routes, it is divided into: (1) patient-controlled intravenous analgesia (PCIA); (2) patient-controlled epidural analgesia (PCEA); (3) patient-controlled nerve block analgesia (PCNA); (4) patient-controlled subcutaneous analgesia (PCSA), etc.

8.7.3.3 Regional Analgesic Techniques

Peripheral regional analgesic technique is commonly used. In general, the analgesic effect of epidural and peripheral regional analgesic techniques (especially when local anesthetics are used) is better than that of systemic application of opioids. However, there are risks associated with the use of these techniques, and clinicians should evaluate the pros and cons for each patient to determine the most appropriate peripheral regional analgesic technique. Oral- and maxillofacial-related analgesic needs are limited by the analgesic area, which precludes the use of intralesional analgesia. Therefore, peripheral regional analgesia techniques (nerve tissue) are often used when performing regional analgesia techniques to provide analgesia for dentistry patients.

8.7.3.4 Other Techniques

Other non-pharmacological techniques such as transcutaneous electrical nerve stimulation (TENS), acupuncture, and psychological therapies can be used to relieve postoperative pain.

8.7.3.5 Preventive Analgesia

Preventive analgesia refers to analgesic treatment that extends from the preoperative to postoperative period by using continuous, multimodal analgesia to achieve elimination of pain caused by surgical stress trauma and to prevent and suppress central and peripheral sensitization. For those predicted to have high-level surgical pain (prolonged major surgery, knee arthroplasty, etc.), preoperative with chronic pain or severe pain, the use of prophylactic analgesia can reduce the amount of perioperative analgesic drugs and mitigate adverse drug reactions.

8.7.3.6 Perioperative Multimodal Analgesia

It refers to the combined application of analgesic drugs, adjuvant drugs, and analgesic techniques with different mechanisms of action throughout the perioperative period to cope with postoperative pain produced by different mechanisms, to achieve the best efficacy of reducing postoperative pain and to reduce the occurrence of analgesia-related complications. The principles of multimodal analgesia include: preoperative, intraoperative and postoperative analgesia; multilevel analgesia, i.e., including terminal, peripheral nerve, spinal cord level, and cerebral cortex; use of multiple drugs and analgesic techniques; and full use of various drugs and techniques in joint programs to achieve the purpose of complementing each other's strengths and weaknesses so that patients can move early, resume gastrointestinal nutrition early, shorten hospitalization time and promote rapid recovery.

It is often implemented clinically through multiple approaches, methods, techniques, and medications. Emphasis is placed on pain prediction and assessment, advocating preventive analgesia, especially for patients with preoperative pre-existing pain, intraoperative individualized analgesia for the intensity of surgical stimulation, and timely and effective postoperative analgesia to prevent the transformation of surgical acute pain to chronic pain and achieve satisfactory analgesic effects. Through multimodal analgesia, the goal of a safe and pain-free perioperative period, pain-free movement, pain-free sleep, and pain-free resting is achieved.

8.7.4 Treatment of Chronic Pain

Chronic pain refers to pain that lasts longer than the general course of an acute disease or longer than the general time required for injury healing or recurrent pain lasting more than 3 months [18]. Chronic pain can be divided into five categories according to the causes: traumatic pain; neuropathic pain; inflammatory pain; psychogenic pain; and cancer pain, etc. [19]. The common treatment methods are as follows.

8.7.4.1 Drug Treatment

Drug treatment is the most basic and commonly used method of pain treatment. Generally, patients with chronic pain require medication for a longer period, and to maintain a minimum effective plasma drug concentration, medication should be administered at regular intervals. Medication at the onset of pain often needs a larger dose, the maintenance of time is shorter, and the effect is not ideal. Commonly used drugs are NSAIDs, opioids, sedative-hypnotics, antiepileptics, and antidepressants.

8.7.4.2 Nerve Block

Nerve block is the main treatment for chronic pain. Long-acting local anesthetics are generally used. For intractable headaches such as trigeminal neuralgia, anhydrous ethanol or 5–10% phenol can be used for nerve destruction treatment to achieve long-term analgesia. Commonly used nerve blocks include brachial plexus nerve block, cervical plexus nerve block, and intercostal nerve block. In addition, the pain of many diseases is related to sympathetic nerves and can be treated by sympathetic nerve block. The commonly used sympathetic nerve block methods include stellate ganglion block and lumbar sympathetic ganglion block.

8.7.4.3 Trigger Point Injection

Each painful spot is injected with 1% lidocaine or 0.25% bupivacaine 1–4 mL, plus prednisolone suspension 0.5 mL (12.5 mg), 1–2 times a week, 3–5 times a course of treatment.

8.7.4.4 Physiotherapy

There are many kinds of physiotherapy, such as electrotherapy, phototherapy, magnetic therapy, radiofrequency thermal coagulation therapy, and paraffin therapy, which are widely used in the treatment of pain. The main functions are anti-inflammatory, analgesic, antispasmodic, improving local blood circulation, softening the scar, etc.

8.7.4.5 Spinal Cord Electrical Stimulation and an Intrathecal Morphine Pump

Spinal cord electrical stimulation and intrathecal morphine pump can be used for patients who have failed to respond to conventional treatment.

8.7.4.6 Psychological Treatment

Psychological factors play an important role in chronic pain. The supportive therapy in the psychological treatment method is that the medical personnel use explanation, encouragement, and comfort to help the patient eliminate the adverse psychological factors such as anxiety, depression, and fear, to mobilize the patient's subjective motivation, change the patient's sensitivity to pain and actively cooperate with the treatment. In addition, there are hypnosis and suggestion therapy, cognitive therapy, and biofeedback therapy.

8.7.4.7 Occupational Therapy

Occupational therapists guide patients to overcome the limitations of activities caused by pain and to achieve the goals of daily activities. The main purpose of treatment is to encourage meaningful family, social, and work relationships through non-pharmacological means, to help patients reduce pain, to facilitate the return of optimal daily living, to enhance patients' self-esteem, to restore self-care, and to enable them to overcome pain and achieve optimal performance in work and entertainment.

8.7.5 Cancer Pain Treatment

Pain is one of the most common symptoms of cancer patients, and cancer pain seriously affects the quality of life of cancer patients. The incidence of pain in primary cancer patients is about 25%; the incidence of pain in advanced cancer patients is about 60–80%, and 1/3 of them have severe pain. If not relieved, it can aggravate patients' anxiety, depression, fatigue, insomnia, loss of appetite, and other symptoms, which can seriously affect patients' self-care ability, social interaction ability, and overall quality of life. The causes of cancer pain include: pain directly caused by cancer development, pain caused by diagnosis and treatment of cancer, and painful diseases complicated by cancer disease entry.

8.7.5.1 Treatment Principles of Cancer Pain

Cancer pain should be treated based on the principle of comprehensive treatment. According to the patient's disease and physical condition, analgesic treatment should be effectively applied to eliminate pain continuously and effectively, prevent and control the adverse drug reactions, and reduce the psychological burden caused by pain and treatment, to maximize the patient's quality of life.

8.7.5.2 Treatment Methods

The treatment methods of cancer pain include: etiological treatment, pharmacological analgesic treatment, and non-pharmacological treatment.

Etiological Treatment

The main causes of cancer pain are the primary diseases and complications. Therefore, anti-cancer treatment such as surgery, radiotherapy, or chemotherapy can effectively relieve cancer pain.

Drug analgesic Treatment

1. Principles.

   According to the World Health Organization (WHO) guidelines, the five basic principles of use of analgesics for cancer pain are as follows.

   (a) *"By mouth"*: Analgesics should be given via the mouth whenever possible. Rectal suppositories are an effective mode of administration for patients with dysphagia, uncontrollable vomiting or gastrointestinal obstruction. Alternatively, for these patients, the drug can be administered by continuous subcutaneous infusion. Continuous subcutaneous infusion is an alternative route of administration to rectal suppositories. There is a wide range of mechanical and battery powered portable infusion pumps that can be selected.

   (b) *"By the clock"*: Analgesics should be administered "over time," i.e. at regular time intervals. The dose of analgesic is determined according to the patient's pain level. In other words, the dose is gradually increased until the patient is comfortable. Re-administration of analgesia should begin before the effect of the previous analgesic dose has completely worn off, in order to achieve the goal of continuous pain relief.

   Some patients require "rescue" doses of analgesia, mostly to urgently handle episodic (intermittent) and breakthrough pain situations. The dose at this point should be 50–100% of the regular 4-h dose and identified as an addition to the regular schedule.

   (c) *"By the ladder"*: The order of their use is shown in Fig. 8.6. The first step is the use of non-opioid drugs. If pain is not

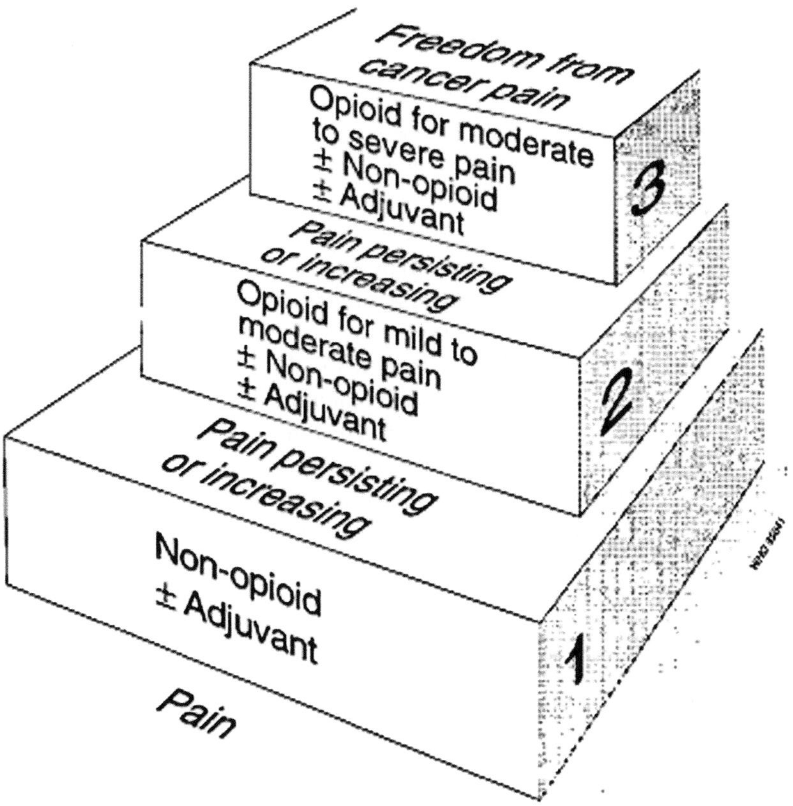

Fig. 8.6 Use of Analgesics by The Ladder

relieved, the treatment moves to the next level, adding opioids for mild to moderate pain. When the first and second steps of medication combined still do not provide pain relief, proceed to the third step, where the opioid currently taken is discontinued and replaced with an opioid used to treat moderate to severe pain. It should be noticed that only one drug in each group should be used together. Adjunctive medication should be given according to the specific indication.

If one of the drugs in the same group is no longer effective, do not turn to an alternative drug of similar efficacy (e.g. from codeine to dextropropoxyphene). Switching from one drug to another drug in the same group is inadvisable. The appropriate choice is to prescribe another more potent drug (e.g. morphine).

(d) *"For the individual"*: There is no standard dose for the use of opioids. The correct dose to use is the one that mitigates the patient's pain. This means that the standard dose of opioids varies from person to person. For instance, doses of oral morphine range from 5 mg every 4 h to over 1000 mg. However, opioids used for mild to moderate pain are prescribed in practice with dose limits that take into account formulation reasons (e.g., in combination with ASA or paracetamol, which are toxic at high doses) or a disproportionate increase in adverse effects at high doses (e.g., codeine).

(e) *"Attention to detail"*: Analgesics should be given at regular intervals and oral morphine should be given every 4 h. The time of the first and last dose of the day should be correlated with the patient's waking time and bedtime. The best times of the day to administer analgesics are usually 10:00, 14:00, and 18:00, and by following this schedule, the duration of the analgesic effect and the severity of adverse effects can be balanced.

Preferably, the doctor should write out the whole patient's medication regimen for easy reference by the patient and their family. The regimen should specifically include the name of the drug, the reason for use (e.g. "for pain," "for bowel movement"), the dose (number of milliliters, number of tablets) and the number of times per day. The patient should be informed of possible adverse reactions.

2. Choice of Analgesic.

According to the degree and nature of pain, the treatment being received and the concomitant diseases of cancer patients, analgesic drugs and adjuvant drugs should be reasonably selected, and the dosage and frequency of drug administration should be individually adjusted to improve the analgesic effect and prevent adverse reactions.

(a) *Non-steroidal anti-inflammatory drugs*: they are the basic drugs for cancer pain treatment. Different non-steroidal anti-inflammatory drugs have a similar mechanism of action and have analgesic and anti-inflammatory effects, and are often used to relieve mild pain or combined with opioids to relieve moderate and severe pain. In the treatment, attention should be paid to peptic ulcer, platelet dysfunction, renal or hepatic impairment, etc.

(b) *Opioids*: They are the drugs of choice for the treatment of moderate and severe pain. At present, the short-acting opioids commonly used in cancer pain treatment are morphine immediate-release tablets and long-acting opioids are morphine extended-release tablets and fentanyl transdermal patches. For the treatment of chronic cancer pain, opioid agonists are recommended. For long-term use of opioid analgesics, oral administration is preferred, and transdermal patch administration or temporary subcutaneous injection can also be used. Intrathecal drug delivery system (IDDS), or spinal morphine pump, is a special analgesic method for cancer pain and chronic intractable pain.

(c) *Adjuvant drugs*: including anticonvulsants, antidepressants, corticosteroids, N-methyl-D-aspartate receptor (NMDA) antagonists, and local anesthetics. Adjuvant medications can enhance the analgesic effect of opioids or produce direct analgesia. Adjuvant analgesics are often used as an adjunct to the treatment of neuropathic pain, bone pain and visceral pain.

3. Non-Pharmacological Treatment.

   Non-pharmacological treatments for cancer pain treatment mainly include: interventional therapy, acupuncture, physiotherapy such as transcutaneous electrical stimulation, cognitive-behavioral training, psychosocial support therapy, and so on. Appropriate application of non-pharmacological therapy can be a useful supplement to pharmacological analgesic treatment and can increase the effect of analgesic treatment when used in combination with analgesic drug therapy.

8.8 Special Pains in Oral and Maxillofacial Area

8.8.1 Temporomandibular Disorders

Temporomandibular disorders (TMD) is a general term for a group of disorders involving the temporomandibular joint and/or the occlusal system, causing joint pain, popping and mouth opening restriction, etc. TMD is a common and frequent disease, mostly seen in adults around 45 years old, with a higher prevalence in women than in men. It may be related to the following factors: (1) occlusal factors: Patients mostly have significant disorders of occlusal relationship; (2) overload on the joint: frequent biting of hard food, grinding of teeth at night, and clenching of teeth during tension increase the load on the joint; (3) anatomical factors: small condyles and excessive joint movement make dislocation easy to occur, etc.; (4) immune factors: local autoimmunity causes progressive destruction of joint cartilage and bone; (5) trauma, micro trauma; (6) psychosocial factors: TMD can be a psychosomatic disease, and psychological factors can affect the development and treatment of TMD. Patients are often accompanied by emotional irritability, mental tension, agitation, insomnia and other symptoms.

The prevalence of TMD in the elderly is as high as 56.3%, and 86.9% are accompanied by pain.

8.8.1.1 Clinical Manifestations

TMD has a long course, usually several years to a dozen years, and can recur. The progression of TMD is divided into three stages: (1) the early functional change stage; (2) the middle stage of structural changes; and (3) the late stage of organic joint destruction.

Pain, joint popping and joint dysfunction are the main clinical manifestations of TMD: (1) pain: joint pain and peri-articular pain, especially pain during chewing and mouth opening, may be accompanied by mild or severe temporomandibular joint pressure pain; (2) abnormal jaw movement: common movement obstruction is restricted mouth opening, jaw deviation during mouth opening, restricted jaw movement to the left and right side, etc.; (3) joint clicking: normal joint movement without clicking sound and noise. In case of abnormality, clicking sounds appear in mouth opening. The sound can occur at different stages of jaw movement, and can be a crisp popping sound, crushing sound and friction sound.

Some TMDs have complex clinical manifestations, and may present with headache, ear symptoms, neck symptoms, or even systemic symptoms, and a few TMDs may present with clinical manifestations of trigeminal neuralgia.

8.8.1.2 Auxiliary Examinations

X-rays (Schuyler's and transpharyngeal lateral views) can reveal sclerosis, bone destruction, osteophytes, cystic changes and other joint space changes and bone changes.

Arthrography can detect joint disc displacement, perforation, and changes of joint disc attachment.

MRI and endoscopic examination of the joint can detect early TMD.

8.8.1.3 Diagnosis and Differential Diagnosis

In 2014, the International Academy of Dental Research published the classification and diagnostic criteria for the most common TMD (DC/TMD) based on symptom questionnaires and clinical examinations. The DC/TMD classification and diagnostic criteria classify the clinical diagnosis of TMD into two major categories: painful diseases and joint diseases.

Painful Disorders

Including muscle pain (limited myalgia, myofascial pain, involved myofascial pain) joint pain (pain on one or both sides of the face, solar plexus, inner or preauricular area, pain on jaw movement plus clinical examination to confirm a pain in the mandibular joint area, familiar pain on palpation or jaw movement in the joint area) TMD headache (headache in the solar plexus area, increased pain on jaw movement. Clinical examination confirms headache in the temporal muscle area, temporal muscle palpation or mandibular movements can trigger a familiar headache in the temporal region).

Joint Disease

Including reducible disc displacement, reducible disc displacement with interlocking, and irreducible disc displacement with restricted opening.

To make an accurate and comprehensive diagnosis or final diagnosis, imaging must be combined. A comprehensive assessment of the patient's somatic disease and psychosomatic status can be performed using the TMD dual-axis diagnostic method (Axis I for clinical diagnosis and Axis II for pain, function and psychological status evaluation) in patients with prolonged chronic pain. Depressive mood can be evaluated by the Patient Health Questionnaire 9, anxiety by the GAD-7, and somatic status by the Patient Health Questionnaire 15.

TMD needs to be differentiated from the following diseases.

Tumors: deep maxillofacial tumors can cause difficulty in opening or closing the teeth, such as benign tumors of the temporomandibular joint, tumors of the infratemporal fossa, tumors of the posterior wall of the maxillary sinus, and nasopharyngeal carcinoma, etc. Imaging can help in the diagnosis.

Acute septic arthritis of the jaw joint: acute onset, pain, and swelling in the joint area, significant pressure pain in the joint area, and changes in the relationship such as misopening of the posterior teeth due to fluid accumulation in the joint cavity. The joint space is clear on the Schuyler film, and intra-articular puncture can aspirate the purulent fluid. (3) Traumatic arthritis: acute traumatic arthritis is manifested as swelling, pain and opening restriction in the joint area: chronic traumatic arthritis can be manifested as soreness in the occlusal muscles, murmur in the joint, opening restriction, pain in the joint area and face.

8.8.1.4 Treatment Principle

The purpose of TMD treatment is to eliminate pain, reduce adverse load, restore function, and improve quality of life. A reversible, non-invasive, and comprehensive approach is used to restore the normal function of the patient's oromandibular system. The principles should be followed: (1) remove various causative factors, personalized treatment, conservative treatment, early treatment and minimally invasive treatment; (2) improve the general condition and the patient's mental state, and perform psychotherapy; (3) follow a reasonable and comprehensive treatment procedure; (4) the treatment procedure should start with conservative treatment, and irreversible surgical treatment should be considered only after all reversible non-surgical treatments have failed; (5) health education: to make patients understand the nature of the disease, hair factors, so that patients increase confidence and cooperate with doctors.

Treatment of the Cause

For occlusal joint disorder syndrome caused by occlusal relationship, the dentist will use occlusal treatment, including reversible occlusal treatment such as occlusal plate and irreversible occlusal treatment such as adjustment, restoration, orthodontics, and extraction.

Conservative Treatment

Daily diet: Encourage patients to eat soft food, bite food in small bites, and chew slowly.

Physical therapy: When the pain in the joint area is significant, physical therapy such as heat, ultra-short wave, ion guide, electrical stimulation acupuncture low degree hydrogen atmosphere laser irradiation, and magnetic therapy can be used to relieve pain, which is more effective for endogenous causes of TMD such as muscle spasm, myositis, and anterior muscle pain.

Drug therapy: Drug therapy is an important part of the comprehensive treatment of MD. It includes non-steroidal anti-inflammatory drugs (NSAIDs), anti-anxiety drugs, muscle relaxants, antidepressants, and antihistamines. Early application of acetaminophen and NSAIDs (such as celecoxib, diclofenac sodium, ericiclib, etc.) can reduce pain; anxiolytics (o-methylphenidate citrate) or antidepressants (amitriptyline), etc., can also achieve better results in the treatment of TMD. (4) Opening training: mandibular motor training includes active training (correction of jaw movement trajectory) and passive training (improvement of maximum opening). (5) Muscle therapy: such as muscle massage, jaw posture exercises, etc. (6) Psychotherapy such as health education and psychological counseling.

Temporomandibular Joint Cavity Injection Treatment

It can relieve joint pain, lubricate the joint, and promote the modification of joint structure. Generally, the injected drugs are large mucopolysaccharides such as hyaluronic acid or gibberellins, local anesthetics, and glucocorticoids. Three consecutive injections are a course of treatment. One injection is given 2 weeks apart and no more than three times a year. Joint cavity irrigation can reduce pain by removing some inflammatory mediators, immune substances, and some cartilage debris flocculent in the joint fluid by irrigation. The efficacy of joint cavity injection of sodium hyaluronate for TMD is better than joint cavity irrigation alone.

Psychological and Cognitive-Behavioral Therapy

The role of psychological and behavioral therapy in the treatment of TMD is emphasized, and cognitive education and behavioral therapy are targeted to the patient's psychology.

Surgical Treatment

Surgical treatment is required for TMD with severe structural disorders and osteoarthrosis that do not respond well to conservative treatment, or that seriously affect joint function and normal life, including joint irrigation, arthroscopic surgery, and open surgery.

Extracorporeal Shockwave Therapy

There are many types of traditional physiotherapy, such as polarized light irradiation, ultrasound therapy, shortwave therapy, and manual release, etc. Although they are effective, they have the disadvantages of long treatment course, poor treatment experience, poor results, and high recurrence rate. The main reason for this is that there is no consensus or guideline for TMD treatment at home and abroad to guide clinical work. Extracorporeal shockwave therapy (ESWT) is a new physical therapy method, which is non-invasive, safe and effective, and has been widely used in the clinical treatment of bone and muscle diseases, and in 2016, the International Society of Medical Shockwave Therapy included oral and maxillofacial diseases such as periodontal disease and jaw joint disorders into its indications.

TMD is not a diagnosis of a single disease, but a general term for a group of diseases with similar clinical symptoms involving the masticatory muscles and/or the temporomandibular joint. At present, there is no unified theory on the etiology and pathogenesis of TMD at home and abroad, and there are successive theories of factors, psychosomatic factors, trauma factors, autoimmune factors, anatomical factors, etc. There is a close relationship between TMD and neck and shoulder pain. On the one hand, masticatory muscles such as the occlusal muscles, internal pterygoid muscle, external pterygoid muscle, temporalis muscle and the back muscles of the head, neck, shoulder, and back are a unified functional whole. Therefore, when the aseptic inflammation of the back of the head, neck, and shoulders stimulates the high cervical nerve, it will also form conduction pain at the temporomandibular joint, so many patients are thought to have cervicogenic headache, cervical spondylosis, migraine, etc. in the early stage, but patients with TMD can mostly find sensitive pressure points locally, i.e. trigger points, indicating that secondary lesions can easily form here, and the inflammation stimulates the occlusal muscle groups causing The inflammation stimulates the occlusal muscle groups causing muscle spasm, which in turn causes pain and affects the occlusal function.

Shock wave is a kind of sound wave with mechanical properties that causes rapid or extremely rapid compression of the medium through vibration, high-speed motion, etc. to gather energy, which is different from the traditional sound wave and can cause jumping changes in the physical properties of the medium such as pressure, temperature and density, thus causing a series of biological effects on the target organ tissue. The mechanism of action may be: after the shock wave enters the body, it produces mechanical stress and unique cavitation effect at the interface, causing elastic deformation and relaxation among soft tissues, and can stimulate vasodilation and generation in the local area, improving microcirculation, and reducing tissue inflammatory response. In addition, the shock wave can stimulate the local nerve endings, so that the sensitivity of nerves is reduced and the transmission of nerve conduction is blocked, thus relieving pain.

8.8.2 Burning Mouth Syndrome

Burning mouth syndrome (BMS) is a group of syndromes with the tongue as the main site of onset, with burning-like pain as the main manifestation, mostly accompanied by dry mouth, taste changes, headache, mood changes, often not accompanied by mucosal disease and other clinical signs, without characteristic histopathological changes. Female onset is more frequent than sexual, with a high prevalence in menopausal women. Currently, the pathogenesis is unclear, and some studies suggest co-morbidity with psychosocial and sperm abnormalities. Whether secondary burning mouth syndrome caused by local lesions (candidiasis, lichen planus, salivation) or systemic diseases (drug hair, anemia, diabetes mellitus, vitamin B_2 or folic acid deficiency, Sjogren's syndrome) should be treated as an independent disease remains controversial.

8.8.2.1 Clinical Manifestations

The painful part of the tongue, the anterior part of the hard palate and the mucosa of the lower lip, most often involving the tip of the tongue or bilateral tongue edges. Some patients have light symptoms in the morning, gradually worsen in the afternoon, and disappear in the evening, and may have subjective dry mouth, sensory dullness and altered sensation. Some patients have nervousness, depression, anxiety, irritability, insomnia, and other mental manifestations.

8.8.2.2 Physical Examination

There is no abnormality in the color, quality, morphology and function of the patient's tongue and oral mucosa.

8.8.2.3 Auxiliary Examinations

The dopamine D_1/D_2 receptor ratio was decreased in the patient with BMS, and there was cerebral hypofunction on functional MRI, and there was microcirculation disorder in the oral mucosal vessels.

8.8.2.4 Diagnosis and Differential Diagnosis

According to the International Classification of Headache, third edition (beta) (ICHD-3) the diagnostic criteria of burning mouth syndrome.

A. The oral pain meets criteria B and C.
B. Recurrent attacks lasting more than 2 h per day for more than 3 months.
C. The pain meets all two of the following:
    1. Burning-like in nature.
    2. Sensation appears on the surface of the oral mucosa.

Normal appearance of the oral mucosa and normal clinical examination including sensory testing.

Cannot be better explained by other diagnoses in the ICHD-3.

Burning mouth syndrome should be differentiated from the following diseases.

Trigeminal neuralgia: Severe electric shock-like, knife-like, or tearing pain occurring in the distribution area of the trigeminal nerve. There are primary and secondary trigeminal neuralgia. In primary trigeminal neuralgia, most of them have "trigger points" and no neurological signs. Secondary trigeminal neuralgia is pain in the area of trigeminal nerve distribution caused by various lesions invading the trigeminal nerve root and the semilunar ganglion. It is often accompanied by signs of trigeminal nerve damage, such as sensory impairment in the affected trigeminal nerve distribution area, diminished or absent corneal reflex, weakness, and atrophy of the occlusal muscles. Sometimes there may be signs and symptoms of nerve structure damage, such as facial palsy, hearing loss, vertigo, nystagmus, ataxia, etc. Intracranial lesions can be detected by cranial MRI or CT examination. Oral carbamazepine for trigeminal neuralgia is effective in treating most patients.

Glossopharyngeal neuralgia: transient and sudden severe pain mainly in the glossopharynx and deep ears, the "trigger point" of pain is often at the root of the tongue or tonsils, throat, ear screen and earwax, and the pain is triggered by swallowing, opening the mouth, cold drinks and coughing. The pain can be relieved by local anesthetic throat wall spray during painful episodes. Oral carbamazepine treatment is effective in some patients.

Tongue pain of other causes: endocrine metabolic disorders, liver diseases, oral Candida albicans infection, lichen planus, alcoholism, immune diseases, etc.

8.8.2.5 Treatment Principle

At present, there is no special method for the treatment of BMS. The treatment principles include: removing suspected causes, avoiding adverse stimuli, stopping bad habits, stopping suspected drugs (such as certain anti-hypertensive drugs, angiotensin II receptor blockers, diuretics), eliminating depression, anxiety and fear.

1. Psychological and psychotropic treatment.

   To eliminate depression, anxiety, fear and other adverse psychology: for those with obvious depression, anxiety and fear, Valium, alprazolam, fluoxetine hydrochloride, duloxetine and other treatments are available. Combining cognitive therapy with pharmacotherapy can improve the efficacy.
2. Estrogen replacement therapy.

   For menopausal women, hormone replacement therapy is mainly used to continuously supplement estrogen.
3. Lingual nerve block treatment.

   Using vitamin B_1, vitamin B_{12} and local anesthetics for bilateral nerve block at the base of the tongue.
4. Physical therapy.
5. Other therapies.

Actively treat the relevant systemic diseases (such as anemia, diabetes, etc.), rinse the mouth with alkaline solution for Candida albicans infection, and use sensitive antibiotics for certain bacterial infections; maintain denture hygiene, correct bad habits such as cheek biting, tongue spitting and tongue licking.

References

1. Chanpong B, Haas DA, Locker D. Need and demand for sedation or general anesthesia in dentistry: a national survey of the Canadian population. Anesth Prog. 2005;52(1):3–11. https://doi.org/10.2344/0003-3006(2005)52[3:nadfso]2.0.co;2.
2. Hermes D, Matthes M, Saka B. Treatment anxiety in oral and maxillofacial surgery. Results of a German multi-centre trial. J Craniomaxillofac Surg. 2007;35(6–7):316–21. https://doi.org/10.1016/j.jcms.2007.03.004. Epub 2007 Sep 21
3. Zagli G, Viola L. Critical care sedation: the concept. In: De Gaudio A, Romagnoli S, editors. Critical care sedation. Cham: Springer; 2018. https://doi.org/10.1007/978-3-319-59312-8_1.

4. Lilly PM, Flohr RT. Intraoperative management. In: Rutherford's vascular surgery and endovascular therapy. 9th ed. Philadelphia, PA: Elsevier; 2019.
5. Courtney M, Townsend JR. Anesthesiology principles, pain management, and conscious sedation. In: Sabiston textbook of surgery; 2022.
6. Reves JG. An essay on 35 years of the society of cardiovascular anesthesiologists. Anesth Analg. 2014;119(2)255–65. https://doi.org/10.1213/ANE.0000000000000273.
7. Dayton PG, Sanders JE. Dose-dependent pharmacokinetics: emphasis on phase I metabolism. Drug Metab Rev. 1983;14(3):347–405. https://doi.org/10.3109/03602538308991394.
8. Dawson R, von Fintel N, Nairn S. Sedation assessment using the Ramsay scale. Emerg Nurse. 2010;18(3):18–20. https://doi.org/10.7748/en2010.06.18.3.18.c7825.
9. Chernik DA, Gillings D, Laine H, Hendler J, Silver JM, Davidson AB, Schwam EM, Siegel JL. Validity and reliability of the observer's assessment of alertness/sedation scale: study with intravenous midazolam. J Clin Psychopharmacol. 1990;10(4):244–51.
10. Ely EW, Truman B, Shintani A, Thomason JW, Wheeler AP, Gordon S, Francis J, Speroff T, Gautam S, Margolin R, Sessler CN, Dittus RS, Bernard GR. Monitoring sedation status over time in ICU patients: reliability and validity of the Richmond agitation-sedation scale (RASS). JAMA. 2003;289(22):2983–91. https://doi.org/10.1001/jama.289.22.2983.
11. Medlej K. Calculated decisions: Richmond agitation-sedation scale (RASS). Emerg Med Pract. 2021;23(Suppl 3):CD3–4.
12. McCormack H, Horne DL, D., & Sheather, S. Clinical applications of visual analogue scales: a critical review. Psychol Med. 1988;18(4):1007–19. https://doi.org/10.1017/S0033291700009934.
13. Chisholm CJ, Zurica J, Mironov D, Sciacca RR, Ornstein E, Heyer EJ. Comparison of Electrophysiologic monitors with clinical assessment of level of sedation. Mayo Clin Proc. 2006;81(1):46–52. https://doi.org/10.4065/81.1.46.
14. Roche D, Mahon P. Depth of anesthesia monitoring. Anesthesiol Clin. 2021;39(3):477–92. https://doi.org/10.1016/j.anclin.2021.04.004; Epub 2021 Jul 12
15. Orr PM, Shank BC, Black AC. The role of pain classification systems in pain management. Crit Care Nurs Clin North Am. 2017;29(4):407–18. https://doi.org/10.1016/j.cnc.2017.08.002; Epub 2017 Sep 21.
16. Bacchi S, Palumbo P, Sponta A, Coppolino MF. Clinical pharmacology of non-steroidal anti-inflammatory drugs: a review. Antiinflamm Antiallergy Agents Med Chem. 2012;11(1):52–64. https://doi.org/10.2174/187152312803476255.
17. Apfelbaum JL, Chen C, Mehta SS, Gan TJ. Postoperative pain experience: results from a national survey suggest postoperative pain continues to be undermanaged. Anesth Analg. 2003;97(2):534–40. https://doi.org/10.1213/01.ANE.0000068822.10113.9E.
18. Wylde V, Dennis J, Beswick AD, Bruce J, Eccleston C, Howells N, Peters TJ, Gooberman-Hill R. Systematic review of management of chronic pain after surgery. Br J Surg. 2017;104(10):1293–306. https://doi.org/10.1002/bjs.10601; Epub 2017 Jul 6.
19. Merskey H, Bogduk N. Classification of chronic pain. 2nd ed. Seattle: IASP Task Force on Taxonomy. IASP Press; 1994. http://www.iasp-pain.org/Education/content.aspx?ItemNumber=1698

9 Complications Associated with Anesthesia: In Oral and Maxillofacial Surgery

Ming Xia

9.1 Introduction

Timely identification and management of problems at the immediate end of surgery may save lives. The likelihood of a patient developing complications depends on the nature of the procedure, anesthesia technique, coexisting diseases, and preoperative medical evaluation and optimization measures.

Most patients undergoing general, regional or monitored anesthesia are generally monitored in the PACU prior to discharge or transfer to a ward. The exceptions are critically ill patients and patients with tracheal intubation, who may have to go directly into the ICU to recover. Most medical monitoring in the PACU is the responsibility of the anesthesiology department.

Postoperative complications can be divided into several categories. According to different anesthetic techniques and methods, the complications can be divided into local anesthesia complications and general anesthesia complications. It should be noted that postoperative complications may either connect with anesthesia or surgery or related to both. This chapter will mainly illustrate complications associated with anesthesia in oral and maxillofacial surgery.

M. Xia (✉)
Department of Anesthesiology, Shanghai Ninth People's Hospital Affiliated to Shanghai Jiao Tong University School of Medicine, Shanghai, China
e-mail: xiaming1980@xzhmu.edu.cn

9.2 Complications Associated with Local Anesthesia in Oral and Maxillofacial Surgery

To mitigate or eliminate pain associated with invasive procedures, local anesthetic drugs have been used in clinical dentistry since the nineteenth century. In oral and maxillofacial operations, local anesthetics are used routinely since its reliability and efficiency are well-recognized. Yet, they are not riskless. Complications associated with this type of drugs can be evaluated systemically and locally. It is reported that systemic reactions after using local anesthetics are psychogenic reactions, systemic toxicity, allergy, and methemoglobinemia. Local complications commonly reported are pain at injection, needle fracture, prolongation of anesthesia and various sensory disorders, lack of effect, trismus, infection, edema, hematoma, gingival lesions, soft tissue injury, and ophthalmologic complications. In this part, the two kinds of complications will be illustrated in detail.

9.2.1 Classification and Chemical Structure of Local Anesthetics

Local anesthetic agents can be classified according to their chemical structure, rate of onset, potency, and duration. According to their chemical structure, there are two types of local anes-

H. Jiang, M. Xia (eds.), *Anesthesia for Oral and Maxillofacial Surgery*,
https://doi.org/10.1007/978-981-19-7287-4_9

thetics, namely, amino esters and amino amides. The ester group includes cocaine, procaine, chloroprocaine, tetracaine, and benzocaine. They are hydrolyzed in the plasma by pseudocholinesterase into para-aminobenzoic acid (PABA) and other derivatives, whereas amide-type local anesthetics are metabolized by the liver. The toxicity of an anesthetic is related to the rate of hydrolysis. Allergic reactions that may be induced by esters are related to para-aminobenzoic acid, which is a major metabolic product of many ester local anesthetic agents. The amide group include lidocaine, mepivacaine, prilocaine, bupivacaine, etidocaine, dibucaine, and ropivacaine. Among them, lidocaine, mepivacaine, etidocaine, and bupivacaine have similar rate of biotransformation. Exceptionally, articaine contains both amide and ester, so it is metabolized in both the liver and blood.

Normally ester local anesthetics are not as popular as amide when used as local anesthetics in dental procedures considering ester local anesthetics' poor efficacy, potential for allergenicity, and the advantages of amide local anesthetics [1–4].

9.2.2 Systemic Reactions Due to Local Anesthesia

9.2.2.1 Psychogenic Reactions

The psychogenic reactions are connected to the body counterbalance of the patient to an anxiety-inducing situation or adrenaline secreted by the vasoconstrictor agent. Heart rate, respiratory rate, and blood pressure are changed along with patient's mood. Sometimes, blush and erythema are confused with allergic reactions, hyperventilation, nausea, and vomiting [5]. Considering that patients' relax and calm mood during the injection of anesthetics may prevent psychogenic reaction, it is necessary to communicate with patients to dispel their misgivings. Other solutions can also be sought, such as using oral sedatives. Oral sedatives can be effective in alleviating the patient's fears during dental treatment. The initial dose of sedatives should be determined by the patient's health status, age, weight, and the duration of the procedure. For healthy adult patients undergoing a short-term surgery, 50 mg antihistamine benzhydramine can be given 1 h before the procedure. For patients in the same condition but with a moderately long procedure (1–2 h), 0.125–0.5 mg benzodiazepines, triazolam should be given 1 h before the procedure. For patients with a longer procedure (2–4 h), benzodiazepines such as 1–4 mg lorazepam can be given 1–2 h before surgery or 30–60 min before sublingual preparation. Depending on the patient's anxiety level, sedatives may be used for dental patients with mild and moderate anxiety, while general anesthesia may be an option for patients with extreme anxiety or fear to ensure a smooth procedure [6, 7].

9.2.2.2 Systemic Toxicity

Local anesthetics have the adverse effect of inducing toxicity in patient's body when the toxic concentration of anesthetics in the blood level reaches to the central nervous system and cardiovascular systems.

Symptoms featured by central nervous system signs include excitation, convulsions, following which are loss of consciousness and respiratory arrest. Meanwhile, cardiovascular signs such as hypertension, tachycardia, and premature ventricular contractions may present. In addition, the common clinical signs and symptoms are quick talking, flicker, and tremor in the extremities [8, 9].

Predisposing factors are associated with age, weight, using of other drugs, gender, the preexisting disease, genetics, vasoactivity, concentration, dose, route of administration, the rate of injection, vascularity of the injection site, and the presence of vasoconstrictors [4].

The patient should be evaluated before injection of local anesthetics, to prevent systemic toxicity. And the above mentioned predisposing factors should be treated very carefully. Preventing from a toxic dose complication, it should be evoked that for healthy adults, the suggested maximum safe dose of 2% lignocaine in 1:80,000 adrenalines is four-and-a-half cartridges of 2 or 2.2 mL (180–198 mg lignocaine); for 3% prilocaine and felypressin 0.03 IU/mL, the maximum safe dose is 400 mg (six 2 mL cartridges) [10].

The practice of local anesthesia in the outpatient setting normally includes airway support, administration of 100% oxygen, supine position, prevention of seizures leading to injury, and treatment of convulsions (administration of benzodiazepines or sodium thiopental; propofol is contraindicated in patients with unstable blood pressure and heart rate) [11]. If patients with cardiac arrhythmias develop severe hypotension, they should be infused with 1.5 mL/kg 20% lipid emulsion for approximately 1 min and then switch to a continuous infusion at 0.25 mL/kg/min = 1000 mL/h. Studies have reported a resuscitation effect when the total dose of lipid emulsion infused was ≤10 mL/kg; therefore, 12 mL/kg can be the approximate estimate for the maximum dose. The dose of adrenaline applied should be referred to resuscitation guidelines, such as the American Heart Association guidelines [9].

9.2.2.3 Allergy

Allergy, also known as hypersensitive reactions, is initiated by immunological mechanisms acquired through exposure to a specific allergen. However, complications caused by allergy only take up less than 1% of the total complications. Many of the complications doubt to be allergic are, in fact, caused by anxiety [12]. Moreover, as introduced in the previous paragraphs that local anesthetics are classified as ester- and amide-type local anesthetics, ester local anesthetics are more allergenic than amide local anesthetics. Therefore, amide local anesthetics are used more widely, especially lidocaine.

Allergic reactions may display mild symptoms, such as urticaria, erythema, and intense itching, and severe reactions in the form of angioedema and/or respiratory distress. It may involve more severe life-threatening anaphylactic responses, including symptoms of apnea, hypotension, and loss of consciousness [12].

The skin prick test is the most endorsed method to diagnose allergies. When the test results are determined to be negative, intradermal testing should be performed for patients who have a history of allergy to local anesthetics [12, 13].

For patients who show allergic reactions, treatments should be adopted. The first step is removing the causative agent. Then, if the patient's allergic symptom is mild, oral or intramuscular antihistamine diphenhydramine should be given. Besides, hydrocortisone cream may be prescribed to relieve skin itching or erythema. If it is a life-threatening case, the patient should be provided with basic life support, intramuscular or subcutaneous epinephrine and hospitalization if necessary. Anaphylaxis is a life-threatening allergic reaction, the clinical symptoms of which are related to the patient's organ function. Risk factors for anaphylaxis contain uncontrolled coexisting asthma, mast cell disorders, and patients with specific allergens. For anaphylaxis, adrenaline is the first and most important treatment, and it should be administered as soon as anaphylaxis is recognized. Moreover, it should be administered by intravenous (IV) route only in the case of profoundly hypotensive patients or patients who develop a cardiopulmonary arrest or those who fail to respond to multiple doses of IM adrenaline because of the potential cardiovascular adverse effects of IV administration of adrenaline [14, 15]. In addition, antihistamines and glucocorticoids are claimed to be effective in treatment of anaphylaxis, though their use is controversial. Overall, the first step treatment should be adrenaline and antihistamines and glucocorticoids may be used to treat severe systemic reactions.

9.2.2.4 Methemoglobinemia

Methemoglobinemia is a condition of elevated methemoglobin in the blood. It may be inherited or acquired [16]. The risk of methemoglobinemia increased in infants, the elderly and patients with underlying health problems such as liver cirrhosis, underdeveloped hepatic and renal function, heart disease, and pulmonary disease. Moreover, it is a unique dose-dependent reaction.

Symptoms may include headache, dizziness, fatigue, shortness of breath and tachycardia, nausea, poor muscle coordination, and cyanosis that can be observed in nail beds and mucous membrane.

Prompt recognition of the condition and initiation of treatment, as indicated (especially in acquired methemoglobinemia), are critical in the management of methemoglobinemia. Once the diagnosis is confirmed, management should be instituted as indicated. Initial care includes administration of supplemental oxygen (100%) and removal of the offending oxidizing substance. Methylene blue may be given to a symptomatic patient. It should be administrated in 1–2 mg/kg doses, given as 0.1 mL/kg of a 1% solution (10 mg/mL) intravenously over 5–10 min every hour up to a 7 mg/kg maximum. For severe cases, hyperbaric oxygenation may also be used if available. After the initial dose, repeated doses should be given within 30–60 min [17, 18].

9.2.3 Local Complications Associated with Local Anesthesia

9.2.3.1 Pain on Injection

Some patients may experience pain during injection. Possible causes of pain on injection are related to the temperature of the solution, the speed of injection, blunt needles, needles with barbs, or inserting too aggressively, which damage soft tissues, blood vessels, nerves or periosteum. For example, local injections of lidocaine produce a strong burning sensation. When the needle pierces a nerve, patients may react as if getting an electric shock, they may suddenly move the head, increasing the risk of self-inflicted wound. In addition, the speed of the injection and the acidity of the solution are possible factors in inducing the burning sensation.

To avoid causing discomfort to the patient, it is best to warm the anesthetics to body temperature and use a smaller gauge needle (27 gauge) when administering local anesthetics. When multiple injections must be given in the same lesion or when multiple sites need to be injected, each injection should be given with a new needle and at a slow rate and low pressure, which will mitigate pain. The recommended rate of injection of the solution is 30 s/mL. Inadequate injection sites can result in blunting of the intramuscular or intradural injection needle [19–21].

9.2.3.2 Prolongation of Anesthesia and Various Sensory Disorders

After dental local anesthetic blocks, prolonged anesthesia, paresthesia, or neuralgia may occur, but this may last for few days, weeks or months and after that sensation will return or it may last forever [22]. This mostly involves nervus lingualis or nervus mandibularis or both [23]. The nerve may be damaged during injection by direct injury, or the needle may damage the intraneural blood supply, resulting in a hematoma, or the needle may traumatize the medial pterygoid muscle which results in trismus. In addition, neurotoxicity is another nerve damage caused by local anesthetics [24]. In this aspect, procaine and tetracaine cause more damage than bupivacaine or lidocaine [25]. Generally, paresthesia or neuralgia complication is temporary, but in the case of injecting anesthetic solution directly into the nerve, it may also be permanent. Consequently, patients may also have symptoms such as tongue biting, drooling, loss of taste, and speech impediment. Piccinni et al. published an analysis of reports to the FDA Adverse Event Reporting System, in which about 573 cases of paresthesia and dysesthesia after using local anesthetics between 2004 and 2011 were recorded. Accordingly, they noted that when using prilocaine, articaine, or both of them, there is higher risk of paresthesia [26].

When during dental local anesthesia a nerve gets injured, the first thing to do is managing the pain. Importantly, the nerve injury should be prevented which can be achieved through reducing concentration of anesthetic agent for inferior alveolar nerve blocks, and avoiding iterative injections. It is suggested to use a low daily dose of multivitamin B to regain nerve healing and function [27, 28].

9.2.3.3 No Effect

Sometimes, the effect of local anesthesia may not be achieved after injection of local anesthetics. The underlying causes may relate to anatomical variants, pathological and psychological factors, anesthesia techniques and methods, and among others [20]. Anatomical factors consist of accessory nerve supply, alteration in foramen location, atypical development of the nerves and bone density [29, 30]. Pathological reasons for the failure of anesthesia are trismus, infection, inflammation, and previous surgery or trauma. Among all these reasons, inflammatory diseases that influence the pharmacokinetics and pharmacodynamics of local anesthetics weaken the response and strengthen unfavorable effects [31]. Conditions with inflammations such as pulpitis and apical periodontitis acute periodontal abscess or pericoronitis may lead to anesthetic failure or difficulty [32]. Psychological factors, for example, angst and anxiety, may also cause local anesthesia failure [29]. In addition, anesthetists' poor technique may bring the effect of mandibular anesthesia instead of the anesthesia within oral and maxillofacial operation area. The effect of local anesthesia depends on the position where the needle is inserted. If the needle is inserted and advanced too deep or deviated, the terminal branches of the facial nerve within the deep lobe of the parotid gland may be impacted. Direct anesthesia to the facial nerve can force a rapid onset that occurs while the anesthetic agent is being injected; reflex vasospasms of the external carotid artery can lead to ischemia of the facial nerve, inducing facial nerve palsy. Thus, the patient is unable to perform a series of facial gestures, such as wrinkle the forehead, raise the eyebrow, close the upper eyelid, retract the commissure of the lips to smile, and turn down the lower lip on the affected side [33, 34].

In most cases, paralysis occurs immediately after mandibular anesthesia injection, but there are also some cases in which paralysis starts later than expected. In a case report for late paralyses, a patient's tooth was extracted easily, without any complication incurred; whereas, in a day he returned complaining a weakness of the muscles of his left side face. When examining the patient, clinicians detected Bell's palsy sign on the patient's left side face that is expressionless, but there was no pathologic change in the wound or any herpetic lesions. They consulted with the Department of Ophthalmology and the Department of Physical Therapy and Rehabilitation and adopted the treatment of lubricant eye drop (4 × 1), tobramycin ophthalmic solution (4 × 1), and lanolin eye ointment (during night) supported by eye patch. In the next 4 weeks, galvanic stimulation of the facial nerve of the affected side was conducted. After another 2 weeks all of the symptoms disappeared [35]. Moreover, the auriculotemporal nerve may also be damaged and bring "numbness" sensation to the ear.

9.2.3.4 Trismus

Trismus refers to the restriction or even the inability of mouth opening, and it is also called lockjaw. It is caused by multiple injections at the same position in a short period of time, intramuscular injections, trauma to the lateral pterygoid muscle or the temporal muscle thereby causing the formation of hematoma and fibrosis, needle fracture during insertion into the muscles of the odontoid process, inaccurate needle positioning during inferior nerve blocks or posterior maxillary injections or inflammation of the masseter muscle and other masticatory muscles, and infection [36]. The hemorrhage induces great pain which results in muscle contraction and restricted movement.

Fortunately, most trismus cases are temporary and can be cured or alleviated by medications such as analgesics, anti-inflammatory drugs, antibiotics and muscle relaxants, physical therapy, soft diet, and other treatments. Paying attention to anatomical landmarks and muscles such as palpation of the bony anterior process of the temporal muscle and the pterygomandibular fold of the pterygopalatine muscle, and anticipating the appropriate angle of needle-bone contact prior to injection are useful in preventing trismus through local anesthesia. The intraoral Vazirani-Akinosi nerve block technique, the closed mandibular nerve block technique or extraoral techniques can be used to provide anesthesia for patients with trismus.

9.2.3.5 Infection

Infection complications are rare due to the use of disposable needles and glass syringes. Infection may extend to the tissues due to needle penetration of contaminated tissues. On the other hand, a latent viral infection may be reactivated due to the trauma of the procedure, which may be the cause of neural sheath inflammation.

The area to be penetrated should be cleaned with a topical antiseptic prior to needle insertion. The use of antiseptic mouthwash solutions, such as chlorhexidine gluconate, should be considered for all regional techniques. Local anesthetics should not be injected through the infected area.

In the presence of infection, injection of local anesthesia is important to raise the pH of the anesthetics, as infected tissue is more likely to be acidic. This process is known as anesthetic buffering and affects patient's comfort during the injection, rapid onset of anesthesia, and reduction of tissue damage. Recommendations for treatment of infection are antibiotics (penicillin V 500 mg every 6 h for 7–10 days), analgesics, heat therapy, drainage, and physical therapy [22, 37, 38].

9.2.3.6 Edema

Tissue swelling may be caused by trauma during injection, infection, allergy, bleeding, and injection of irritating solutions. The management of edema depends on its cause. Treatment of allergy-induced edema includes intramuscular epinephrine as described above, in addition to antihistamines and corticosteroids, and consultation with an allergist to determine the exact cause of the edema. Edema caused by trauma should be treated as a hematoma. To treat edema caused by infection, antibiotics should be administered [39].

9.2.3.7 Hematoma

As a complication of local anesthesia, a hematoma forms as a result of a venous or arterial laceration; elevated intra-arterial blood pressure causes blood to leak into the surrounding soft tissues. At the time of injection, the presence of high pressure may warn of an injection against bloodstream. The size of the hematoma depends on the density and solidity of the affected tissue. Hematomas do not necessarily occur when a ruptured vein is involved. Discoloration of the affected area and bruising may accompany the hematoma [40].

From an anatomical point of view, different nerve actions can lead to hematomas in specific areas, such as anterior superior alveolar (infraorbital) nerve block below the lower eyelid, incisive (mental) nerve block in the chin area, buccal nerve block or any palatal injection in the oral cavity, and extraoral posterior superior alveolar nerve block in the inferior buccal region of the mandible, and intraoral block distal to the maxillary tuberosity.

Hematoma formation can be prevented by aspiration prior to the injection of anesthetic solution, using a short needle and minimal needle insertion into the tissue. When swelling forms immediately after the injection, local pressure should be applied for at least 2 min. This will stop the complication.

Swelling and discoloration usually subsides within 10–15 days. Ice packs should be adhered to for the first 24 h after surgery, after which they can be addressed with intermittent hot wet compresses and massage therapy with heparin cream. If the hematoma is large, antibiotics should be used to prevent the development of wound infection [11, 41].

9.2.3.8 Gingival Lesions

Gingival lesions comprise of recurrent aphthous stomatitis, and herpes simplex can occur intraorally after the injection of a local anesthetic or any trauma to the intraoral tissues. Any trauma to tissues by a needle may activate the latent from of the disease process that was present in the tissues with previous injection, though the precise mechanism under it remains unknown.

Before any severe pain is felt, it is unnecessary to manage the lesions. Administering topical anesthetic solutions on affected areas may be useful to relieve the pain. A concoction of identical amounts of diphenhydramine and milk of magnesia rinsed in the mouth effectively covers the ulcerations and provides relief from pain. Triamcinolone acetonide without corticosteroid can remedy pain [11, 39].

9.2.3.9 Soft Tissue Injury

In children with special needs or disabled patients, the numbness following local anesthesia in the mouth can cause them to bite their lips or tongue [42]. This problem can be addressed by choosing a shorter-acting local anesthetic, such as plain mepivacaine, and telling the patient or their custodian to test the residual effects of anesthesia by eating, drinking hot liquids, and gently biting the lips or tongue. To prevent chewing, cotton rolls can be placed between the teeth and soft tissues. To speed up the recovery of sensation, phentolamine mesylate, an alpha-adrenergic receptor, can be injected. The dose of the injection varies from person to person; the recommended dose for adult patients is 1–2 cartridges (0.4–0.8 mg), while for pediatric patients the recommended dose is 0.5–1 cartridge (0.2–0.4 mg) [42–44].

The swelling will gradually resolve after 2–3 days. Healing of the lesion takes 10–14 days. For patients whose pain remains significant, analgesics may be prescribed or a local anesthetic may be applied topically to the area.

9.2.3.10 Ophthalmologic Complications

The most common ophthalmologic complications related to local anesthesia are diplopia (dual vision), ophthalmoplegia (paralysis or weakening of eye muscles), ptosis, and mydriasis (dilatation of pupil). Amaurosis (partial/total blindness) may also present though very rarely. Fortunately, all these complications are transient and patients will recover once the anesthetic effects are interrupted [45].

The sympathetic fibers running along the internal maxillary artery to the orbit may be stimulated by intra-arterial injection or perforation of the vessel wall; thus, an intravenous injection of anesthetic may be preferred. The intravenous injection may reach the cavernous sinus through the pterygoid plexus and anesthetize the oculomotor, cochlear or dorsal nerves.

During inferior dental nerve block, the anesthesia may trigger Horner's syndrome since local anesthetic penetration through the lateral pharyngeal and anterior vertebral spaces, causing obstruction of the stellate ganglion [46, 47].

A systematic review of ophthalmic complications arising after local anesthesia in dentistry was conducted by Alamanos et al. in 2016, which included 66 reports and 89 cases. It was found that mandibular block anesthesia using the Gow-Gates technique was only associated with diplopia; inferior alveolar nerve blocks were more likely to cause visual impairment compared to posterior superior alveolar nerve blocks, and few studies reported blindness with the posterior superior alveolar nerve block technique. The majority of patients mentioned in the literature who developed ocular complications were injected with lidocaine [48].

To minimize the occurrence of possible complications, the regional anatomy should be observed in detail prior to the injection of local anesthetic, and multiple suctions should be performed at the time of injection and in at least two planes.

9.2.4 Conclusion

Local anesthetics may lead to the occurrence of adverse events or complications. To prevent them, a detailed assessment of the patient's medical history and attention to the patient's mood should be routinely performed. The dose of local anesthetics administered should refer to the patient's weight, while taking care not to exceed the maximum recommended dose. When administering anesthesia, painless injections should be performed to avoid causing direct intravascular or intramuscular or nerve trauma. The anesthesiologist should closely monitor new developments in the patient's body to minimize the incidence of complications that may be associated with local anesthesia.

9.3 Common Complications After General Anesthesia in Oral and Maxillofacial Surgery

The incidence of postoperative complications is affected by a variety of factors, including surgical ones, such as the type of surgery, and may additionally be closely related to the patient's physical condition, such as physical health, but less so to the type of anesthesia. Patients with unhealthy habits or chronic diseases such as smoking, hypertension, obesity, diabetes, stroke, seizures, obstructive sleep apnea, any condition involving kidney, lung and heart disease, drug allergies, history of anticoagulants and allergies to GA, and malnutrition may all exacerbate the risk of complications after anesthesia [49].

Postoperative complications after general anesthesia varies from mild distress to long-term squeal to death or permanent disability. Fortunately, such major catastrophic sequelae are scarce. Whereas, minor morbidity such as nausea, vomiting, sore throat, myalgia's pain, headache, damage to teeth and intraoral soft tissues, and morbidity associated with throat packs and nasal intubation affect the body function and have significant impact on recovery [49]. Some of these are common complications following general anesthesia. This section will discuss restrictedly the oral and maxillofacial related injuries, including damage to teeth and intraoral soft tissues, and morbidity associated with throat packs and nasal intubation.

9.3.1 Etiology of Dental Injury During Anesthesia

Although the majority of dental injuries during anesthesia are reported after laryngoscopy, endotracheal or nasotracheal intubation, about 25% occur during emergence and the injury is commonly associated with extubation or the use of oropharyngeal airways, laryngeal masks, bite blocks, or suction catheters [50–52]. Emergence dental injuries may commonly be associated with lower teeth and may be easily ignored by the anesthetist [53]. Diagnostic laryngoscopy or the instrumental assisted passage of a nasogastric tube in an anesthetized patient may lead to sustained abnormally applied force, resulting in dental or soft tissue trauma.

The upper left central incisors are the most vulnerable teeth to damage during anesthesia [51, 52]. The preponderance of left-sided injuries is considered to reflect the fact that most anesthetists are right-handed. Particularly, although not exclusively, dental damage is usually limited to a single tooth [50]. Teeth have different dental axes depending on their function. Incisors are monotooted teeth with a forward dental axis and small cross-sectional area designed to withstand considerable biting forces along their axis. Upper premolar and molar teeth have two or three roots, respectively, and are designed to withstand substantial aligned forces along a vertical dental axis. Lower premolar and molar teeth have one or two roots, respectively. Any alteration in the vector of the force applied, such as strong vertical forces applied to incisors, causes them more vulnerable to damage.

An appreciation of normal developmental dental anatomy is necessary for an understanding of the mechanism of dental injury during anesthesia. Human's 20 deciduous teeth, also known as "milk" or "baby" teeth, would be replaced by 32 permanent teeth by the second decade of life. In patient with normal dentition, when the teeth are brought together, the lower mandibular teeth will lie symmetrically and slightly lingually to the upper maxillary teeth. A slight incisor overbite is normal, with about one-third of the upper incisors covering the lower incisors. The upper and lower teeth are designed to meet during mastication. Molars, which have up to three roots, are in the position of maximal mechanical advantages adjacent to the power muscles of mastication. Teeth tolerate substantial applied axial forces in the intended physiological vector better than lesser abnormally applied lateral forces [50].

In general anesthesia, dental injuries are caused by direct contact of the upper anterior teeth with the rigid blade of the laryngoscope. Apart from predisposing patient factors, dental injury is associated with the characteristics of the laryngoscope blade in use and the skill of the anesthetist [54]. The proximity of the upper anterior incisors to the laryngoscope blade in optimal view of the vocal cords has been studied. The forces exerted on the upper teeth vary with the design of the laryngoscope. As a result, modifications to laryngoscope blades with the intention of minimizing contact with the upper teeth have been proposed [55]. Alternative protective strategies have included the application of compressible adhesive tape and foam cushions to the upper surface of the laryngoscope blade [56]. The use of plastic-bladed scopes may confer some protective advantage [57]. Electronic warning devices for the prevention of dental injury during laryngoscopy have been developed but have not been widely accepted [58].

The inadvertent use of the upper incisors as a fulcrum during difficult intubation is a well-recognized pre-sequel to dental injury, although when intubation is difficult this is regarded as inevitable by some. Forces of 30–65 N (Newtons) or greater exerted on the maxillary incisors during laryngoscopy have been recorded but the sensitivity of the measuring devices was questioned following subsequent reports of mean axial forces of 20 N [50]. Regardless, the applied forces are substantial. Putting this into perspective, a gallon of water exerts a force of 37 N. The patient's body mass index, height, weight, and Mallampati score appear to correlate with the overall force applied when using a Macintosh blade, but less so with the McCoy modified blade [50]. Patients of increasing age required less applied force for intubation.

9.3.2 Oropharyngeal Airways

Oropharyngeal airways have been implicated in 20% of anesthetic related dental injuries. Masseter spam and teeth clenching are commonly seen following anesthesia with volatile agents [59]. During emergence, the masseter muscles can exert considerable forces (of up to 80 N) which are normally absorbed by the multi-rooted molar and premolar teeth. In the presence of a midline placed oropharyngeal airway, the molar teeth are unable to meet, resulting in the transfer of the vertical jaw clenching forces forward through the anterior mono-rooted incisors [60]. The common practice of using an oropharyngeal airway as a bite guard to protect an endotracheal tube or laryngeal mask airway may therefore put incisor teeth at an increased risk of fracture or impaction [60]. A similar mechanism of injury could also result from biting hard on a midline placed suction catheter. Placing a bite block between the premolar or molar teeth, rather than adjacent to the incisor teeth, would in theory be less likely to result in dental damage.

9.3.3 Predisposing Factors and Anesthetic Related Dental Injury

9.3.3.1 Localized Infection and Inflammation

Healthy teeth are robust and capable of withstanding considerable force and pressure. Although factors predisposing to dental injury during anesthesia are multifactorial, a prime contributory factor is pre-existing dental or intraoral disease, which increases the risk of injury five-fold [50]. Dental caries resulting in enamel loss, dentine softening, cavity formation, and previous injury can all weaken teeth, making them susceptible to fracture or dislodgement even with minimal applied force.

Apart from dental caries, periodontal and gingival disease are the most prevalent worldwide diseases in adults. Bacterial plaque which has accumulated in the crevices between the teeth and gums can give rise to inflammation of the gums and loss of the supporting underlying alveolar bone. Patients with abnormal dentition are especially prone to plaque accumulation. If left unattended plaque can thicken, become mineralized, and provide a localized anaerobic environment in which bacteria can proliferate. Periodontitis, which is invariably painless, is caused by an aggressive immune and inflammatory response to the bacteria resident on the tooth's surface. Released collagenases destroy the adjacent bony support, predisposing to dental avulsion. Avascular root-filled teeth become brittle and devitalized, leading to root fracture or dislodgement, even with minimal force. Associated risk factors include poorly controlled diabetes, osteoporosis, arteriosclerosis, smoking, and an individual genetic predisposition. Patients whose anterior segments have significant decay, advanced periodontitis, or are shedding deciduous teeth are the most prone to anesthetic related damage [50].

9.3.3.2 Systemic Diseases with Intraoral Manifestations

Many systemic diseases have intraoral manifestations that exacerbate periodontal disease; thus weakening the teeth and gums, and making them susceptible to damage during anesthesia [61–63]. The mechanisms by which systemic disease can influence the pathogenesis of periodontal disease are unclear but may involve a modification of the host's normal immune response. Adequate saliva production is a prerequisite for optimal dental health. Conditions in which saliva production is diminished or absent are often associated with dental disease and a vulnerability to injury during anesthesia.

9.3.4 Medication and Dental Disease

Chronic medication can result in dental discoloration, structural damage or intraoral manifestations that predispose to dental injury during anesthesia. The drugs most implicated are those formulated in sugar-containing vehicles and drugs which lower the intraoral pH such as aspirin and powdered antiasthmatic medication. Anticholingergics, antidepressants, and antipsychotics all result in decreased saliva secretion, predisposing to periodontitis. Over one-third of patients on the immunosuppressant cyclosporine, nifedipine, and anticonvulsants such as phenytoin will experience gingival overgrowth which may undergo subsequent local inflammatory changes. Localized irradiation can also result in a loss of bony support.

Patients who chronically misuse illegal drugs have a high incidence of periodontal disease. Cocaine and methamphetamine mixed with saliva creates a highly acidic environment, resulting in erosion of enamel and dental caries, often in a very short period of time. Heroin causes a craving for sweet and sugary foods, and ecstasy induces xerostomia, a prerequisite to periodontal disease. Patients on supervised withdrawal programs are often prescribed methadone. In order to make methadone palatable, it is formulated in concentrated sugary syrup which partly explains why such patients often have very poor dental health and frequently require a dental clearance. For a comprehensive discussion of this topic, the reader should consult Tredwin et al. [63].

9.3.4.1 Age

Between the age of 6 and 12 years, a child's deciduous teeth are progressively replaced by permanent adult teeth and children of this age will have mixed dentition present. Deciduous teeth have shorter roots than adult teeth. As the erupting permanent tooth develops, the root of the overlying deciduous tooth undergoes resorption, leading to a loss of structural bony support. Adult teeth take up to 3 years before they are fully embedded and reach optimal strength [50]. As a result, children between the ages of 5 and 10 are at the greatest risk of inadvertent dental damage during anesthesia. Ignoring damage to deciduous teeth because deciduous teeth will be replaced is a wrong conception. Damage to a deciduous tooth may easily destroy the developing underlying permanent tooth. Losing teeth may lead to premature eruption of the permanent teeth, inducing crowding and dental misalignment that need orthodontic treatment in the future. Anesthetists should treat deciduous teeth with the same respect they show permanent teeth [50].

Although the elderly is at greater risk of dental injury [53], such condition is not frequently reflected in the literature as many patients in the past would have been wholly or partially edentulous. Although the forces applied during laryngoscopy appear to be less with increasing age, the overall incidence of dental injury is high, reflecting the increased incidence of dental and periodontal disease in the elderly. Bony support of teeth declines with age. With greater health education and the availability of dental services, a significant number of elderly patients have retained some or all of their teeth, putting them at greater risk than before.

9.3.4.2 Abnormal Oral and Maxillofacial Anatomy

The anatomical relationship between the upper and lower incisors can have a significant effect on their tolerance to applied forces. Misaligned teeth resulting in malocclusion are more likely to be exposed to abnormal forces [64]. Traditionally there are three classes of dental malocclusion as described by Angle's classification, the details of which can be found in any standard dental textbook, Class II relationships, or retrognathia, are of greatest concern to the anesthetist [65]. Malocclusion, retarded mandibles, prominent anterior teeth, anterior crowding, and high dental arches can all increase the risk of dental damage during anesthesia. Where the upper incisors are severely proclined or irregular, visualization of the vocal cords during laryngoscopy can be very difficult, encouraging the inadvertent use of the incisors as a lever fulcrum. Patients with malocclusion are also more susceptible to dental and periodontal disease on account of the difficulties in providing effective dental hygiene.

Isolated teeth, which lack the support of adjacent teeth and may have the same pathological condition as the missing teeth, are vulnerable to damage or dislodgement during laryngoscopy by the passage of the endotracheal tube and positioning of a laryngeal mask [64, 66].

9.3.4.3 Prosthetic Dental Restorations

The anesthetist may encounter several forms of dental restoration, such as single or multiple crowned teeth, fixed bridges, surface veneers, removable partial or complete dentures, and dental implants. Pathologically weakened teeth, either from disease or previous restoration, are unable to withstand the forces tolerated by healthy teeth. Although modern dental resins and porcelain are very robust, excessive pressure from a laryngoscope blade or via an oropharyngeal airway can result in fragmentation. Gold, as a restorative material, seems to be more robust, with fewer patients reporting dental damage following anesthesia. In one retrospective study, previously filled teeth accounted for 50% of those damaged during anesthesia [67].

While the cosmetic result of dental restorations may be pleasing to the patient, the prosthetic tooth is unable to withstand the forces accommodated by a normal healthy tooth. The commonest site for crowned restorations is the upper incisors, further compounding the risk [60], especially during recovery from an anesthetic. Prosthetic dental restorations, such as crowned teeth, involve cavity preparation which removes some of the tooth's original structure and replacement with resins and metal supporting posts. The remaining tooth structure, while restored, may not be optimally healthy to withstand axial loading forces along the line of the tooth such as those experienced in chewing. Applied lateral or shearing forces are tolerated poorly. The type of restoration can also influence the consequences of the injury. Where a crowned tooth has a long metal supporting post within the tooth cavity, excessive applied force can cause vertical splitting of the tooth. Crowns with short metal retaining posts are more prone to dislodgement if excessive non-axial force is applied, while both restorations are vulnerable to root factures.

In consequence of the minimal preparation involved, the cosmetic application of thin veneers to visible teeth has become welcomed. Veneers are 0.5–1 mm thick laminates of porcelain, ceramic or a composite of both materials, the former overweighing the later due to its enhanced strength. The veneer is bound to either the tooth enamel or underlying dentine and the tooth enamel makes a more stable bond [68]. As veneers are bonded only to healthy teeth, abnormally applied forces, especially of a levering nature, will have the risk of chipping the veneer or shearing the comparatively weaker bond between the tooth and the overlying veneer. Bridges, which involve prosthetic teeth being interconnected with supporting bands of metal, are particularly at risk of displacement if excessive shearing force is applied [68].

9.3.5 Classification of Dental Injury

Dental injuries are classified into six classes according to the level of the damage (Table 9.1). Classes I, II, and VI constitute the majority of iatrogenic anesthetic related injuries which are invariably associated with underlying dental and periodontal disease [50].

9.3.6 Prevention of Anesthetic Related Dental Injury

Prevention of anesthetic related dental injury should begin with an attempt to achieve optimal dental and gingival health. Routine pre-anesthetic dental examination of all patients has been proposed but dismissed as unworkable. Whenever possible, any remedial and restorative dental treatment should be undertaken prior to elective anesthesia and surgery. In reality, this is often unattainable and unrealistic. Patients who present with poor dental health will invariably have a long history of dental neglect and poor intraoral hygiene which is unlikely to be changed during the immediate preoperative period. Lack of availability of dental care lead to a greater incidence

Table 9.1 Classification of dental injury during anesthesia

Class	Site of injury	Features	Dental treatment
Class I	Fracture through dental enamel	Commonest injury. Damage to tooth surface. Painless and may go unnoticed by the anesthetist. Patients may complain of feeling a new irregular tooth edge with their tongue	May require filing to smooth tooth edge or prosthetic capping non-urgent dental referral
Class II	Facture into dentin	Invariably painful especially to extremes of temperature as the sub-enamel layer is exposed. Exposed dentin is porous and renders the pulp susceptible infection, especially in children who only have a thin layer of dentine	Dental emergency. Requires prompt dental referral
Class III	Fracture into tooth pulp	Exquisitely painful as fracture penetrates the densely innervated tooth pulp. Typically, anterior teeth involved. Exposed pulp at risk of infection	Requires urgent dental referral and treatment. Treatment can be complex necessitating root canal education followed by metal post insertion and overlying crown placement or restoration
Class IV	Fracture of tooth root	Typically associated with an unstable tooth as a result of periodontal disease	Surgical extraction of damaged tooth
Class V	Subluxation (displacement) of a tooth	Tooth becomes loose and dislodged although retained within the alveolar bone. Subluxation can interrupt the blood supply to the teeth	Provided the tooth still has periodontal support it can be stabilized by splinting into original position. If support is lost then surgical extraction may be necessary
Class VI	Avulsion of entire tooth	Complete dislodgement of the tooth representing a serious aspiration risk. Essential to recover tooth. Invariably associated with periodontal disease	Dental emergency. Prompt reimplantation may be possible provided there is no significant coexisting periodontal disease

Among all these classes, Class I, II and VI are the most common injuries of anesthetic related dental damage, and this may induce concerns [52]. Patients attending anesthetic pre-assessment clinics should have their oral cavity and teeth carefully inspected for risk factors such as dental caries, loose teeth, and periodontal disease [51, 69]. When risk factors are identified, an explanation of your concerns should be given to the patient and, time permitting, they should be encouraged to attend their dentist for treatment.

9.3.7 Protective Mouth Guards

Protective mouth guards have long been used to reduce dental injury to upper incisors while performing laryngoscopy and intubation. It was reported that 90% of dental injuries were preventable if the patient's dental state had been correctly assessed before surgery and a mouth guard had been used. Apart from this, in light of the fact that using mouth guards makes laryngoscopy and intubation difficult impedes the routine practice of mouth guards by anesthetists [70].

The most popular anesthetic mouth guards are bulky and commercially manufactured to a standard design. A performed custom-made mouth guards fitting the patient's dentition accurately is less popular but more alternative. The thinner performed mouth guards affect intubation weakly and have been proved to dissipate the forces applied to teeth during laryngoscopy successfully [69]. Whereas, the measured protective effect correlated with the increasing bulk of the mouth guard refutes any advantage. Thus, using mouth guards does not eradicate the risk of dental injury during anesthesia [69]. Consequently, their efficacy and routine use has been questioned [50]. Meanwhile, though their use may protect against superficial chipping of dental enamel, the avulsion of loose teeth cannot be prevented.

9.3.7.1 Immediate Management of a Damaged Tooth During Anesthesia

The anesthetists should communicate and explain to the patient about the tooth damaged during anesthesia, and record the details in the patient's notes.

The degree of the injury as classified in Table 9.1 decides whether there should be immediate management of damaged teeth. If the damage is superficial, namely injuries belong to Class I, a routine dental appointment is enough. For injuries that are Class II–VI, considering there are risk of secondary infection, they should be treated by professionals in 24 h. Class II and III injuries can be extremely painful, so the patient should be urged to seek treatment.

Subluxed deciduous teeth should not be replaced in their sockets as they are prone to fuse with alveolar bone in an abnormal manner. Subluxed or avulsed permanent teeth, however, require urgent treatment if the tooth is to remain viable. Once a subluxed tooth has been repositioned, the tooth socket should be pressed firmly between the thumb and forefinger for 1 min and the tooth temporarily splinted back into position to avoid further movement [71]. Movement may induce blood supply, resulting in an avascular tooth. The patient should be referred to a dental surgeon for definitive stabilization urgently.

If a deciduous tooth has been avulsed, it is unnecessary to take other action except for informing the parents. Conversely, and avulsed permanent tooth can be regarded as a dental emergency. Usually, dental caries and periodontal disease coexist. Despite, an attempt should be made to salvage the tooth and preserve the periodontal ligament. A tooth deprived of its blood supply becomes increasingly unviable after 30 min. Prompt treatment is paramount.

Reimplantation is only possible if the tooth remains viable. The avulsed tooth and socket should be immediately lavaged in sterile isomolar normal saline (nerve water) and inspected. Provided the tooth is intact and there are no root fractures, the tooth should be immediately returned to the socket by holding the crown and taking great care to avoid touching the root. When immediate reimplantation is not feasible, the tooth should be restored in sterile isomolar saline or milk and the patient referred urgently to a dental surgeon. Reimplantation of a tooth in a patient partially recovered from a general anesthetic always carried the risk displacement and aspiration.

An unaccounted dislodged tooth or fragment of tooth can be life-threatening if it was inhaled during extubation [50]. Recovering the tooth and any fragments is vital. If a tooth, or part of a tooth, is unaccounted for, the clinicians should seek imaging technologies such as X-rays to detect it.

Damage or dislodgement to prosthetic teeth and fittings should be paid attention to within several days of injury. Ensuring that all detached fragments being recovered is significant. The fact that some prosthetic materials are not radiolucent, making the location of fragments difficult.

9.3.8 Oral Soft Tissue Injuries

Damage to intraoral soft tissue as a consequence of general anesthesia is common. Although such damage is not likely to be life-threatening in most cases, significant problems may develop after a period of time. Injuries are not only associated with laryngoscope and endotracheal intubation, but also may be related to laryngeal mask airways (LMA), Guided airways, bite blocks, suction catheters, and throat packs. The incidence of oral trauma caused by anesthesia and endotracheal intubation was once as high as 18% [72]. Later, a study conducted by Chen et al., revealed that the incidence of damage to dentition before or after anesthesia using endotracheal tube was 12.1%. In the survey of Lockhart et al., the incidence of trauma to dental structures during tracheal intubation was 1:1000 [73].

Among dental trauma, lip injuries are most commonly caused by laryngoscopy, including hematomas, lacerations, and generalized oedema which, although usually self-limiting, leads to inconvenience and discomfort. A mal-positioned or overinflated LMA can compress the lingual artery, causing cyanosis of the tongue and loss of taste. Similarly, a well-recognized symptom during overzealous laryngoscopy is loss of tongue sensation secondary to compression of the lingual nerve. Gross tongue swelling or macroglossia have been reported in multiple cases, some of which have resulted in life-threatening airway obstruction; thus requiring lengthy intubation [50]. Underlying causes include positioning of the patient, prolonged procedures, and anything that causes compression on the base of the tongue resulting in arterial and venous compromise and massive oedema. Therefore, prolonged intraoral surgery and the use of pharyngeal packs and bite blocks are risk factors.

The compression of an oral or nasal endotracheal tube, LMA or suction may cause injury to the uvula, leading to oedema and subsequent necrosis. There are several case reports of injury to the uvula secondary to suctioning the tip of the uvula into the Yankauer sucker, which is usually associated with heavier suction power. Suctioning with a narrower-tipped Yankauer with smaller side holes than the traditional wide-tipped, larger side holed catheter has also been reported to have caused soft tissue injury to the tonsillar pillars, and pharyngeal soft tissue with bleeding and aspiration of small amounts of tissue. Ideally, suctioning would always be under direct vision but this is not practical immediately prior to extubation when airway reflexes and muscle tone have returned. Care should always be taken to use the lowest power of suction that achieves optimal results.

There were cases reported death caused by pharyngeal perforation after mediastinitis, though such cases are rare [74]. Laryngoscopy and difficult passage of endotracheal tubes make up most cases, but both nasogastric tube placement and suctioning have been implicated, particularly in the pediatric setting [75].

After surgery, damage to the laryngeal muscles and suspensory ligaments or minor lacerations and abrasions to the cords may result in hoarseness. Severe injuries are often associated with difficult and traumatic intubation with the use of adjuncts such as stylets and bougies. Symptoms often resolve without intervention, yet hoarseness can be perpetual after unilateral cord paralysis which is considered to be the result of compression on the repeated laryngeal nerve from the cuff of a poorly placed endotracheal tube in the subglottic larynx [76]. While, soft tissue injuries may occur during induction, maintenance, and emergence of anesthesia, resulting in a wide range of pathologies.

9.3.8.1 Injuries Associated with Throat Packs

Throat packs are commonly used in dental, maxillofacial, and ENT surgery to pack the oropharynx and nasopharynx. The pack itself usually comprises of variable amounts of coarse green gauze which is moistened and supplied in rolls 180 cm long and 10 cm wide. It is used to absorb any blood which is not adequately aspirated, to prevent drainage of this blood into the stomach and leaking of blood around the cuff of an endotracheal tube (ETT) with subsequent contamination of the trachea. It was found that a cuffed ETT cannot provide 100% protection from aspiration and so prolonged pooling of blood in the pharynx is undesirable [77]. There are different ways to place pharyngeal packs, such as Magill forceps and digital insertion. To avoid tearing the frenulum, particularly during blind insertion, the tongue should always be displaced. The insertion of throat packs is implicated in grazes to the soft and hard palate, and tears to the frenulum and posterior pharyngeal wall. Injuries as a consequence of the above conditions are often ignored as direct laryngoscopy is not routinely performed [78]. Therefore, studies have revealed a high incidence of sore throat associated with pharyngeal packs. Fine et al. [79] found an 80% incidence of sore throat in patients with pharyngeal packs and a zero incidence with no packing. Whereas, this study was limited in sample size. Another study by Tay et al. [80] reported conflicting results with no difference in the incidence or severity of sore throat when throat packs were used. Basha et al. [81] studied 100 patients receiving nasal surgery and found a higher incidence of sore throat in those with a throat pack, though the discharge was not postponed and the incidence of postoperative nausea and vomiting (PONV) was unaffected by the presence of a throat pack.

Pharyngeal packs may damage the pharyngeal plexus and have resulted in macroglossia due to compression ischemia and subsequent oedema as previously discussed. Neglecting to remove the pharyngeal pack after the completion of the anesthetic can be the most catastrophic hazard, which could lead to airway obstruction and asphyxiation following extubation.

The risk of complications resulting from using throat packs must be minimized though careful attention. A throat pack is not necessary in all oral, maxillofacial, dental, and ENT surgeries. Risk-benefit assessment should be made for each patient before deciding to insert a throat pack. Concern over the lack of uniform practice as regards ensuring removal of packs has been discussed at a Royal College of Anesthetists Safety Conference. Several methods have been recommended, including visual checking systems such as labeling the airway device, tying the pack to the airway device, or leaving part of the pack protruding. Noticeably, no method can suit all situations. For instance, intraoral surgery may not allow either tying the pack to the airway or leaving part outside the mouth. Other methods concluded from documentary were discussed as well, including a two-person checking system on insertion and removal. A solution that involve the throat pack in the surgery and introduce a uniform practice is expected.

9.3.8.2 Injuries Associated with Nasal Intubation

Nasotracheal intubation is a common anesthetic technique which enables access during oral, dental, and maxillofacial surgery. Complication of both oral and nasotracheal intubation are well illustrated in researches, and some of them have been described in previous sections associated with soft tissue injuries. Nevertheless, there are injuries specifically pertinent to nasotracheal intubation that need to be explored. Moreover, modern dedicated nasotracheal tubes are intentionally made of a softer and more pliable material; thus they are more vulnerable to extraneous compression and kinking during oral and maxillofacial surgery.

Indications for nasal ETT include maxillofacial surgery, oropharyngeal, and dental surgery, as well as being useful in rigid laryngoscopy and microlaryngeal surgery. Awake fiberoptic intubation always concerns the nasal route and can be useful in a wide variety of situations when the difficult direct laryngoscopy exists.

The nasal airway assessment is critical if clinicians try to prevent local injuries. Patients with nasal septal deviations and hypertrophied turbinates are commonly seen. Yet recognition of patency problems through patient's medical history, particularly asking airflow obstructive symptoms may not provide reliable prediction of the most suitable nostril to intubate [82].

Nasendoscopy is used to identify asymptomatic nasal abnormalities. Whereas, anesthetists who are able to use it as part of routine practice are rare. Therefore, the prediction of the most suitable nostril is hard [83].

9.3.8.3 Epistaxis

Epistaxis is the most common injury happened during nasal intubation and is often caused by mucosal tears in the anterior part of the nasal septum, namely Little's area [84]. Avulsion of polyps, especially in asthmatics, trauma to tonsils, adenoids, or the posterior pharyngeal wall can lead to bleeding and worse still, may be torrential and life-threatening. The reported incidence of epistaxis varies widely from 18% to 66% [85, 86], though the majority of these cases were minor bleeding, with some classifying blood-tinged saliva as a significant event.

The risk of epistaxis may increase when a larger nasotracheal tube is used. When applying excessive force as the clinicians experienced difficulty during navigating the tube through the nasal passage, repeated attempts are required [87].

Several solutions have been proposed to alleviate epistaxis, for example, thermosoftening of the tube, change of tube materials and the use of vasoconstrictors. Lubricating the tube end and administering vasoconstrictors such as phenylephrine, ephedrine, cocaine or oxymetazoline used together with lidocaine, to the nostril are common measures adopted. Nevertheless, literature provides no solid evidence to reveal significant difference in efficacy between these agents in lowering the incidence of epistaxis after intubation [88]. Recently, Yu et al. [89] found that nasal packing with bupivacaine can reduce epistaxis and nasal pain more effectively as compared to cases without pretreatment with this anesthetic. In addition, there are controversial proposals to reduce epistaxis such as the introduction of sequential nasopharyngeal airway [50].

Regardless of these attempts to minimize the risks, significant nasal bleeding may arise as well. Blood within the airway not only obscures vision but blocks the airway, particularly when large clots have formed, which may result in bronchospasm, laryngospasm and obstruct sufficient ventilation. The situation may worsen and be disastrous when direct laryngoscopy is suboptimal. A case report emphasized the hazardous scenario where epistaxis occurred happened during advancing the nasal ETT through a vasoconstricted nostril [90]. An unpredicted Cormack and Lehane grade 4 view was displayed through direct laryngoscopy. Copious blood accumulated in the airway, resulting in ventilation difficult and hindering the use of a fiberoptic scope to facilitate endotracheal intubation. Emergency cricothyroidotomy was necessary to facilitate oxygenation. Visualization of the larynx and fiberoptic intubation was only then achievable after the hemorrhage was brought under control by nasal tamponade. Prior laryngoscopy to assess the adequacy of the laryngeal view before introducing a nasotracheal tube has been proposed as a means of reducing the risk of the aforementioned situation. Having evaluated the airway, fiberoptic devices can then be used if required without the risk of blood obscuring the view. These also allow the anesthetist to make a judgment that, if nasal hemorrhage does occur, laryngeal intubation will be readily achievable.

Epistaxis resulting from nasotracheal intubation is usually self-limiting and can invariably be controlled by either the pressure of the nasal tube or though insertion of an absorbent nasal tampon and sitting the patient upright. More persistent hemorrhage may necessitate inserting a Foley catheter and applying a tamponade by means of inflating the cuff.

9.3.8.4 Structural Injuries Associated with Nasotracheal Intubation

Avulsion of nasal polyps, inferior and middle turbinates, and tumor have all been reported as resulting in airway and nasotracheal tube obstruction. Less common injuries include submucosal placement and creating false submucosal passages, usually when there have been repeated attempts to pass the tube through the nose. This can lead to retropharyngeal abscess formation. The use of antibiotics should be considered when a pharyngeal tear is recognized [91]. Likewise, applying prophylactic antibiotics in susceptible patients with valve replacements should be considered as nasotracheal intubation, which may be associated with a bacteremia [92].

Lengthy nasal intubation can result in pressure necrosis of the nostrils and septum, retropharyngeal abscess formation, and paranasal sinusitis.

9.3.8.5 Eye Injuries During Oral and Maxillofacial Surgery

Although a detailed discussion of eye injuries associated with general anesthesia is beyond the scope of this chapter, patients undergoing oral and maxillofacial surgery are at an increased risk from such injuries [93]. While implementing surgery, though patient's eyes are usually covered by operative drapes, considering that they are close to the surgical field, they are prone to suffer both physical insult and careless instillation of antimicrobial skin preparations. The eyes are at particular risk during laser surgery. It has been reported that eye injury made up 3% of all compensatory claims against anesthetists, of which 35% relate to corneal abrasions. Soothingly, most of those injuries can recover without permanent visual impairment.

Techniques to protect the eyes during oral and maxillofacial surgery contain taping the eyes shut, with or without protective ointment, protective ointment alone, methylcellulose drops, and goggles [50].

9.3.9 Conclusion

Damage to the oral and maxillofacial structures are common iatrogenic anesthetic related complications reported. No matter how minor the injuries are, they can bring discomfort and inconvenience to the patient. In this case, teeth and intraoral soft tissues' injuries during laryngoscopy are primary. Above all, anesthetists should be acquainted with different risk factors that may prompt injuries of the oral cavity and maxillofacial region during anesthesia so that the risk of injuries could be minimized.

References

1. MacKenzie TA, Young ER. Local anesthetic update. Anesth Prog. 1993;40(2):29–34.
2. Kocak Berberoglu H, Gurkan Koseoglu B, Kasapoglu C. Dis Hekimliginde lokal anestezi. Istanbul: Quintessence; 2007. p. 142–60. ISBN:9944564137.
3. Giovannitti JAJR, Rosenberg MB, Phero JC. Pharmacology of local anesthetics used in oral surgery. Oral Maxillofac Surg Clin North Am. 2013;25(3):453–65.
4. Becker DE, Reed KL. Essentials of local anesthetic pharmacology. Anesth Prog. 2006;53(3):98–108.
5. Haas DA. An update on local anesthetics in dentistry. J Can Dent Assoc. 2002;68(9):546–51. https://doi.org/10.1111/ors.12252.
6. Donaldson M, Gizzarelli G, Chanpong B. Oral sedation: a primer on anxiolysis for the adult patient. Anesth Prog. 2007;54(3):118–28.
7. Appukuttan DP. Strategies to manage patients with dental anxiety and dental phobia: literature review. Clin Cosmet Investig Dent. 2016;8:35–50. https://doi.org/10.2147/CCIDE.S63626.
8. Sekimoto K, Tobe M, Saito S. Local anesthetic toxicity: acute and chronic management. Acute Med Surg. 2017;4(2):152–60.
9. Safety Committee of Japanese Society of Anesthesiologists. Practical guide for the management of systemic toxicity caused by local anesthetics. J Anesth. 2019;33:1–8. https://doi.org/10.1007/s00540-018-2542-4.
10. Singh P. An emphasis on the wide usage and important role of local anesthesia in dentistry: a strategic review. Dent Res J (Isfahan). 2012;9(2):127–32.
11. Bosack RC, Lieblich S. Anesthesia complications in the dental office. 1st ed. New York: Wiley-Blackwell; 2014. p. 211–8.
12. Batinac T, Sotosek Tokmadzic V, Peharda V, Brajac I. Adverse reactions and alleged allergy to local anesthetics: analysis of 331 patients. J Dermatol. 2013;40(7):522–7.
13. Lee J, Lee JY, Kim HJ, Seo KS. Dental anesthesia for patients with allergic reactions to lidocaine: two case reports. J Dent Anesth Pain Med. 2016;16(3):209–12.
14. Muraro A, Roberts G, Worm M, Bilo MB, Brockow K, Fern Andez Rivas M, et al. Anaphylaxis: guidelines from the European academy of allergy and clinical immunology. Allergy. 2014;69:1026–45. https://doi.org/10.1111/all.12437.

15. Australasian Society of Clinical Immunology and Allergy guidelines. 2017. www.allergy.org.au/health-professionals/papers/acute-management-of-anaphylaxis-guidelines.
16. Barash M, Reich KA, Rademaker D. Lidocaine-induced methemoglobinemia: a clinical reminder. J Am Osteopath Assoc. 2015;115(2):94–8.
17. Chowdhary S, Bukoye B, Bhansali AM, Carbo AR, Adra M, Barnett S, et al. Risk of topical anesthetic–induced methemoglobinemia: a 10-year retrospective case-control study. JAMA Intern Med. 2013;173(9):771–6.
18. Hegedus F, Herb K. Benzocaine-induced methemoglobinemia. Anesth Prog. 2005;52(4):136–9.
19. Meechan JG. Local anaesthesia: risks and controversies. Dent Update. 2009;36(5):278–80.
20. Säkkinen J, Huppunen M, Suuronen R. Complications following local anaesthesia. Nor Tannlaegeforen Tid. 2005;115:48–52.
21. Kudo M. Initial injection pressure for dental local anesthesia: effects on pain and anxiety. Anesth Prog. 2005;52(3):95–101.
22. Crean SJ, Powis A. Neurological complications of local anaesthetics in dentistry. Dent Update. 1999;26(8):344–9.
23. Pogrel MA. Permanent nerve damage from inferior alveolar nerve blocks-an update to include articaine. J Calif Dent Assoc. 2007;35(4):271–3.
24. Smith MH, Lung KE. Nerve injuries after dental injection: a review of the literature. J Can Dent Assoc. 2006;72(6):559–64.
25. Renton T. Oral surgery: part 4. Minimizing and managing nerve injuries and other complications. Br Dent J. 2013;215(8):393–9.
26. Piccinni C, Gissi DB, Gabusi A, Montebugnoli L, Poluzzi E. Paraesthesia after local anaesthetics: an analysis of reports to the FDA adverse event reporting system. Basic Clin Pharmacol Toxicol. 2015;117(1):52–6. PMID:25420896. https://doi.org/10.1111/bcpt.12357.
27. Sambrook PJ, Goss AN. Severe adverse reactions to dental local anaesthetics: prolonged mandibular and lingual nerve anaesthesia. Aust Dent J. 2011;56(2):154–9. https://doi.org/10.1111/j.1834-7819.2011.01317.x.
28. Vasconcelos BC, Bessa Nogueira RV, Maurette PE, Carneiro SC. Facial nerve paralysis after impacted lower third molar surgery: a literature review and case report. Med Oral Patol Oral Cir Bucal. 2006;11(2):175–8.
29. Meyer FU. Complications of local dental anesthesia and anatomical causes. Ann Anat. 1999;181(1):105–6. PMID:10081571.
30. Wolf KT, Brokaw EJ, Bell A, Joy A. Variant inferior alveolar nerves and implications for local anesthesia. Anesth Prog. 2016;63(2):84–90. https://doi.org/10.2344/0003-3006-63.2.84.
31. Siddiqui A, Shenoi R, Sharma HU, Harankhedkar N, Shrivastava A, Vats V, et al. Causes of failure of dental local anaesthesia—a review. Int J Contemp Med Res. 2015;2(2):415–9.
32. Wong MK, Jacobsen PL. Reasons for local anesthesia failures. J Am Dent Assoc. 1992;123(1):69–73. https://doi.org/10.14219/jada.archive.1992.0004.
33. Blanton PL, Jeske AH, ADA council on scientific affairs, ADA division of science. Avoiding complications in local anesthesia induction anatomical considerations. J Am Dent Assoc. 2003;134(7):888–93.
34. Ogle OE, Mahjoubi G. Local anesthesia: agents, techniques, and complications. Dent Clin N Am. 2012;56(1):133–48. https://doi.org/10.1016/j.cden.2011.08.003.
35. Cakarer S, Can T, Cankaya B, Erdem MA, Yazici S, Ayintap E, et al. Peripheral facial nerve paralysis after upper third molar extraction. J Craniofac Surg. 2010;21(6):1825–7. https://doi.org/10.1097/SCS.0b013e3181f43dcf.
36. Yalcin BK. Complications associated with local Anesthesia in oral and maxillofacial surgery. In: Whizar-Lugo VM, Hernández-Cortez E, editors. Topics in local Anesthetics. London: IntechOpen; 2019. https://doi.org/10.5772/intechopen.87172. https://www.intechopen.com/chapters/67979.
37. Cummings DR, Yamashita DD, McAndrews JP. Complications of local anesthesia used in oral and maxillofacial surgery. Oral Maxillofac Surg Clin North Am. 2011;23(3):369–77.
38. Fonseca RJ, Frost DE, Hersh EV, Levin LM. Oral and maxillofacial surgery. Philadelphia, PA: Saunders; 2009.
39. Malamed SF, Reed K, Poorsattar S. Needle breakage: incidence and prevention. Dent Clin N Am. 2010;54(4):745–56. https://doi.org/10.1016/j.cden.2010.06.013.
40. Baiju A, Krishnakumar K, Panayappan L. Anaesthesia complications: an overview. J Bio Innov. 2018;7(4):526–34.
41. Biočić J, Brajdić D, Perić B, Đanić P, Salarić I, Macan D. A large cheek hematoma as a complication of local anesthesia: case report. Acta Stomatol Croat. 2018;52(2):156–9. https://doi.org/10.15644/asc52/2/9.
42. Bendgude V, Akkareddy B, Jawale BA, Chaudhary S. An unusual pattern of self-inflicted injury after dental local anesthesia: a report of 2 cases. J Contemp Dent Pract. 2011;12(5):404–7. https://doi.org/10.5005/jp-journals-[10024-1067].
43. Jung RM, Rybak M, Milner P, Lewkowicz N. Local anesthetics and advances in their administration—an overview. J Pre-Clin Clin Res. 2017;11:94–101.
44. Malamed SF. Handbook of local anesthesia. 5th ed. St Louis, MO: Elsevier Mosby; 2004. p. 621–55.
45. Pandey R, Dixit N, Dixit KK, Roy S, Gaba C. Amaurosis, an unusual complication secondary to inferior alveolar nerve anesthesia: a case report and literature review. J Endod. 2018;44(9):1442–4. https://doi.org/10.1016/j.joen.2018.05.005.
46. Peñarrocha-Diago M, Sanchis-Bielsa JM. Ophthalmologic complications after intraoral local anesthesia with articaine. Oral Surg Oral Med Oral Pathol Oral Radiol Endod. 2000;90(1):21–4.

47. von Arx T, Lozanoff S, Zinkernagel M. Ophthalmologic complications after intraoral local anesthesia an analysis of 65 published case reports. Swiss Dent J. 2014;124:784–95.
48. Alamanos C, Raab P, Gamulescu A, Behr M. Ophthalmologic complications after administration of local anesthesia in dentistry: a systematic review. Oral Surg Oral Med Oral Pathol Oral Radiol. 2016;121(3):39–50.
49. Kehlet H, Dahl JB. Anaesthesia, surgery, and challenges in postoperative recovery. Lancet. 2003;362:1921–8.
50. Shaw I, Kumar C, Dodds C. Oxford textbook of anaesthesia for oral and maxillofacial surgery. Oxford: Oxford University Press; 2010.
51. Kok PHK, Kwan KM, Koay CK. A case report of a fractured healthy tooth during use of Guedel oropharyngeal airway. Signapore Med J. 2001;42:322–4.
52. Watts J. NHS dentist shortage may have adverse effects for anesthetists. Anesthesia. 2008;63:1377.
53. Givol N, Gershtansky Y, Hlamish-Shani T, et al. Perianesthetic dental injuries: analysis of incident reports. J Clin Anesth. 2004;16:173–6.
54. Hastings RH, Hon ED, Nghiem C, Wahrenbrock EA. Force and torque vary between laryngoscopists and laryngoscope blades. Anesth Analg. 1996;82(3):462–8.
55. Lee J, Choi JH, Lee YK, et al. The Callander laryngoscope blade modification is associated with a decreased risk of dental contact. Can J Anaesth. 2004;51(2):181–4.
56. Owen H, Waddel-Smith I. Dental trauma associated with anaesthesia. Anaesth Intensive Care. 2000;28:133–45.
57. Itoman EM, Kajioka EH, Yamamoto LG. Dental fracture risk of metal vs. plastic laryngoscope blades in dental models. Am J Emerg Med. 2005; 23(2):186–9.
58. Ho AMH, Hewitt G. Warning devices for prevention of dental injury during laryngoscopy. J Clin Monit Comput. 2000;16(4):269–72.
59. Quinn JB, Schulthesis LW, Schumacher GE. A tooth broken after laryngoscopy: unlikely to be caused by the force applied by the anesthesiologist. Anesth Analg. 2005;100:594–6.
60. Tolan TF, Westerfield S, Irvine D, Clark T. Dental injuries in anesthesia: incidence and preventive strategies. Anesthesiology. 2000;93(3; SUPP/2):A1133.
61. Kinane DE, Marshall GJ. Periodontal manifestations of systemic disease. Aust Dent J. 2001;46(1):2–12.
62. Swinson B, Witherow H, Norris P, Lloyd T. Oral manifestations of systemic diseases. Hosp Med. 2004;65(2):92–9.
63. Tredwin CJ, Scully C, Bagan-Sebastian J-V. Drug induced disorders of teeth. J Dent Res. 2005;84(7):596–602.
64. Owen H. Anesthesia and dental trauma. Anesth Intensive Care Med. 2002;3:253–5.
65. Houston WJB, Stephens CD, Tulley WJ. The classification of occlusion and malocclusion. In: A textbook of orthodontics. 2nd ed. Oxford: Wright Butterworth Heinemann; 1992. p. 42–53.
66. Skeie A, Schwartz O. Traumatic injuries to teeth in connection with general anesthesia and the effect of use of mouthguards. Endod Dent Traumatol. 1999;15:33–6.
67. Burton JF, Baker AB. Dental damage during anesthesia and surgery. Anesth Intensive Care. 1987;15:262–3.
68. Abraham R, Kaufman J. Dental damage during anesthesia. In: Kaufman L, Ginsburg R, editors. Anesthesia reviews 15, chapter 12. Edinburgh: Churchill Livingtone; 1999. p. 158–200.
69. Monaca E, Fock N, Doehn M, Wappler F. The effectiveness of performed tooth protectors during endotracheal intubation: an upper jaw model. Anesth Analg. 2007;105:1326–32.
70. Whitley S, Shaw IH. Dental throat packs and airway protection. Anaesthesia. 1992;47:173.
71. Welbury R. Dental pain, infection, hemorrhage and trauma. In: Hawkesford J, Banks JG, editors. Maxillofacial and dental emergencies. Chapter 2. Oxford: Oxford University Press; 1994. p. 7–34.
72. Chen J-J, Susetio L, Chao CC. Oral complications associated with endotracheal general anesthesia. Anesth Sinica. 1990;28:163–9.
73. Yasny JS. Perioperative dental considerations for the anesthesiologist. Anesth Analg. 2009; 108(5):1564–73.
74. Domino KB, Posner KL, Caplan RA, Cheney FW. Airway injury during anesthesia: a closed claims analysis. Anesthesiology. 1999;91:1703.
75. Patnaik S, Raju U, Arora M. Neonatal pharyngeal perforation. Med J Armed Forces India. 2007;63:275–6.
76. Hagberg C, Georgi R, Krier C. Complications of managing the airway. Best Pract Res Clin Anesthesiol. 2005;19:641–59.
77. Seraj MA, Ankutse MN, Khan FM, Siddiqui N, Ziko AO. Tracheal soiling with blood during intranasal surgery. Mid East J Anesthesiol. 1991;11:79–89.
78. Parry MG, Glaisyer H, Enderby DH. Prevention of trauma associated with throat pack insertion. Anesthesia. 1997;54:444–53.
79. Fine J, Kaltman S, Bianco M. Prevention of sore throat after nasotracheal intubation. J Oral Macillofac Surg. 1998;46:946–7.
80. Tay JY, Tan WK, Chen FG, Koh KF, Ho V. Postoperative sore throat after routine oral surgery; influence of the presence of a pharyngeal pack. Br J Maxillofac Surg. 2002;40:60–3.
81. Basha SI, McCoy E, Ullah R, Kinsella JB. The efficacy of pharyngeal packing during routine nasal surgery—a prospective randomized controlled study. Anesthesia. 2006;61:1161–5.
82. Smith JE, Reid AP. Identifying the more patent nostril before nasotracheal intubation. Anesthesia. 2001;56:258–62.
83. Williamson R. Nasal intubation and epistaxis. Anesthesia. 2002;57:1033–4.
84. Kido K, Shindo Y, Miyashita H, Kusama M, Sugino S, Masaki E. Acute management of mas-

sive epistaxis after nasotracheal extubation. Anesth Prog. 2019;66(4):211–7. PMID: 31891291; PMCID: PMC6938169. https://doi.org/10.2344/anpr-66-02-09.
85. Watanabe S, Yaguchi Y, Suga A, Asakura N. A bubble tip tracheal tube system-its effects on incidence of epistaxis and ease of tube advancement in the subglottic region during nasotracheal intubation. Anesth Analg. 1994;78:1140–3.
86. Kim YC, Lee SH, Noh GJ, et al. Thermosoftening treatment of the nasotracheal tube before intubation can reduce epistaxis and nasal damage. Anesth Analg. 2000;91:698–701.
87. O'Connell JE, Stevenson DS, Stokes MA. Pathological changes associated with short term nasal intubation. Anesthesia. 1996;31:347–50.
88. Katz RI, Hovagirn AR, Finkelstein HS, et al. A comparison of cocaine lidocaine with epinephrine and oxymetazoline for prevention of epistaxis on nasotracheal intubation. J Clin Anesth. 1990;2:16–20.
89. Yu HK, Park J, Kang Y, Park HB, Bae SI, Lee SH, Ok S, Jeong S, Park M. Nasal packing with bupivacaine during nasotracheal intubation can reduce intubation-related epistaxis. Oral Biol Res. 2021;45:107–14.
90. Piepho T, Thierbach A, Werner C. Nasotracheal intubation: look before you leap. Br J Anesth. 2005;6:859–60.
91. Divatia JV, Bhowmick K. Complications of endotracheal intubation and other airway management procedures. Ind J Anesth. 2005;4:308–18.
92. Valdes C, Tomas I, Alvarez M, et al. The incidence of bacteremia associated with tracheal intubation. Anesthesia. 2008;63:588–92.
93. Anderson DA, Braun TW, Herlich A. Eye injury during general anesthesia for oral and maxillofacial surgery: etiology and prevention. J Oral Maxillofac Surg. 1995;53:321–4.

10 Anesthesia for Outpatient Oral and Maxillofacial Surgery

Jue Jiang

10.1 Introduction

Significant advancements in outpatient anesthesia in oral and maxillofacial surgery have been achieved continuously. These advancements are numerous and far reaching, and encompass the agents most frequently used and their method of delivery, as well as perioperative management and monitoring. In this chapter, some of the more significant of these advancements that have taken place during the last decade are explored.

Data from the American Association of Oral and Maxillofacial Surgeons (AAOMS) studies revealed that third molar removal remains to be the most commonly performed surgery [1]. Other oral outpatient surgery mainly includes therapies such as dental caries filling, root canal therapy, pit, and fissure sealing, etc., as well as minor surgeries such as tooth extraction, dental implant, alveolar surgery, and excision of minor oral soft tissue tumors, etc. Patients who cannot cooperate, such as children or patients with dental phobia, need to be given appropriate analgesia, sedation, and even general anesthesia, which is also a basic requirement of comfortable oral diagnosis and treatment.

J. Jiang (✉)
Department of Anesthesiology, Shanghai Ninth People's Hospital Affiliated to Shanghai Jiao Tong University School of Medicine, Shanghai, China

10.2 Pre-anesthetic Preparation

10.2.1 Equipment and Operation Site

Oral outpatient anesthesia belongs to the category of anesthesia outside the operating room, which requires an office equipped with essential and relevant devices and a dedicated room for postanesthesia recovery.

The satisfactory implementation of operation necessarily requires certain equipment, including manifold system, remote gas storage, communication equipment, record keeping/time-out forms, anesthesia machine, venipuncture armamentarium and infusion pumps, airway armamentarium, operating suite, monitors, surgical chair or operating table, oxygen and supplemental gas delivery system, lighting system, suction device, and transport equipment.

1. Manifold System and Remote Gas Storage

   The gas manifold is a kind of centralized gas filling or supply device, which is special equipment that connects multiple cylinders of gas to the manifold through valves and conduits in order to fill these cylinders at the same time; or after decompression and pressure stabilization, it is transported by pipeline to the place of use to ensure the gas source pressure of gas using appliances is stable and adjustable, and to achieve the purpose of uninterrupted gas supply. Most outpatient manifold

H. Jiang, M. Xia (eds.), *Anesthesia for Oral and Maxillofacial Surgery*,
https://doi.org/10.1007/978-981-19-7287-4_10

systems are installed in enclosures away from patient care areas to prevent accidental fires, explosions or sudden gas releases that could cause injury or death. During the soldering of copper tubing, nitrogen must be blown into the tubing to eliminate oxidation by-products within the tubing and to avoid inadvertent transfer of these harmful byproducts to the patient [2].

All gas tanks should be installed with the convenience of office personnel in mind, including checking the pressure gauge and replacing the empty tank in a timely manner. Each manifold system should be equipped with a minimum of two oxygen tanks; thus, when the line pressure drops in one tank, another can be activated. If an automatic changeover system is used, there must be an audible or visible low oxygen pressure warning device. The shut-off valves for each gas should be clearly labeled for accurate use by any staff member in the event of an emergency [2].

2. Airway Devices

   Airway devices that should be prepared include a full face mask (preferably in multiple sizes with connectors); bag-valve-mask device with a pressure manometer, capable of providing positive pressure ventilation; various types of oral and nasopharyngeal airways; various supraglottic airway devices; endotracheal tubes (various pediatric and adult sizes); laryngoscope in both pediatric and adult blades (with extra batteries and bulbs); and a cricothyrotomy kit.

   It should be noticed that the emergency airway equipment, such as cricothyrotomy kit and tracheotomy kit, must be both readily accessible and familiar to anyone providing anesthesia in the office.

3. Monitors

   Monitoring equipment normally contains electrocardiogram, pulse oxygen saturation monitoring, respiratory function monitoring, end-expiratory carbon dioxide partial pressure monitoring, EEG bispectral index monitoring, noninvasive and invasive arterial pressure monitoring, central venous pressure monitoring, cardiac function monitoring, etc.

10.2.2 Anesthetics and Emergency Drugs

Commonly used clinical anesthetics include general anesthetics such as propofol, esketamine, sevoflurane, laughing gas, etc.; sedative drugs such as midazolam, dexmedetomidine, etc.; opioid analgesics such as fentanyl, remifentanil, sufentanil, etc.; muscle relaxants such as rocuronium bromide, cis-atracurium, etc.

Anesthetic adjuncts include atropine, dexamethasone, dolasetron, etc.; cardiovascular-active drugs such as nicardipine hydrochloride, phenylephrine, urapidil hydrochloride, ephedrine; first-aid medicine such as epinephrine, norepinephrine, etc.; various types of crystalloid solution, colloidal fluids, and other fluids.

10.2.3 Pre-anesthetic Visit

Laboratory and auxiliary examinations shall be improved before oral outpatient surgery. Laboratory examinations include routine blood test and test for coagulation function, liver and kidney function, blood electrolytes, hepatitis, rapid plasma regain (RPR), HIV, blood glucose, etc. Auxiliary examinations include electrocardiogram, chest X-ray or chest CT, lung function and heart function, etc. The type of examination is determined according to the patient's age and underlying diseases. The main purpose of preoperative visit is to find out the patient's medical history (current medical history, systemic medical history, family history, etc.), perform the necessary physical examination, check the results of laboratory and auxiliary tests, to get familiarized with the proposed surgical plan and the specific requirements for anesthesia, to formulate the required anesthesia plan according to the patient and surgical needs, to inform the patient of the risks of anesthesia and precautions before anesthesia, and to guide the patient to sign the informed consent of anesthesia. The patient should be informed of the time of arrival at the hospital, the duration of solid food fasting and liquid fasting, the preoperative medication, whether the medication for chronic diseases should be stopped and whether the company of family members is needed.

1. Indications

   Patients with ASAI-II, generally in good condition, tolerant of oral outpatient surgery, whose operation is of short duration with less bleeding.

2. Contraindications

   Premature infants under 36 weeks and children with respiratory diseases, cardiovascular diseases, severe malformations or upper respiratory tract infections; patients with severe systemic diseases and poor compensation; patients with acute respiratory infections; patients with high risk of presenting difficult airway; patients with acute myocardial infarction and cerebral infarction; patients of ASA III-IV; patients in need of long-term postoperative monitoring and treatment, etc.

3. Screening for Difficult Airway

   The presence of oral and maxillofacial diseases, the anesthetist's sharing upper respiratory tract with surgeons in oral outpatient anesthesia and some other factors can lead to a greater need for detailed preoperative assessment of the patient's risk of difficult airway and a pre-arranged plan for difficult airway. Patients with significantly difficult airways are required for admission to the hospital and surgical anesthesia is performed in the operating room.

   Screening items for difficult airway: measurement of mouth opening (the distance between upper and lower incisors when opening the mouth as wide as possible), thyromental distance (the distance from thyroid cartilage to mentum), observation of mandibular movement (whether underbite can be done), cervical mobility, tongue extension, Mallampati score, head and neck imaging, and epiglottis, pharynx, and larynx under electronic laryngoscopy.

10.3 Outpatient General Anesthesia

Outpatient general anesthesia (GA) is used for extraction of dental caries in children and for direct alveolar surgery, such as extraction of impacted teeth, cystectomy, and dental implants in adults. Although local anesthesia is the most common anesthesia method for oral surgery, general anesthesia can be used in special cases, such as when local anesthesia is ineffective, in patients who are uncooperative due to age, fear or anxiety, mental impairment, or physical disability [3]. Therefore, the choice between general anesthesia or moderate sedation and analgesia is determined by the patient's own condition and the need for oral treatment.

Outpatient GA for oral surgery has won patient's satisfaction. When the appropriate anesthesia and surgical protocol is selected based on the patient and the procedure, accompanied by improved perioperative patient monitoring and the use of newer, enhanced recovery anesthetics with fewer side effects, major patient morbidity decreases to a low level.

1. Premedication

   The preoperative medication plan and strategy of oral outpatient surgery patients are the same as those of inpatients. The main purpose of preoperative medication is to sedate, ease pain, prevent or decrease certain side effects of some anesthetics, and reduce the basal metabolism and nerve reflex irritability. The main drugs are sedatives and tranquilizers, analgesics, anticholinergics such as atropine, and H_2 receptor antagonists such as ranitidine.

2. The Establishment of Venous Access

   Peripheral veins are routinely accessed before anesthesia for outpatient oral surgery to support intravenous infusion and drug injection. For special patients, femoral vein puncture and catheterization should be performed when necessary.

3. Monitoring

   The main monitoring items include electrocardiogram, pulse oxygen saturation, blood pressure, body temperature, respiration, etc. General anesthesia also requires monitoring of airway pressure, tidal volume, end-expiratory carbon dioxide partial pressure, concentration of inhaled anesthetics at the inhalation and expiration ends, oxygen concentration, etc.

4. General Anesthesia
   (a) Induction

      Patients with no risk of difficult airway on preoperative assessment can choose fast induction of oral or nasal endotracheal intubation. Commonly used drugs include propofol, fentanyl, rocuronium, etc. Pediatric and uncooperative patients with open intravenous access can be selected for inhalation induction, in which sevoflurane is often applied. Patients with difficult airway can be sedated and analgesic by intravenous injection of fentanyl, midazolam, etc., and then injected with lidocaine through cricothyroid membrane puncture. Endotracheal intubation is guided by fiberoptic bronchoscope under topical anesthesia when autonomous respiration is kept to avoid hypoxia. Laryngoscope, intubating laryngeal mask airway, retrograde catheterization, blind intubation device, light wand, etc. are also available clinically. Local anesthesia can be achieved by lidocaine oropharyngeal spray, cricothyroid puncture injection of lidocaine, and nebulized inhalation of lidocaine, so as to lessen the adverse stress reaction during tracheal intubation.

   (b) Maintenance

      Combined anesthesia is often used to maintain the depth of anesthesia needed for surgery, which can significantly reduce the side effects caused by overdosing with single drugs. Sevoflurane, propofol, remifentanil, CIS atracurium, etc. are commonly used in the procedure.

10.4 Local Anesthesia

Local anesthetics have a long history of providing dental anesthesia. Cocaine was the first agent used, but its potential adverse reactions and dependence were soon realized. The development of the first synthetic local anesthetic, procaine, allowed dentists to avoid treating patients under general anesthesia. However, the short duration of action and potential for allergic side effects of procaine led to the synthesis of lidocaine in 1944 by Lofgren. This agent has prevailed as a local anesthetic of choice, as it possesses many ideal qualities. It has become the primary agent used in dentistry and oral and maxillofacial surgery. Its relatively fast onset of action, good duration of action (when combined with a vasoconstrictor), and low incidence of side effects has promoted it to be dentistry's prototypical local anesthetic agent [4].

Other local anesthetics are available, but with relatively minor improvements over lidocaine. Bupivacaine, indeed, being more highly protein bound, thus possessing a longer duration of action, is available, but with that comes a longer time for the onset of action (due to a higher acid dissociation constant [pK_a]). Other recently introduced agents, including prilocaine and articaine, are claimed to be more effective than lidocaine, yet there is lack of strong evidence since their differences are hard to test in controlled clinical trials. There also are concerns with the use of these 4% solutions as creating a somewhat higher incidence of neurotoxicity, but that, too, is controversial. These agents are not recommended as nerve block agents, instead, they suit for infiltration use only, though the package insert describes them to be used for nerve blocks [4].

10.5 Sedation and Analgesia

Sedation and analgesia can be divided into deep sedation and analgesia, moderate sedation and analgesia, and minimal sedation.

Deep sedation/analgesia is a drug-induced depression of consciousness during which patients cannot be easily aroused but respond purposefully following repeated or painful stimulation. In this state, patients are unable to maintain spontaneous ventilation. Therefore, they need interventions to keep a patent airway. Their cardiovascular function is still unimpaired.

Moderate sedation/analgesia, also called conscious sedation, is a drug-induced state during which patients' consciousness is depressed, responding purposefully to verbal commands, either alone or with mild physical stimulation. In this condition, patients can rely on the spontaneous ventilation, requiring no interventions to keep a patent airway, while their cardiovascular function is unaffected. Although not defined as anesthesia by ASA guidelines, moderate sedation and analgesia given during oral treatment can lessen stress response, pain, and discomfort, to facilitate examination and treatment. Sedation and analgesia are especially needed for uncooperative patients such as pediatric patients or patients with dental phobias, which is a part of comfort dental care. Before sedation and analgesia, it is necessary to confirm both the patient's physical and psychological tolerance for dental treatment, which sedation method is most suitable for the patient, whether there are contraindications, and whether the patient's condition and medical equipment meet the requirements of anesthesia and surgery [5].

Minimal sedation is a drug-induced state during which patients respond normally to verbal commands. Although cognitive function and coordination may be impaired, ventilator and cardiovascular functions are unaffected. This is also not anesthesia.

The classification of control measures corresponding to pain is shown in Fig. 10.1 (Table 10.1).

1. Behavior-induced Sedation

   Behavior-induced sedation is defined as the relief of patients' anxiety through the behavior of medical personnel, instead of using medications to achieve the purpose of sedation. By appropriate ward management (e.g., lessening patients' fear of turbine sounds by playing music), friendly and mild language, and gentle and painless treatment, a smooth doctor–patient communication bond

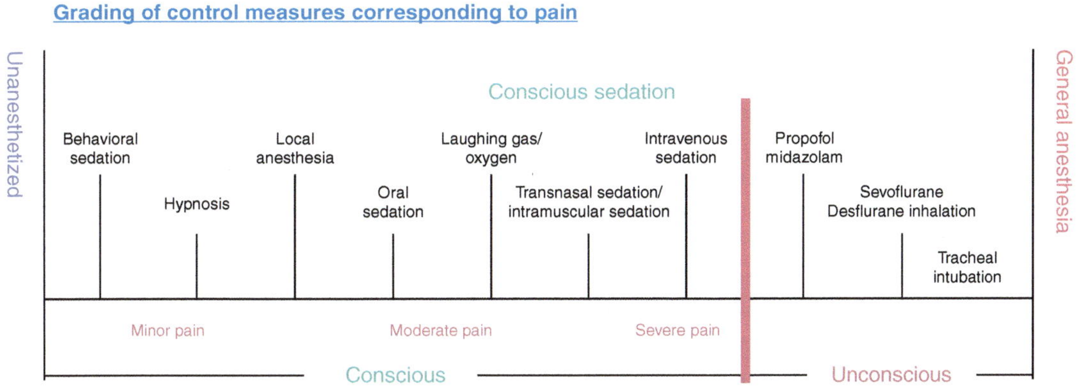

Fig. 10.1 Classification of control measures corresponding to pain

Table 10.1 Degree of sedation and clinical manifestations

	Minimal sedation	Moderate sedation	Deep sedation	General anesthesia
Ramsay sedation score	2–3	4	5–6	
Responses to stimuli	Normal response to verbal stimuli	Responsive to words or touch	Responsive to repetitive or painful stimuli	Cannot be awakened, nor can painful stimuli
Airway patency	Unaffected	No intervention required	Might require intervention	Usually require intervention
Autonomous respiration	Unaffected	Sufficient	Might be insufficient and require intervention	Usually insufficient and often require intervention
Cardiovascular function	Unaffected	Usually can be maintained	Usually can be maintained	Might be damaged

can be established and the patient's need for pharmacologic sedation can be reduced.

2. Sedation and Analgesia for Oral Administration

   Oral sedative and analgesic medication can effectively relieve patients' tension and pain during oral treatment, which makes it the most commonly used way of administration. It costs less, has minor side effects and low incidence rate, can be easily managed and is usually highly accepted with no need for any syringes or other medical equipment. However, there are also disadvantages, for example, it takes effect quite slow, is of long duration and unable to adjust the level of sedation. At present, the routine practice is to apply it in combination with other sedation, analgesia or general anesthesia. Midazolam can be administered orally at a dose of 0.2–0.5 mg/kg in children aged between 4 and 14 with ASA I-II, with a maximum dose of 15 mg. It can provide sedation on the premise of patients' safety with no significant inhibition of intraoperative hemodynamic and respiratory function, which gains high acceptance by parents. The main adverse effect is irritability.

3. Intravenous Sedation and Analgesia

   Sedation and analgesics are administered by single injection or continuous pumping into the cardiovascular system through intravenous access for the purpose of sedation and analgesia. It has the advantages of rapid drug onset, titratable drug concentration, and shorter recovery time than oral and intramuscular drugs. In addition, intravenous access is a guarantee of patients' safety. Disadvantages are: uncertainty in the maintenance of sedation and analgesia, difficulty in regulating the level of sedation and analgesia; overlap of operation area and anesthesia site area, threatening airway safety and increasing the difficulty of airway management; need for close monitoring; risk of respiratory depression, requiring preoperative preparation for emergency assisted respiration or tracheal intubation.

   Midazolam, dexmedetomidine, droperidol, fentanyl, sufentanil, remifentanil, esketamine, etomidate, propofol, etc. are often used as sedatives and analgesics. The dosage can be referred to Table 10.2.

   The loading dose of propofol for deep sedation is 1–2.5 mg/kg for children undergoing tooth extraction with poor compliance, which can be administered in a single or divided dose; the maintenance dose is 75–100 μg/(kg min). Pay attention to whether there is respiratory depression and provide assisted respiration if necessary. The disadvantages include injection pain, extremely deep sedation, unstable effect, etc.

4. Inhalation Sedation

   Laughing gas is the most commonly used inhalation anesthetic in oral treatment, which is a sort of nearly perfect way of sedation. It requires specific anesthetic equipment and a simultaneous inhalation of both laughing gas (N_2O) and oxygen (O_2), the intensity can be adjusted through oxygen flow. When the content of laughing gas in the mixture of laughing gas and oxygen is less than 30%, it has only

Table 10.2 Loading doses and maintenance doses of commonly prescribed drugs

Medication	Loading dose (μg/kg)	Maintenance dose (μg/(kg·min))
Midazolam	30–70	0.25–1.0
Droperidol	5–17	
Propofol	250–1000	10–50
Ketamine	300–500	15–30
Etomidate	100–200	7–14
Fentanyl	1–2	0.01–0.03
Remifentanil	1–2	0.01–0.03
Sufentanil	0.1–0.5	0.005–0.015
Tramadol	500–1000	4–4
Dexmedetomidine	0.5–1	0.2–0.7

sedative effect; when the content of laughing gas reaches 30–50%, it shall work as an analgesic (the concentration in the majority of clinical use); the content of 80% or more can enable it to play an anesthetic role. It is suitable for patients who are anxious and afraid of treatment, have terrible dental treatment experience, unable to be fully affected by local anesthesia, and children who cannot cooperate. It has a rapid onset of action, sedative effect, and is easy to master [6]. The disadvantage is that the patients need to have initiative to inhale, the analgesic effect is not strong enough when applied alone, and the anxiolytic effect is weak.

Sevoflurane is also a commonly used inhalation anesthetic in outpatient oral surgery. The concentration of sevoflurane for induction is 7–8%, and a flexible mask is inserted with a maintenance concentration of 1.5–2.0%. This method preserves the patient's autonomous respiration, but the incidence of agitation and vomiting during awakening period is higher than that of propofol.

10.6 Monitored Anesthesia Care (MAC)

MAC is defined as anesthesia services provided by anesthesiologists and anesthesia specialists (including anesthesia certified registered nurses, anesthesia residents, and licensed anesthesia assistants) to monitor and control the patient's vital signs and administer appropriate anesthetic medications or other treatments as needed during diagnosis and treatment. The primary purpose of MAC is to ensure the comfort and safety of patients during surgery and the smooth performance of diagnostic and therapeutic procedures [7].

In the early days, MAC was only used for patients who were considered to be high risk in surgery and not suitable for general anesthesia, such as patients undergoing palliative surgery. Later, MAC was gradually applied to patients who underwent smaller procedures but were unable to cooperate well due to excessive stress. With the recent development of minimally invasive surgery, procedures that previously required large incisions can now be performed with less trauma, and most of these procedures can be performed under MAC. The main advantages of MAC are that it avoids some of the complications of general anesthesia, reduces the incidence of aspiration pneumonia, shortens postoperative care period, and provides early postoperative analgesia. Surgical and therapeutic or examining operations for which MAC is indicated include head and neck surgery caries extraction, blepharoplasty, ptosis repair, cataract extraction, wrinkle removal, rhinoplasty, endoscopic sinus surgery, laceration suturing, biopsy or excision of neck masses, facial and neck nevus, and keloid excision, etc. [5].

10.7 Risks of Anesthesia in the Oral and Maxillofacial Surgery Setting

1. Shared Airway Between Anesthesia and Oral Therapy

   The office anesthesia team has been described to include the doctor who administers the anesthetic and performs the surgery, known as the operator–anesthetist model. Since anesthesia and oral therapy have to share the same airway of a patient, the anesthesiologist needs to maintain a balance between "minimizing or avoiding their impact on oral therapy" and "keeping the airway unobstructed throughout the treatment." It is deemed that such a model with separate identifiable tasks will maintain a high degree of safety for the patient.
2. Accidental Slippage of Airway or Endotracheal Tube

   During oral treatment, saliva and other liquids may lower the firmness of adhesive tape fixation. Besides, when the body of patient is being moved and the oral operation is being carried out during multi-site treatment, airway accidents may be caused by accidental slippage of airway and endotracheal tube, which is in need of close monitoring and adequate attention.

3. Aspiration

   Anesthesia has an inhibitory action on the protective reflex of the pharynx, while a large amount of cooling water, saliva, blood or pus, debris, and foreign matter shall be produced in oral treatment, which are very likely to cause aspiration-induced asphyxia and pneumonia, hence require timely suction and clearance, enhanced monitoring, and strict precautions.

4. Emergency Treatment of Airway Accidents

   Firstly, make emergency treatment preparations for perioperative airway accidents by having respiratory masks, endotracheal intubation equipment, simple ventilators, cardiopulmonary resuscitation equipment, and emergency drugs, etc. Secondly, once airway accidents occur, check the breathing circuit and oxygen source immediately. Closely monitor the patient's blood pressure, heart rate, heart rhythm, oxygen saturation, and other vital signs. If necessary, remind the oral surgeon to terminate the operation, find out the cause together and deal with it promptly. Be alert to the effects of preoperative comorbidity and other adverse stimuli such as pain and tension that can trigger cardiovascular and cerebrovascular accidents in elderly patients.

10.8 Post-anesthetic Recovery and Discharge

10.8.1 Post-anesthetic Recovery

All the patients need to enter the postanesthesia care unit (PACU) for resuscitation after anesthesia. The recovery of outpatients after anesthesia can be divided into the following stages: (1) Early stage of recovery. From the end of anesthesia to the patient's awakening from anesthesia. It is the high incidence period of post-anesthesia complications. Patients need to lie flat and their vital signs such as blood pressure, heart rate, and oxygen saturation should be closely monitored; (2) Middle stage of recovery. From awakening to reaching the discharge standard; (3) Late stage of recovery. From discharge to complete recovery. If the Steward Score (Table 10.3) is over 4 and Level of consciousness (Table 10.4) is above grade, patients shall leave the operating room or recovery room. Whether a patient can discharge or not shall be assessed by the Postsedation/Anesthesia Discharge Scale (Table 10.5), and a score of 9 or above indicates that the patient can be discharged.

Table 10.3 Steward Score

	2	1	0
Level of consciousness	Complete awakening	Respond to stimuli	No response to stimuli
Airway patency	Cough as directed	Able to keep respiratory tract unobstructed without respiratory support	Support required
Limb mobility	Conscious motion	Unconscious motion	No motion

Table 10.4 Level of consciousness

Level 0	Asleep, no response to voice of calling
Level 1	Asleep, with body movement, eye opening or head and neck movement
Level 2	Awake, the patient can open the mouth and extend the tongue with clinical manifestations of level 1
Level 3	Awake, the patient is able to state his/her name or age with clinical manifestations of level 2
Level 4	Awake, the patient is able to recognize people around or is aware of where he/she is with clinical manifestations of level 3

Table 10.5 Postsedation/Anesthesia Discharge Scale

	2	1	0
Vital signs (blood pressure and heart rate)	Less than 20% of change before operation	21–40% of change before operation	More than 41% of change before operation
Mobility	Stable gait, no dizziness	Assistance needed	Unable to walk, with dizziness
Nausea and vomiting	Minor	Moderate	Severe
Postoperative pain assessment	Minor	Moderate	Severe
Operative hemorrhage	Minor	Moderate	Severe

10.8.2 Discharge Instructions

When the patient has met the discharge criteria, the following instructions should also be taken into consideration.

1. Diet: Start with clear liquid and gradually transition to a normal diet.
2. Advice on medication: analgesics should be included.
3. Leave a contact number: to follow up the patient's postoperative condition and to deal with any complications that exist.

10.9 Complications of Anesthesia in the Outpatient Oral and Maxillofacial Surgery

Commonly seen complications include allergic reactions, toxicity, methemoglobinemia, post-injection pain and trismus, facial nerve paresis, broken needle, and lingual nerve injury [8, 9]. Besides, there is also study reported that postoperative nausea and/or vomiting (PONV) was the most common complication induced by intravenous sedation [10].

The great advancements made by anesthetics in dentistry have changed patient's perspectives of dental procedures. Normally, anesthesia techniques and anesthetic agents used in oral and maxillofacial surgery are safe and effective, yet they do have potential risks. The complications mentioned above have low incidence. Realizing them may help the surgeons, anesthesiologists, and patients minimize the adverse outcomes of using anesthetics.

References

1. Robert RC, Liu S, Patel C, Gonzalez ML. Advancements in office-based anesthesia in oral and maxillofacial surgery. Atlas Oral Maxillofac Surg Clin North Am. 2013;21(2):139–65. PMID: 23981491. https://doi.org/10.1016/j.cxom.2013.05.007.
2. Chung WL. Anesthesia equipment for the oral and maxillofacial surgery practice. Oral Maxillofac Surg Clin North Am. 2013;25(3):373–83. PMID: 23870146. https://doi.org/10.1016/j.coms.2013.03.002.
3. Sim KM, Boey SK. Outpatient general anaesthesia for oral surgery. Singapore Dent J. 2000;23(1 Suppl):29–37. PMID: 11699360.
4. Lieblich S. Providing anesthesia in the oral and maxillofacial surgery office: a look back, where we are now and a look ahead. J Oral Maxillofac Surg. 2018;76(5):917–25. Epub 2018 Feb 24. PMID: 29481773. https://doi.org/10.1016/j.joms.2018.01.026.
5. King BJ, Levine A. Controversies in anesthesia for oral and maxillofacial surgery. Oral Maxillofac Surg Clin North Am. 2017;29(4):515–23. PMID: 28987231. https://doi.org/10.1016/j.coms.2017.07.006.
6. Fauteux-Lamarre E, McCarthy M, Quinn N, Davidson A, Legge D, Lee KJ, Palmer GM, Babl FE, Hopper SM. Oral Ondansetron to reduce vomiting in children receiving intranasal fentanyl and inhaled nitrous oxide for procedural sedation and analgesia: a randomized controlled trial. Ann Emerg Med. 2020;75(6):735–43. Epub 2020 Jan 24. PMID: 31983494. https://doi.org/10.1016/j.annemergmed.2019.11.019.
7. Department of Health & Human Services (DHHS) Certification Centers for Medicare & Medicaid Services (CMS), CMS Manual System, Pub. 100–107 State Operations Provider Certification, Transmittals 59 and 74, May 21, 2010 and December 2, 2011.
8. Ogle OE, Mahjoubi G. Local anesthesia: agents, techniques, and complications. Dent Clin N Am. 2012;56(1):133–48, ix. PMID: 22117947. https://doi.org/10.1016/j.cden.2011.08.003.
9. Cummings DR, Yamashita DD, McAndrews JP. Complications of local anesthesia used in oral and maxillofacial surgery. Oral Maxillofac Surg Clin North Am. 2011;23(3):369–77. PMID: 21798437. https://doi.org/10.1016/j.coms.2011.04.009.
10. Christensen L, Svoboda L, Barclay J, Springer B, Voegele B, Lyu D. Outcomes with moderate and deep sedation in an oral and maxillofacial surgery training program. J Oral Maxillofac Surg. 2019;77(12):2447–51. Epub 2019 Jul 30. PMID: 31449763. https://doi.org/10.1016/j.joms.2019.07.007.

11 Anesthesia for Oral and Maxillofacial Plastic Surgery

Yu Sun

11.1 Introduction

For years, people have never stopped their aspiration for beauty and thus, rather all forms of efforts to seeking for a beautiful self have emerged and intensified along with the boost and flourish of global economy. In recent years, the amount of plastic surgery in China has increased rapidly, and the complexity and diversity of surgery has also been upgraded. It is known that plastic surgery may sometimes be a great challenge for anesthesiologists as it involves a wide range of surgery types and meticulous requirements, especially the anesthesia for head, neck, and maxillofacial plastic surgery, the particular surgical site of which may be vulnerable to complications such as airway obstruction, massive blood loss, and adverse nerve reflex during the operation. Therefore, whether the perioperative anesthesia treatment is correct or not is directly related to the safety of patients and the success of the operation.

11.2 Preoperative Assessment and Preparation

11.2.1 Preoperative Assessment

Preanesthesia assessment aims to check the medical history of patients, especially the existence of problems related to respiratory system, circulatory system, nervous system, endocrine system, urinary system, hematologic and digestive system, and the musculoskeletal and anatomical defects that may hinder airway management and regional anesthesia, as well as their anesthesia history.

Medical examinations are parts of the preoperative assessment. Preoperative physical examination includes vital signs, heart and lung, nerve reflex, etc. Before anesthesia, the airway must be evaluated to determine whether there is any chance to encounter difficult airway. The preoperative laboratory examination includes blood tests, liver and kidney function test, coagulation function test, electrolyte, and blood glucose. Special examinations include chest radiograph, electrocardiogram, etc.

11.2.2 Preoperative Preparation

The preparation of anesthesia normally covers drugs, articles and devices, and equipment. Patients also need to be prepared for the

Y. Sun (✉)
Department of Anesthesiology, Shanghai Ninth People's Hospital Affiliated to Shanghai Jiao Tong University School of Medicine, Shanghai, China

H. Jiang, M. Xia (eds.), *Anesthesia for Oral and Maxillofacial Surgery*,
https://doi.org/10.1007/978-981-19-7287-4_11

anesthesia. Anesthesiologists and surgeons should try to understand the special expectation and fear of patients before plastic surgery. To make patients fully understand the anesthesia process and risks, so that patients are in a good psychological state. When patients have underlying diseases, especially cardiovascular and cerebrovascular diseases, they should receive treatment first, so that their physical condition can meet the criteria of accepting elective surgery. Likewise, if patients have acute diseases before operation, such as upper respiratory tract infection, these diseases should be treated at first. Surgery could only be performed when acute diseases are cured. Appropriate fasting should be followed according to the age and anesthesia methods before operation, so as to avoid asphyxia and aspiration pneumonia caused by reflux aspiration during perioperative period. Preanesthesia medication mainly includes narcotic analgesics, sedatives, anticholinergics, etc. Anesthesiologists should make the anesthesia plan after considering the patient's age, physical and psychological conditions comprehensively.

11.3 Selection of Anesthesia Methods

Commonly used anesthesia methods in head and maxillofacial plastic surgery include local anesthesia, sedation and analgesia anesthesia, and general anesthesia. In general anesthesia, anesthetics can be administered through respiratory tract, vein or muscle injection. When the anesthetic enters the body, it will gradually inhibit central nervous system. Thus, patients temporarily lose consciousness and memory. Their muscles get relaxed, and have no response to external stimuli and pain. As a result, general anesthesia requires endotracheal intubation and mechanical ventilation support after anesthesia induction. Otherwise, the relaxation of respiratory muscles could not guarantee the sufficient oxygen supply. This anesthesia method is suitable for large and complex cosmetic surgery such as orthognathic surgery and costal cartilage rhinoplasty.

Intravenous sedation and analgesia can avoid some adverse reactions of general anesthesia and endotracheal intubation [1]. It is usually applied in superficial small and medium-sized cosmetic surgery and benefits patients who are anxious and nervous. Commonly used drugs include midazolam, dexmedetomidine, opioid analgesics, etc. [2].

Local anesthesia includes surface anesthesia, local infiltration anesthesia, and nerve block anesthesia. Among them, infiltration anesthesia refers to injecting local anesthetic into the subcutaneous operation area extensively, temporarily blocking the local sensory nerve conduction function, while patients remain awake. Convenient and easy to operate, this method is commonly used in minor facial cosmetic surgery. Surface anesthesia is an anesthetic method adopted in epidermal surgery, which applies anesthetic to the skin surface by smearing, and anesthetics act on the peripheral nerves on the skin surface after absorption to achieve analgesic effect. Nerve block anesthesia is to inject local anesthetic directly into the area near the peripheral nerve trunk to temporarily block the sensation of the area dominated by the nerve, and motor nerve may also be blocked in different degrees. It is an anesthesia method commonly used in facial filling, rhinoplasty, and other operations.

In plastic surgery, the choice of anesthesia methods is closely related to patients' safety. In another word, an improper anesthesia method may deprive of patients' life. Therefore, several factors need to be considered while making the choice, such as the patient's physiological condition and the type of surgery. Specifically, factors that need to be considered are roughly as follows.

11.3.1 The Mental State and Willingness of Patients

For patients who are nervous and could not calm down, the surgery which originally can be completed under local anesthesia then can combine with sedation and analgesia. For patients who are too afraid of pain and unwilling to receive surgery in an awake state, general anesthesia may be a better choice.

11.3.2 Age of Patients

Pediatric patients often undergo general anesthesia in surgeries. For teenagers who can tolerate the operation, local anesthesia can be used considering the short surgery time. For adults, local anesthesia is often selected for minor operations on the surface of human body, and major operations can be completed under local anesthesia combined with sedation and analgesia.

11.3.3 Requirements of Surgical Operation

Some operations require the cooperation of patients during surgery. Thus, local anesthesia is appropriate for such situation. In addition, in some surgeries, to observe the surgical effect timely, the surgical region is not allowed to be deformed by local injection of drugs. Under such circumstances, nerve block anesthesia or general anesthesia should be selected.

11.3.4 Surgical Site

If there is inflammation, infection or malignant skin lesions in the operation field, nerve block anesthesia, regional block anesthesia or general anesthesia should be selected, and local infiltration anesthesia is contraindicated [3].

11.3.5 Surgical Wound

For surgery that may cause severe trauma, general anesthesia is applicable.

11.4 General Anesthesia

11.4.1 Anesthesia Induction

The decision on which anesthesia induction protocol and which anesthetic drugs to use for endotracheal intubation is based on the patient's condition, the anticipated degree and risk of a difficult airway, the experience of the anesthesiologist, and the equipment available.

11.4.2 Anesthesia Maintenance and Management

1. Respiratory Management

   Monitor and adjust anesthesia ventilator parameters to maintain respiratory parameters such as partial pressure of end-expiratory carbon dioxide, respiratory rate, tidal volume, minute ventilation and airway pressure in the normal range, and pay attention to observation of clinical signs (breath sounds in both lungs, airway secretions; observation of mucous membrane of mouth and lips, skin, and nails and blood color in the surgical field), and perform arterial blood gas analysis when necessary.
2. Circulatory Management

   It is suggested to open one to two venous accesses according to the type of surgery, and establish central venous access if necessary. The transfusion of blood and fluid, and the application of vasoactive drugs should be reasonable. Smooth hemodynamic status and adequate tissue perfusion should be maintained during anesthesia and surgery.
3. The Depth of Anesthesia

   The depth of anesthesia is usually determined based on a combination of blood pressure, heart rate, respiration, and EEG dual frequency indices, etc. Maintaining a stable circulatory state solely by regulating the depth of anesthesia is unreliable. Intraoperative awareness should be prevented.

11.4.3 Management of Anesthesia Recovery Period

1. Endotracheal Extubation Indications

   The use of sedative, analgesic, and inotropic drugs throughout the anesthesia should be analyzed, including the number, total amount, and time of drug administration. Patients are able to breathe spontaneously and their circulatory system should be stable. Specifically, the tidal volume, minute ventilation, pulse oxygen saturation return to normal level. Cough reflex and swallowing reflex recover to normal status. They can respond to call and open their eyes, and complete movement directions. If necessary, the arterial blood gas analysis could serve as a reference. For patients with difficult airway and who undergo oral and maxillofacial surgery that may potentially affect airway safety, whether the tracheal tube should be retained or not postoperatively should be considered in light of their airway and surgery condition. Above all, ensuring the airway safety is the priority.
2. Extubation

   Before extubation, to prevent accidental aspiration, a gastric tube should be placed to suck the blood in the digestive tract when it is nasal or oral intubation. The secretions or blood remaining in the trachea, mouth, nose, and throat shall be suctioned out, and the suction should not exceed 15 s each time. The suction tube is can be slowly removed together with the tracheal tube or the tracheal tube can be removed when the lung is artificially inflated. During the process, the anesthesiologists should avoid stimulating the patient's airway and causing coughing.
3. Post-extubation Monitoring and Management

   After removal of the tracheal tube, the secretions in the oropharyngeal cavity should be sucked out while the patient's head should be turned aside to prevent vomiting and aspiration. Vital signs such as heart rate, blood pressure, respiration, and pulse oxygen saturation should be continuously monitored after extubation. In oral and maxillofacial plastic surgery, airway obstruction is an urgent situation worthy of attention. Patients are allowed to be transferred to wards after meeting the criteria for leaving the PACU.

11.5 Sedation and Analgesia

11.5.1 Medication

Commonly used sedative drugs include dexmedetomidine, midazolam, propofol, etc.; commonly used analgesic drugs include opioids, ketamine, etc. For light sedation, a sedative drug is usually used for anxiolytic purposes, and for moderate and deep sedation, a combination of sedative and analgesic drugs can be used to facilitate the surgery. Sedative and analgesic drugs should be administered in a titrated manner in elderly patients. When the surgical anesthesia is unsatisfactory, the administration of high-dose sedative and/or analgesic drugs to complete the surgery without airway protection and respiratory monitoring is strictly forbidden and should be promptly changed to general anesthesia [4].

11.5.2 Monitoring and Care During Sedation and Analgesia and Post-anesthesia

ECG, respiration, blood pressure, and pulse oxygen saturation should be monitored routinely. End-expiratory carbon dioxide should be monitored during deep sedation [5].

11.5.3 Common Complications and Their Management

1. Respiratory Depression

   Once respiratory depression occurred, stop the administration of sedative and analgesic drugs immediately. If patients are suspected of airway obstruction caused by glossoptosis, clinicians should perform the jaw thrust, and place the oropharynx or nasopharynx snorkel when necessary. If the pulse oxygen saturation continues to fall, high concentration oxygen should be provided through masks to assist or control ventilation. If necessary, endotracheal intubation or laryngeal mask should be performed and placed.

2. Hypotension

   During sedation and analgesia, if hypotension is caused by cardiovascular central inhibition, the depth of sedation should be reduced, and ephedrine, norepinephrine or norepinephrine should be given repeatedly or through continuous infusion. The rate of infusion could be accelerated if necessary.

3. Bradycardia

   Sinus bradycardia generally requires no special treatment, but the depth of sedation can be adjusted. If the heart rate is less than 50 bpm, atropine can be injected intravenously as appropriate; patients with hypotension can be administered with ephedrine as appropriate.

11.6 Local Anesthesia

11.6.1 Types of Local Anesthetics

Local anesthetics are divided into two categories: ester local anesthetics and amide local anesthetics. Commonly used ester local anesthetics include procaine and tetracaine, and commonly used amide local anesthetics include lidocaine, bupivacaine, and ropivacaine. Pharmacokinetic characteristics of these drugs include onset time, efficacy, action time, and side effects, which are different among different drugs and within different categories. Generally speaking, ester compounds hydrolyze and metabolize rapidly in plasma. On the contrary, the degradation of amides takes place through the liver, which leads to slow metabolism and increases the possibility of accumulation and systemic reaction. And surgeons and anesthesiologists should fully understand the kinetic characteristics of drugs belonging to this category in order to optimize anesthesia and minimize the risks associated with these preparations [6]. Although these are local anesthetics, they still have systemic effects. Whereas, the toxic and allergic reactions are rare if the dosage used is strictly monitored. Anesthesiologists who administer local anesthesia should follow the guidelines on safe maximum dose. The systemic toxicity of local anesthetics may include headache, tinnitus, paralysis of the mouth and tip of the tongue, restlessness, and convulsion, respiratory and circulatory depression in the late stage [7].

11.6.2 Peripheral Nerve Block Anesthesia

1. Sterilization

   Taking the puncture point as the center, the area around it (within the diameter of 15 cm) should be sterilized for three times.

2. Nerve Block Drugs

   Lidocaine, bupivacaine, mepivacaine, ropivacaine, etc.

3. Procedures

   Anatomical position, ultrasound and nerve stimulator can facilitate the nerve block by determining the block position. Seeking all possible techniques to improve the safety of nerve block, such as the visualization technology of ultrasonic location.

4. Intraoperative Monitoring and Support

   These include continuous ECG, blood pressure, respiration, pulse oxygen saturation monitoring, and continuous oxygen inhalation and infusion.

11.6.3 Local Infiltration Anesthesia

1. Sterilization

   Taking the puncture point as the center, the area around it (within the diameter of 15 cm) should be sterilized for three times.

2. Nerve Block Drugs

   Lidocaine, bupivacaine, mepivacaine, ropivacaine, etc.

3. Procedures

   The puncture needle should infiltrate the layers possibly involved in the operation, including muscular layer and deep muscular layer. In the process of anesthesia, it is necessary to withdraw repeatedly to avoid injecting drugs into the blood, and at the same time, pay attention to whether there is skin infection or tumor at the puncture site. In addition, drug overdose should be avoided.

4. Intraoperative Monitoring and Support

   Monitoring the pulse oxygen saturation.

11.6.4 Treatment of Severe Local Anesthetic Toxicity

1. Clinical Symptoms

   After injection of local anesthetic, patients suddenly lose consciousness and concurrently, they may develop convulsion, circulatory collapse, bradycardia, conduction block, cardiac arrest, and ventricular arrhythmia.

2. Treatment

   Firstly, anesthesiologists should stop administering local anesthetics and keep the airway patent. When necessary, the tracheal intubation should be implemented to ensure good ventilation while 100% oxygen should be supplied. Then, patients should be given benzodiazepines, thiopental sodium or low-dose propofol to treat convulsions. Cardiopulmonary-cerebral resuscitation (CPR) in standard mode should be started immediately for cardiac arrest patients. Patients should be injected with 20% fat emulsion with a loading dose of 1.5 mL/kg (the maximum loading dose is 100 mL) for more than 1 min, followed by continuous intravenous infusion at 0.25 mL/kg/min. The loading dose can be repeated until a good and stable circulation is restored, and the total dose should not exceed 12 mL/kg.

11.7 Intraoperative Monitoring

To ensure the safety of patients during operation, intraoperative monitoring should be strengthened. Anesthesia equipment should be set with reasonable alarm limits and continuous activated audible alarm, which can be heard in the whole operating room area. Basic life monitoring includes non-invasive blood pressure, electrocardiogram, pulse oxygen saturation, respiration, end-expiratory carbon dioxide partial pressure, and body temperature. It is expected that invasive arterial blood pressure, central venous pressure, cardiac output, and urine output should be monitored for patients in plastic surgery or with basic diseases, since they may have more blood loss. Patients under general anesthesia should be monitored with their concentration of inhaled oxygen and anesthetics, and respiratory parameters. Anesthesiologists should pay attention to the operation process and bleeding, whether there are any adverse nerve reflexes, massive bleeding, etc., and correct them in time. For local anesthesia, we should closely observe the patient's reaction, namely, whether there is cold sweat, chills, conscious disorders, numbness of lips, slurred speech, etc. Once such symptoms are observed, they should be treated immediately [8, 9].

11.8 Post-anesthesia Management

11.8.1 Post-anesthesia Recovery Management

To ensure the safety of patients after surgery, all patients must recover in appropriate places after anesthesia. Patients receiving general anesthesia with endotracheal intubation or laryngeal mask airway, deep sedation and analgesia, and peripheral nerve block anesthesia should be transferred to PACU for recover after surgery. Patients receiving local anesthesia, mild and moderate sedation, and analgesia should stay in certain recovery area after surgery.

PACU should be equipped with oxygen supply, power supply, negative pressure suction device, ventilator, monitor, simple respirator, emergency airway equipment, defibrillator, thermal insulation equipment, tracheal intubation and emergency airway treatment devices. Drugs such as antihypertensive drugs, antiarrhythmic drugs, cardiotonic drugs, antagonists, diuretics, antiasthmatic and spasmolytic drugs, sedative and analgesic drugs, hormones, etc. should be constantly prepared in PACU.

After patients are transferred to PACU, the chief anesthesiologists and the doctors in the care unit should communicate the anesthesia status of patients during operation, including the general information, the history of using special drugs, the induction and maintenance of anesthesia, whether there are any special conditions such as difficult airway, massive bleeding, the operation region, whether the operation has any potential impact on the airway, whether the tracheal catheter is retained after operation, etc.

After entering PACU, patients should be oxygenated and provided with breathing support and strengthened monitoring, including ECG, blood pressure, pulse oxygen saturation, respiration, body temperature, etc. According to individual patient's situation, the necessary anesthesia antagonism treatment may be carried out. The extubation should depend on the recovery of the patient's consciousness, breathing and muscle tension. Noticeably, the airway risk should be reassessed before extubation. After extubation, patients should inhale oxygen with mask, and vital signs such as respiratory rate, pulse oxygen saturation, electrocardiogram, and blood pressure should still be monitored.

Only patients who meet the discharge criteria of PACU can be transferred to general ward. All patients must be evaluated and recorded by the anesthesiologist in charge of PACU before discharging. The PACU discharge criteria can refer to Steward Awakening Scale (Table 11.1) and Aldrete Scoring System (Table 11.2), while the risk of airway obstruction being excluded, the vital signs such as heart rate, blood pressure, tidal volume, respiratory rate, and pulse oxygen saturation remaining stable for at least 1 h, and the postoperative pain being well controlled.

11.8.2 Postoperative Follow-Up

In order to ensure patient safety, postoperative follow-up visits should be strengthened and should be taken charge of by a qualified anesthesiologist or anesthesiology nurse. The postoperative follow-up is usually completed at the first day after surgery, and visits and treatment are

Table 11.2 Aldrete Scoring System

Score item	Answer choices (points)
Consciousness	Fully awake (2)
	Arousable on calling (1)
	Not responding (0)
Mobility—On command	Able to move four extremities (2)
	Able to move two extremities (1)
	Able to move 0 extremities (0)
Breathing	Able to breathe deeply (2)
	Dyspnea (1)
	Apnea (0)
Circulation	Systemic BP ≠ 20% of the preanesthetic level (2)
	Systemic BP between 20% and 49% of the preanesthetic level (1)
	Systemic BP ≠ 50% of the preanesthetic level (0)
SPO_2	Maintain $SpO_2 > 92\%$ in ambient air (2)
	Maintain $SpO_2 > 90\%$ with O_2 (1)
	Maintain $SpO_2 < 90\%$ with O_2 (0)

Note: Results vary between 0 and 10. Patients with scores of 9 and 10 can be safely discharged from PACU

Table 11.1 Steward Post-anesthetic Recovery Score System

Patient Sign	Criterion	Score
Consciousness	• Awake	2
	• Responds to stimuli	1
	• Does not respond to stimuli	0
Airway	• Actively crying or coughing on command	2
	• Maintain airway patency	1
	• Requires assistance to maintain airway patency	0
Movements	• Moves limbs purposefully	2
	• Moves limbs randomly	1
	• Not moving	0

Note: The total score of the above three items is 6. Patients with score above 4 can be safely discharged from PACU done at any time in special emergencies. During postoperative follow-up, anesthesiologists should closely observe patients' vital signs such as consciousness, circulation, respiration, postoperative analgesic effect, the presence of postoperative nausea and vomiting, and other adverse reactions, so that they can timely manage the anesthesia-related complications, learn about the preoperative long-term treatment of hypertension and other diseases, and collect and handle problems related to patient satisfaction with anesthesia and other psychological problems.

11.8.3 Postoperative Pain Management

Postoperative analgesia should be adopted early in order to improve patient comfort and movements, following the principle of voluntary and informed consent. Individualized, multimodal postoperative analgesic measures should be taken according to the patient's condition, such as surgery types, underlying disease, etc. Postoperative nausea and vomiting and other adverse reactions should be actively prevented and treated. Monitoring should be strengthened and respiratory depression should be prevented during postoperative analgesia. When patient-controlled analgesia is used, patients should be fully informed the operation procedures and precautions of the device. Medical and nursing staff specializing in pain treatment work should be designated to follow-up and record the changes in patients' vital signs, analgesic effects, adverse reactions and treatment methods and results before and after analgesia, and to evaluate and record the treatment effects.

11.9 Airway Management for Cosmetic Head, Neck, and Maxillofacial Surgery

11.9.1 Airway Assessment

For patients undergoing head, neck, and maxillofacial plastic surgery, more emphasis should be placed on airway assessment during the preanesthetic visit. Anesthesiologists ask for the medical history regarding the airway and review relevant anesthesia records, to learn if patients have difficult airway history, if necessary. Physical examination includes modified Mallampati classification, mouth opening, thyromental distance, relation of maxillary and mandibular incisors, atlantoaxial joint extension, and Cormack-Lehane classification.

11.9.2 Airway Devices

Each anesthesia department should have an anesthesia cart or equipment box prepared for difficult airway management which should be equipped with devices such as direct laryngoscopes with various types and sizes of lenses, visual laryngoscopes, stylets, laryngeal masks, and fiberoptic bronchoscope. At least one type of emergency airway tool (laryngeal mask, cricothyroid puncture ventilation device) should be equipped. The cart should be regularly checked, replenished, and replaced by a special staff, so that all instruments are in standby and placed in fixed position.

11.9.3 Management of Anticipated Difficult Airway

Patients who are anticipated that may have difficult airway in the anesthesia should be informed of the risk so that they and their family members could fully understand the situation and cooperate with hospital staffs. During the surgery, there should be at least one senior anesthesiologist experienced with difficult airway management responsible for airway management and an assistant involved in the process. A preferred plan and an alternative choice for establishing the airway should be identified prior to anesthesia, and the alternative option should be performed promptly when the preferred one fails. The operator should adopt familiar techniques and devices, and minimally invasive approaches are preferred. When necessary, awake tracheal intubation with the preservation of patients' voluntary breathing could be an option. After three times of unsuccessful intubation attempt, the operator should consider postponing or abandoning anesthesia and surgery [10].

11.9.4 Unanticipated Difficult Airway

For patients who are successfully ventilated but have difficulty in laryngoscopy and intubation, visual laryngoscope or fiberoptic bronchoscope can be selected to facilitate intubation. For those who have difficulty with ventilation, immediate assistance should be sought. Using an oropharyngeal airway, tightening the mask, lifting the jaw, and performing pressure ventilation by two clinicians to deal with the situation. If an anesthesiologist experienced in using laryngeal mask airway is present, a laryngeal mask airway should be placed immediately. If the above methods are not effective, an emergency surgical airway should be established, and waking the patient and canceling the procedure to ensure the patient's life should be considered.

11.9.5 Intraoperative Airway Management

It should be noted that the risk of intraoperative dislodgement of anesthetic equipment and line connectors, twisting and displacement of the endotracheal tubes in oral and maxillofacial plastic surgery is higher than that of general surgery, which may result in hypoxia and serious consequences for the patient, given the proximity of the tracheal intubation tube and anesthesia lines to the surgical field of head, neck, and maxillofacial plastic surgery. Before surgical sterilization, anesthesiologists should check and confirm that the tracheal tube is correctly positioned and securely fixed, and that the anesthesia line connector is tightly connected. Intraoperatively, the position of the tracheal tube and the tightness of the anesthesia line should be closely observed, and the respiratory parameters such as end-expiratory carbon dioxide, airway pressure, and pulse oxygen saturation should be monitored.

11.9.6 Postoperative Airway Management

It should be noted that head, neck, and maxillofacial plastic surgery, especially mandibular, chin, oral, and nasal surgery, are the most common procedures leading to postoperative airway obstruction and asphyxia and require adequate attention. Bleeding from surgical sites or the formation of hematomas in airway may lead to airway obstruction. Injury to the deep branch of the middle artery of the occlusal muscle, which can bleed up to 1500 mL or more and is difficult to be stopped, is a major cause of postoperative local hematoma and airway obstruction in mandibuloplasty. Oropharyngeal tissue edema and submucosal bleeding occurred in surgery should not be ignored. In addition, improper placement or strength of the dressing and drainage after maxillofacial plastic surgery causes local compression affecting the patient's cough and swallowing, which may induce nausea and vomiting and aspiration, increasing the risk of airway obstruction. Therefore, the tracheal tube should be removed only after airway problems are ruled out, and oxygen should be given at the same time. For surgery with difficult airway, the need for retaining the tube should be considered according to the patient's postoperative airway and surgery condition with the purpose of ensuring airway safety.

11.10 First Aid Treatment of Crisis in Plastic Surgery

11.10.1 Airway Obstruction

Symptoms	First aid treatment
Glossocoma to the pharynx obstructing the upper airway	Tilt the head back, lift the jaw, and place the oropharynx or nasopharynx to achieve ventilation.
Secretions, purulent sputum, blood, foreign body obstructing the airway	Check the oral cavity and remove the foreign body from the airway.
Reflux and aspiration	Turn the head down to one side, suck the airway, and relieve bronchospasm.

Symptoms	First aid treatment
Allergic laryngeal edema	Provide anti-allergic treatment, oxygen administration by mask pressure. In severe cases, perform tracheal intubation.
Laryngospasm	Remove local irritation and administer pressure oxygen by mask. In severe cases, give muscle relaxants and perform tracheal intubation.

11.10.2 Anaphylaxis

1. Symptoms
   In addition to symptoms on skin, hypotension, tachycardia or bradycardia, and arrhythmia, or even cardiac arrest may occur as well.
2. First Aid Treatment
   (a) Stop giving suspicious drugs immediately.
   (b) Stabilize the circulation, rapidly infuse electrolyte solution, and promptly inject small doses of epinephrine intravenously, 30–50 μg repeatedly in 5–10 min, or continuously infuse 1–10 μg/min if necessary. If the circulation is severely depressed, phenylephrine, norepinephrine, vasopressin, and glucagon can also be infused continuously through intravenous.
   (c) Relieve bronchospasm, provide pure oxygen inhalation; perform endotracheal intubation and mechanical ventilation if necessary, let patients inhale salbutamol or ipratropium bromide.
   (d) Intravenous infusion of adrenocorticotropic hormone, preferably hydrocortisone or methylprednisolone. Hydrocortisone succinate 1–2 mg/kg can be given intravenously, which can be repeated after 6 h but not exceeding 300 mg in 24 h; methylprednisolone 1 mg/kg can also be given intravenously, not exceeding 1 g in total.
   (e) Skin testing should be completed 4–6 weeks after incision healing to determine the allergen and inform the patient and family of the results, and at the same time fill out an allergic reaction warning card for record purposes.

11.10.3 Fat Embolism Syndrome

1. Symptoms
   Hypoxemia with arterial partial pressure of oxygen less than 60 mmHg and fat particles found in blood, urine and sputum.
2. First Aid Treatment
   (a) Provide oxygen therapy and respiratory support treatment. Perform early mechanical ventilation when dyspnea is obvious and pulse oxygen saturation is less than 90%.
   (b) Provide circulatory support. Continuous intravenous infusion of appropriate amount of vasoactive drugs such as dopamine, norepinephrine, or phenylephrine to maintain circulation.
   (c) Hormone therapy, preferably hydrocortisone or methylprednisolone [11].

11.10.4 Malignant Hyperthermia

1. Triggers and Symptoms
   It is mainly induced by inhaled anesthetics or depolarizing muscle relaxants such as succinylcholine. The clinical manifestations are masseter muscle spasms, developing to muscle spasms of the whole body, which cannot be relieved by muscle relaxants. The partial pressure of end-tidal carbon dioxide and body temperature rises sharply. The temperature of the absorbent canister increases and burns. The complication may rapidly progress to multi-organ failure with high mortality.
2. First Aid Treatment
   (a) Immediately stop the inhalation of anesthetics and succinylcholine and suspend surgery.
   (b) Replace the anesthesia machine's tubes and absorbent canister, hyperventilate with pure oxygen to expel carbon dioxide.
   (c) Enhance monitoring and transfer to an intensive care unit or a general hospital capable of treating such complications.
   (d) Correct metabolic acidosis with sodium bicarbonate and monitor arterial blood gas.

(e) Actively apply all possible methods to lower the body temperature, and adopt extra corporal circulation if necessary.
(f) Correct hyperkalemia and abandon calcium.
(g) Correct cardiac arrhythmias by inotropes and vasoactive drugs.
(h) Replenish blood volume to maintain hemodynamic stability; using diuretic and monitor urine output.
(i) Infuse dantrolene, a potent antagonist, as early as possible.
(j) Strengthen the prevention and treatment of disseminated intravascular coagulation and renal failure [12].

11.10.5 Cardiac and Respiratory Arrest

1. Symptoms.

   It is manifested as cardiac arrest, ventricular fibrillation, and cardiac electromechanical dissociation, which may be transformed into each other.
2. First Aid Treatment:
   (a) In case of perioperative respiratory arrest, cardiopulmonary resuscitation should be performed immediately, while calling other medical personnel to help resuscitate the patient.
   (b) Quickly prepare defibrillator and emergency vehicle to provide basic life support, which includes immediate application of chest cardiac compressions, tracheal intubation for patients who have not been intubated and opening two intravenous accesses if necessary.
   (c) Advanced life support includes electrical defibrillation and pacing, restoration of autonomic circulation, stabilization of blood pressure, monitoring, recognition, and treatment of arrhythmias, and restoration of respiration. Adrenaline is the drug of choice.
   (d) Continued life support includes the maintenance of effective ventilation, circulation and acid-base equilibrium, the prevention of cerebral edema, and the active cerebral resuscitation.
   (e) Treat the primary disease to prevent acute functional failure and secondary infection.
   (f) Participants in resuscitation should closely cooperate with each other, be organized, strictly check and keep records in a timely manner, and keep ampoules and bottles of all drugs to record the process of resuscitation accurately and factually [13, 14].

References

1. Failey C, Aburto J, de la Portilla HG, Romero JF, Lapuerta L, Barrera A. Office-based outpatient plastic surgery utilizing total intravenous anesthesia. Aesthet Surg J. 2013;33(2):270–4. Epub 2013 Jan 18. PMID: 23335648. https://doi.org/10.1177/1090820X12472694.
2. Shapiro FE. Anesthesia for outpatient cosmetic surgery. Curr Opin Anesthesiol. 2008;21:704–10.
3. May DM. Ambulatory anesthesia for cosmetic surgery in Brazil. Anesthesia outside the operating room. Curr Opin Anesthesiol. 2016;29:493–8.
4. Taub PJ, Bashey S, Hausman LM. Anesthesia for cosmetic surgery. Plast Reconstr Surg. 2010;125(1):1e–7e. PMID: 19910860. https://doi.org/10.1097/PRS.0b013e3181c2a268.
5. Allak A, Conderman CP. Analgesia and conscious sedation. In: Wong BJF, Arnold MG, Boeckmann JO, editors. Facial plastic and reconstructive surgery. Cham: Springer; 2021. https://doi.org/10.1007/978-3-030-45920-8_1.
6. Suresh S, Ecoffey C, Bosenberg A, et al. The European Society of Regional Anaesthesia and Pain Therapy/American Society of Regional Anesthesia and Pain Medicine recommendations on local anesthetics and adjuvants dosage in pediatric regional anesthesia. Reg Anesth Pain Med. Pediatric Analgesia. 2018;43(2):211–6.
7. Suresh S, Ecoffey C, Bosenberg A, et al. The Third American Society of Regional Anesthesia and Pain Medicine Practice Advisory on local anesthetic systemic toxicity. Reg Anesth Acute Pain. 2018;43(2):113–23.
8. Gelb AW, Morriss WW, Johnson W, et al. World Health Organization-world Federation of Societies of anaesthesiologists (WHO-WFSA) international standards for a safe practice of Anesthesia. Can J Anesth. 2018;65:698–708.
9. Luba K, Apfelbaum JL, Cutter TW. Airway management in the outpatient setting. Clin Plast Surg. 2013;40:405–17.

10. American Society of Anesthesiologists Task Force on Management of the Difficult Airway. Practice guidelines for management of the difficult airway: an updated report by the American Society of Anesthesiologists Task Force on Management of the Difficult Airway. Anesthesiology. 2013;118:251–70.
11. John FB. Morgan & Mikhail's clinical anesthesiology. 5th ed. New York: McGraw-Hill Education/Medical; 2013.
12. Riazi S, Kraeva N, Hopkins PM. Updated guide for the management of malignant hyperthermia. Can J Anesth. 2018;65:709–21.
13. Wilton CL. Clinical anesthesia procedures of the Massachusetts General Hospital. 8th ed. Philadelphia: Lippincott Williams and Wilkins; 2010.
14. Ronald DM. Miller's anesthesia. 8th ed. Chicago: Saunders; 2014.

12 Anesthesia for Oral and Maxillofacial Head and Neck Infections

Jie Chen

12.1 Introduction

Odontogenic infection is the main cause of oral and maxillofacial infection. The existence of sinuses, cavities, and other structures in the oral and maxillofacial region forms a vulnerable environment, which has special tissues such as teeth, with a superficial location, and rich sweat glands, hair follicles, and sebaceous glands in the facial area, with abundant blood circulation, and a large number of microorganisms in the oral cavity. When the body's resistance to diseases is lessened or the body has suffered stress, injury or surgical trauma, the micro-ecological balance in the body is dislocated, further leading to the occurrence of oral and maxillofacial infections. Oral and maxillofacial infections are mainly mixed infections caused by aerobic and anaerobic bacteria. There is a network of many potential spaces in the maxillofacial bones, which are filled with loose connective tissues. Therefore, once infection occurs, the tissues are likely to spread to each other and cause diffuse infection. Oral and maxillofacial infections can spread downward through the deep cervical fascia to the anterior tracheal space, the vascular fascial space, or even lead to cervical or mediastinal abscesses of greater severity [1, 2].

12.2 Origins and Manifestations of Oral and Maxillofacial Infections

Oral and maxillofacial infections can be divided into the following categories according to the origins: odontogenic, hematogenous, adenogenic, traumatic, and iatrogenic infections. The acute phase is a typical manifestation of inflammation: redness, swelling, warmth, pain, and dysfunction. When the infection involves the masseter muscles and masseteric space, it may lead to restricted mouth opening; when the infection affects the soft tissues of the buccal bottom, parapharyngeal spaces, and neck, it may lead to difficulty in eating and swallowing, and even dyspnea; when the infection involves the tissue space, the gas produced by bacteria might cause localized crepitus. When abscesses appear in the infected tissues, the properties of the pus may vary if the infecting organism is different. When oral and maxillofacial infections become chronic, local proliferative fibrous connective tissue replaces normal tissue to form chronic sinuses and fistulas. Severe oral and maxillofacial infection may be accompanied by systemic poisoning symptoms and even toxic shock.

J. Chen (✉)
Department of Anesthesiology, Shanghai Ninth People's Hospital Affiliated to Shanghai Jiao Tong University School of Medicine, Shanghai, China

H. Jiang, M. Xia (eds.), *Anesthesia for Oral and Maxillofacial Surgery*,
https://doi.org/10.1007/978-981-19-7287-4_12

12.3 Common Oral and Maxillofacial Infectious Diseases

12.3.1 Pericoronitis of Third Molar

Pericoronitis of third molar is an inflammation of the soft tissues surrounding the tooth crown of a wisdom tooth with incomplete eruption or obstruction as the etiology of the disease, and clinically it is mostly seen in mandibular third molar. The mandibular third molar is the last tooth to erupt, also known as the wisdom tooth. The crown of third molar is partially or completely covered by the gingival flap due to its insufficient eruption position, which is prone to have bacteria and food embedded in it. Pericoronitis may occur when the gums on the crown of the third molar are injured while chewing food or when the body's resistance is reduced.

Pericoronitis of third molar usually has no obvious systemic symptoms. Swelling and discomfort may appear in the molar area, with pain arising during chewing and movement. If the condition further worsens and the masticatory muscles are involved, mouth opening may be limited to varying degrees. Systemic symptoms shall appear in severe cases.

In the acute phase, pericoronitis of third molar should be treated with anti-inflammatory therapy and incisional drainage as soon as possible. When it comes to chronic stage, pericoronary gingival flap removal under local anesthesia is required. If the third molar is malposed or not erupted, or even with facial fistula in severe cases, third molar extraction and fistula resection can be performed under local or general anesthesia.

12.3.2 Oral and Maxillofacial Interstitial Infections

Oral maxillofacial interstitial infections are mainly of odontogenic or glandular origin, while other ways of infections are less common [3]. Oral maxillofacial and cervical areas are surrounded by fascia and there are loose connective tissues within fascia. Since oral maxillofacial interstitial infections are mostly caused by the combination of aerobic and anaerobic bacteria, in early stage, it is mainly manifested as cellulitis. When the adipose tissue is involved, it will lead to fat liquefaction and abscess necrosis. When the infection involves multiple interstitial spaces in the maxillofacial and cervical areas, diffuse cellulitis or abscess can be formed. In severe cases, cavernous sinus thrombophlebitis, brain abscess, mediastinal infection, and systemic poisoning symptoms can be caused. The infections can be classified as follows according to the interstices of infection:

1. Infection of Infraorbital Space

   Infraorbital space is the space among the infraorbital area, the anterior wall of the maxilla, and the facial expression muscles. When infection occurs in the infraorbital space, it often involves multiple areas of skin, including the inner canthus, eyelids, and cheekbones. In severe cases, orbital cellulitis and cavernous sinus thrombophlebitis may occur.

   Low incision and drainage of the abscess is feasible in the early stage of treatment, which is supplemented with systemic anti-inflammatory medication. After the inflammation is kept down, the focal tooth shall be extracted.
2. Buccal Cavity Infection

   A buccal cavity infection refers to the infection of the space between the buccal skin of and the buccal mucosa, or in a narrower sense, the buccal space infection between the masseter and buccal muscles.

   The treatment consists of intraoral or facial incision and drainage depending on the site of the abscess.
3. Infection of Temporal Space

   Infection of temporal space is the infection of both superficial and deep temporal space. There is edema, compression pain, and restriction of mouth opening in the lesion area. The temporal muscles are solid, thus chronic abscesses can cause temporal osteomyelitis, and the infection might also spread from the squamotemporal sutura into the brain, forming brain abscesses, and meningitis, etc.

For treatment, incision and drainage should be performed according to the depth of the abscess site. If osteomyelitis of skull occurs, sequestrum and lesion removal should be actively applied to avoid intracranial infection.

4. Infection of Infratemporal Space

   Temporomandibular space infection mainly refers to the infection spread from the adjacent space. Clinically, it is often manifested as varying degrees of limited openings, accompanied by swelling of relevant areas, eye movement disorders, headache, nausea, etc.

   For treatment, intraoral or extraoral incision and drainage shall be performed, accompanied by antibiotics.

5. Masseter Space Infection

   Masseter space infection is one of the most common maxillofacial space infections, which mainly originates from pericoronitis of mandibular of third molar, alveolar abscess or adjacent space infection. The clinical manifestations are swelling, compression pain, and limitation of mouth opening in the masseter area. If the inflammation becomes chronic, osteomyelitis at the edge of mandibular branch might be developed.

   The principle of treatment is to apply general antibiotics. If there is any local abscess, timely incision and drainage is required. In case of osteomyelitis, lesion curettage should be performed early and the sequestrum should be removed.

6. Pterygomandibular Space Infection

   The infection of pterygomandibular space is caused by the spread of pericoronitis of third molar and premolar inflammation to the inside of mandible and the outside of medial pterygoid muscle. Clinically, it often starts with toothache, followed by restriction of mouth opening and abscesses deep in the pterygomandibular region, which in severe cases, can spread further into the adjacent space in severe cases.

   The treatment shall include incision and drainage of intraoral and extraoral abscess and systemic anti-inflammatory therapy.

7. Infection of Sublingual Space

   The sublingual space is the space between the tongue and the floor of mouth, and most of the infections are odontogenic. The clinical manifestations are limitation of tongue movement, elevation of the floor of mouth, difficulty in eating and swallowing with pain.

   The treatment is incision and drainage of abscess in the swelling area of the floor of mouth.

8. The Infection of Parapharyngeal Space

   The parapharyngeal space is located lateral to the pharyngeal cavity, in a potential area among the cephalopharyngeus, deep lobe of the parotid gland, and the medial pterygoid muscle. The infections are also mostly odontogenic, with clinical manifestations of redness and swelling of the lateral wall of pharynx and palatal tonsil protrusion. When accompanied by infection of pterygomandibular space or other adjacent spaces, there might be redness and distending pain in the neck, hoarseness, difficulty in eating, swallow pain, and in severe cases, expiratory dyspnea. If the infection spreads further to the parapharyngeal and submandibular spaces, it is often likely to form mediastinal abscess due to breathing and negative pressure in the thoracic cavity.

   The treatment includes incision and drainage by intraoral and extraoral approaches and systemic anti-inflammatory therapy.

9. Infection of Submandibular Space

   The submandibular space is a loose connective tissue located in the submandibular triangle. Infections in the submandibular space are mostly odontogenic, with clinical manifestations of swelling in the submandibular area, enlarged lymph nodes. Once the infection spreads, tongue swelling, exercise pain, and dysphagia may occur.

   For treatment, incision of drainage of abscess and systemic treatment should be applied.

10. Submental Space Infection

    The submental space lies between the submental triangle and the suprahyoid region. The infection is mostly generated from lymph nodes and is limited to lymph nodes in the early stage. However, in severe cases, the swelling extends to the submental triangle with local congestion and flare.

    This infection should be treated by local incision and drainage of submental triangle.

11. Cellulitis of the Floor of the Mouth

    Cellulitis of the floor of the mouth involves multiple sublingual, submandibular, and submental spaces when the infection spreads further to the deep cervical fascia and mediastinum, which is particularly fatal.

    The clinical manifestation of cellulitis of the floor of mouth is anthorisma, local redness, swelling, and thermal pain, accompanied by hardening of skin tissue. When deep muscle tissue is necrotic, fluctuation may occur, and sometimes massive crepitus can be detected. The patient experiences elevation of the tongue, limited tongue extension, slurred speech, and difficulty in swallowing due to the swelling of the floor of mouth. When the inflammation spreads to the root of the tongue and the deep part of the pharyngeal cavity, there may be symptoms such as dyspnea, irritability, and even "three concave sign," which can be life-threatening due to asphyxia. When the infection spreads to the mediastinum, the patient may develop high fever, dyspnea, and toxic shock.

    Antibiotic therapy should be adopted in the early stage, meanwhile extensive incision and drainage should be applied ensuring airway patency. However, if the infection has spread to the mediastinum and formed a mediastinal abscess, negative pressure drainage of the mediastinal cavity must be performed, and symptomatic supportive treatment of systemic conditions is also very important.

12.4 Osteomyelitis of Jaw

Osteomyelitis of jaw is a sort of inflammation of jaws caused by bacterial or physicochemical factors. Osteomyelitis of jaw is mostly caused by odontogenic infection, the most common route of infection for osteomyelitis of jaw is odontogenic infection. According to the pathogenesis, osteomyelitis of jaw can be classified as pyogenic osteomyelitis of the jaws and specific jaw osteomyelitis. In addition, factors such as radiotherapy can also cause osteomyelitis of the jaws and osteonecrosis. According to the cause of infection, the specific classification is as follows.

1. Pyogenic osteomyelitis of the jaws

   Staphylococcus aureus is the most common pathogen of pyogenic osteomyelitis of the jaws, and odontogenic infection is the main route of infection. In the acute phase of osteomyelitis of jaw, there can be severe pain in the teeth of lesion area, while the chronic phase presents with abscesses, diabrosis, and restriction of mouth opening in the lesion area. The chronic phase of central osteomyelitis of jaw starts at 2 weeks after the onset of the acute phase and is mainly characterized by the formation of massive inflammatory granulation tissue, sequestrum, and fistula in the oral cavity and skin. Marginal jaw osteomyelitis is also mostly an odontogenic infection, with symptoms like those of subpteral space infection and masseter muscle infection in the acute phase and often accompanied with restriction of mouth opening and dysphagia in the chronic phase [3, 4].

   The infections shall be treated with surgery and systemic supportive treatment. Surgical treatment includes removal of infectious lesions and drainage of pus.

2. Osteomyelitis of Jaw in Newborn

   Osteomyelitis of jaw in newborn usually refers to pyogenic central jaw osteomyelitis in infants and children within 3 months of birth, which is mainly associated with blood-borne or mother-to-child factors. Clinical manifestations include redness and swelling of the skin in the lesion area, eyelid swelling, formation of sequestrum, and fistula formed after pus overflow.

Osteomyelitis of jaw in newborn shall be treated with systemic anti-inflammatory therapy, incision, and drainage should be applied in the early stage.

3. Radiation Osteomyelitis of Jaw

   Radiation osteomyelitis of the jaw is a sort of osteomyelitis induced by secondary infection after jaw necrosis due to radiation factors. The clinical course of the disease is long, patients are characterized by emaciation and anemia. There is severe pinprick-like pain in the early stage, with muscle atrophy and fibrosis, ulcerations, defects, and deformities at the lesion site.

   Systemic anti-inflammatory therapy should be applied, sequestrum needs to be removed by local surgery.

4. Chemical Jaw Necrosis

   Chemical jaw necrosis is defined as osteonecrosis of the jaw caused by the application of bone resorption inhibitor or anti-angiogenesis drugs. Clinical manifestations are local swelling and pain, oral and gingival infections, apocenosis, and formation of fistulas and sinus tracts.

   Chemical Jaw Necrosis should be treated with systemic anti-inflammatory therapy and debridement and drainage surgery.

12.5 Other Oral and Maxillofacial Infections

1. Lymphadenitis of Face and Neck

   Lymphadenitis of the face and neck can originate from oral and maxillofacial infections or facial skin infections. For children, it can be caused by upper respiratory tract infections and tonsillitis. Clinical manifestations are local lymphadenopathy, pain, and local inflammatory infiltrative masses, which may be accompanied by mild or severe systemic symptoms. Tuberculous lymphadenitis is characterized by "cold abscess" in the lymph nodes and the formation of sinus tracts or fistulas.

   The treatment includes systemic anti-inflammatory therapy and incision and drainage.

2. Facial Furuncle and Carbuncle

   Facial furuncle and carbuncle is the inflammation of skin, hair follicles, and other adnexa. Furuncle refers to the infection of single hair follicles and relevant adnexa, while infection of most adjacent hair follicles and their adnexa is called a carbuncle. The clinical manifestation is induration of redness, swelling, flare, and pain. If the inflammation spreads, systemic poisoning symptoms may occur.

   Systemic and local therapy should be combined for treatment.

3. Maxillofacial Tuberculosis, Syphilis, Actinomycosis

   Oral and maxillofacial tuberculosis is mostly hematogenous. In the early stage, there is only a systemic low-grade fever and anthorisma of soft tissue. In the later stage, sinus tracts, cold abscesses, and systemic symptoms may appear at the lesion site. There should be anti-tuberculosis therapy and surgical removal of sequestrum from the lesion.

   Maxillofacial actinomycosis is a chronic granuloma of facial soft tissue caused by actinomyces infection. Clinically, patients are predominantly male and present with tissue hardening, multiple abscesses or fistulas, and sulfur-like granules within the abscesses. The principle of treatment is to focus on antibacterial drugs, with surgery if necessary.

   The main clinical manifestations of maxillofacial syphilis are oral and lip chancre, syphilis rash, and gum-like swelling. Systemic treatment is preferred and after the syphilis lesion is basically controlled, surgery can be considered for the repair of the remaining tissue defects and deformities.

12.6 Characteristics of Anesthesia Management

1. Severe infection of the oral and maxillofacial regions can lead to maxillofacial swelling and restriction of mouth opening. The displacement of the floor of mouth and neck tissue is often accompanied by dysphagia and dyspnea. The difficulty of intubation needs to be fully assessed before induction of anesthesia, and a comprehensive assessment of 3D airway reconstruction can be applied if available. If there is acute upper respiratory tract obstruction and loss of consciousness, tracheotomy should be performed immediately.
2. Patients with severe multi-space infections involving the floor of mouth or the neck are often in a critical condition, and most of them are undergoing emergency surgeries with a full stomach. The anesthesiologist should immediately clarify the patient's airway obstruction, deal with it presuming a full stomach, prepare for difficult airway intubation. Meanwhile, emergency tracheotomy device should be prepared at the bedside.
3. Patients with oral and maxillofacial infections accompanied by systemic toxic symptoms may develop hypovolemia and circulatory failure induced by infectious shock during perioperative period, which should be taken seriously and corrected in time before anesthesia.
4. After the operation of oral and maxillofacial infections, the swelling and bleeding of the surgical wound can easily involve the airway. Therefore, it is necessary to cautiously judge whether an indwelling tracheal tube should be kept after surgery. If necessary, the tracheal tube should be indwelling and the patient should be admitted to the monitoring room for further observation and treatment, and the tracheal tube shall be removed after the swelling of the oropharynx has subsided.

12.7 Anesthesia in Common Use

12.7.1 Pre-anesthetic Visit and Preparation

Anesthetists usually visit patients the day before surgery. However, since a large proportion of patients with oral and maxillofacial infections require emergency treatment under general anesthesia, which often involves complex airway management, the standard procedure of orotracheal or nasotracheal intubation presents significant challenges. Therefore, anesthetists are required to complete an accurate evaluation of the surgery patient's general condition and airway status in limited time and prepare for the procedure.

1. A detailed airway assessment must be carried out before anesthesia is administered. Swelling of the neck with a "woody" sensation when pressing and an opening of less than 4 cm are often associated with difficult mask ventilation. The following signs and symptoms suggest a difficult airway: Head turning pain; restriction of mouth opening; voice changes; dysarthria; dysphonia; tongue swelling; elevated floor of the mouth; dysphagia; drooling. When a patient shows neck crepitus, wheezing, dyspnea, and " three concave sign," it often indicates that the patient has an obstructed airway and airway crisis may appear at any time. General anesthesia under rapid sequence induction may lead to complete airway collapse, resulting in difficulty in mask ventilation and tracheal intubation. The awake intubation technology under fiberoptic bronchoscope can ensure airway safety to the greatest extent. Nevertheless, since this technique requires certain operation experience of the anesthetists, it is not risk-free, and in some cases, a rupture of parapharyngeal abscess may occur during intubation. Therefore, a preoperative preparation with a video laryngoscope, cricothyroid membrane

puncture kit, and emergency tracheotomy device is recommended.

2. Adequate imaging examination must be arranged to determine the depth and degree of infection in the cervical space, the degree of displacement and obstruction of pharyngeal portion, and whether there is any deviation in the position of the trachea, etc. Enhanced reconstruction of neck and maxillofacial CT and airway three-dimensional CT can help to accurately display the extent of head and neck infection, displacement of anatomical structures, etc.
3. The risk of awake intubation induced by fiberoptic bronchoscope will be increased in the presence of aggravated oral and maxillofacial infections, bacteremia, and sepsis. If the patient has severe systemic toxic symptoms, preoperative supportive therapy is recommended to maintain circulatory stability and correct acid-base and water-electrolyte imbalance.

12.7.2 Pre-anesthetic Medication

1. Topical surface anesthetics. Lidocaine is frequently-used for preoperative surface anesthesia. Lidocaine (1–2 mg/kg) can be administered intravenously 1–2 min before intubation to inhibit airway reflex. 4% Lidocaine spray can be used for surface anesthesia near the glottis after cricothyroid membrane puncture, and for surface anesthesia of nasopharyngeal and oropharyngeal cavities. Since lidocaine can cause burning pain when encountering infected tissue and take effects slow, sodium bicarbonate shall be used clinically to improve the pH value of lidocaine. Preoperatively, 4% lidocaine is recommended for local spray (nasopharyngeal cavity, oropharyngeal cavity, supraglottis) or oral nebulized lidocaine (like "respiratory nebulizer"). However, if the infection involves deep cervical portion and the anatomy of the neck is unclear, traditional methods such as supraglottic nerve blocks and cricothyroid membrane puncture for injections of topical anesthetics may lead to further spread of the infection.
2. Sedations and analgesics. Sedations and analgesics can increase the comfort for patients undergoing awake tracheal intubation. The benzodiazepine midazolam can be used for awake endotracheal intubation, but sedative drugs must be used with caution, for they can inhibit the central nervous system. It is used at a dose of 0.02–0.04 mg/kg as appropriate depending on the patient's age, severity of illness, and degree of airway obstruction prior to induction. Intravenous injection or drip of analgesic opioids can inhibit autonomous respiration and may aggravate the symptoms of airway obstruction in patients with severe oral and maxillofacial infections. Therefore, opioid analgesics are not recommended or must be used very carefully in patients with potential or definite airway crisis. On the premise that airway safety has been fully evaluated, the use of fentanyl at doses of 1–2 μg/kg by slow injection is recommended. Dexmedetomidine is recommended for patients with oral and maxillofacial infections and can be used as an adjunct for preoperative sedation of awake fiberoptic bronchoscopic endotracheal intubation. Dexmedetomidine will not damage protective reflexes, respiratory inhibition, or affect hemodynamics, hence is recommended to be administered at a dose of 0.7–1 μg/kg by slow intravenous injection or of 0.2–0.7 μg/(kg h) by intravenous infusion before induction.
3. Anticholinergic agents: In the absence of preoperative contraindications, preoperative administration of atropine 0.01–0.03 mg/kg or scopolamine 0.005–0.01 mg/kg is recommended for intramuscular injection 0.5 h before surgery.
4. Inhalation anesthetics: Slow inhalation of sevoflurane for induction before intubation can also rapidly influence the depth of anesthesia, maintain cardiovascular stability and

autonomous respiration, thus sevoflurane induction is recommended for pediatric patients. When used in adult patients, the process of sevoflurane induction is often complex and slow, accompanied by the occurrence of apnea and hypoxemia. Since sudden airway obstruction may still occur, it is not recommended for adults.

12.7.3 The Practice of Anesthesia

The option of induction position: The patient is ideally placed in a 45-degree head-high semi-recumbent position with a thin pillow under the head in the sniffing position to maximize the opening of the oropharyngeal airway, to facilitate the placement of the nasopharyngeal airway.

The selection of induction modality: Standard direct laryngoscope exposure often fails in patients with deep cervical or floor of mouth multi-space infections. However, due to the complex and diverse symptoms, manifestations and aggravating factors of oral and maxillofacial infection, the correct method of airway management has not reached a consensus. If the patient is evaluated as potentially difficult airway, the following three intubation techniques are recommended: (1) awake nasotracheal or orotracheal intubation via fiberoptic bronchoscopy; (2) awake blind nasotracheal intubation; (3) tracheotomy. At present, it is still not clear which of the three induction intubation techniques mentioned above is the best [5].

1. Awake Nasotracheal or Orotracheal Intubation via Fiberoptic Bronchoscopy

   This operative technique requires the anesthetist to have extensive clinical experience and operation skills, and the ability to apply appropriate amounts of preoperative sedations and analgesics (e.g., midazolam, dexmedetomidine, fentanyl, etc.) to perform endotracheal intubation with preserved consciousness and autonomous respiration. Sophisticated surface anesthesia shall reduce the stress response of the sympathetic and endocrine systems as well as adverse memories by reducing intubation stimulation, and can ease the patient's pain, which is the key to accomplish the intubation.

   Specific operation: Put the tracheal tube on the fiberoptic bronchoscope rod, first insert the fiberoptic bronchoscope through the nose or mouth to the pharyngeal cavity, use the lever to rotate the handle, change the direction of the front of the scope rod. After finding the epiglottis and glottis, send the scope rod back into the glottis according to the principle of endoscope operation. Afterwards, send the tracheal tube into the trachea along the fiberoptic bronchoscope static rod, and finally withdraw the scope rod to complete intubation. Or insert the endotracheal tube to the pharyngeal cavity through the nose or mouth, and then insert the fiberoptic bronchoscope into the endotracheal tube, followed by the same method as above.

2. Awake Blind Nasotracheal Intubation

   Pre-intubation preparation is the same as above.

   Specific operation: For nasal intubation, after the completion of surface anesthesia, drop vasoconstrictor through the nose, deliver the selected catheter into the nasal cavity. Rotate the catheter at the same time when advancing and retreating the catheter, and adjust the head position (hypsokinesis—prostration—anteflexion) to accomplish the intubation. Or a new blind tracheal intubation device (the whole set of device includes esophagotracheal guiding tube, optical cable, and power box) pioneered by our hospital shall be used, which has changed the previous method of intubation and completes the intubation by entering the trachea under the guidance of esophagus and light guide, instead.

3. Tracheotomy

   For more information, please refer to relevant chapter on difficult airway management.

   Since tracheotomy may result in the connection of a neck abscess and the adjacent tissue space, and awake fiberoptic bronchoscopy has less impact on the degree of distortion of the neck anatomy, hence is less invasive and may be safer. When awake fiberoptic bronchoscopy intubation is performed, the risks and pros and cons of tracheotomy must be reported and discussed preoperatively. The advantages of tracheotomy are that it allows for early transfer of patients from the intensive care unit to the general ward, reduces costs and conserves more medical resources. However, tracheotomy presents risks of abscess spread, bleeding, scarring, pneumothorax, and long-term tracheal stenosis, etc. Therefore, there is a current preference to avoid tracheotomy if possible.

12.7.4 Intraoperative Monitoring and Management

1. Respiratory monitoring and management: Since the patient's head and neck belongs to the surgical area and the head position often needs to be changed during the surgery, the anesthetist must pay close attention to the observation of whether there are irregular issues such as folding and dislodging of the tracheal tube, so that it can be dealt with in a timely manner. When the tracheal intubation is completed, the type of maintenance anesthetics should be selected according to the patient's general condition and surgical stimulation. The patient's vital signs should be closely monitored during the operation, and meanwhile whether the surgical procedure affects or involves the airway should be observed. After the operation, the patient should be further observed for swelling, blood oozing, and head and the condition of facial bandages, in order to predict and evaluate whether the patient needs further indwelling of tracheal tube for observation and treatment. Patients with systemic poisoning symptoms may be accompanied by hypoxemia, imbalance of water-electrolyte and acid-base disturbance, resulting in disorder of the internal environment. Blood gas analysis should be monitored preoperatively and intraoperatively.
2. Circulation monitoring and management: Generally, incision and drainage play the major part in the surgery of oral and maxillofacial infections, and the operation time is relatively short. Certain oral and maxillofacial infections are often accompanied by systemic toxic symptoms and can even spread to the mediastinum, and such patients would require inter-disciplinary diagnosis and surgery. in addition to incision and drainage of the infected area of the head and neck, further flushing and drainage of the thoracic and mediastinal abscess is required, hence monitoring and management of circulation cannot be neglected. ECG, pulse oxygen saturation, and blood pressure should be monitored routinely, intraoperative fluid intake and output should be recorded and bleeding volume should be accurately estimated, and crystalloid and colloid fluids should be supplemented in time.

12.7.5 Recovery from Anesthesia

In the recovery room, the anesthetist in charge is supposed to do a good handover with the anesthetist of post-anesthesia care unit. In particular, it is necessary to explain the preoperative airway evaluation, endotracheal intubation method, the condition of postoperative wound swelling, blood oozing, etc. In addition to routine monitoring, close observation of the surgical area should be paid attention to. If abnormal circumstances such as wound pus and blood draining from soaking the surgical dressing, rapid swelling of the wound, fresh blood being drawn from the negative pressure drainage tube or even a decrease in blood pressure and an increase in pulse rate are found, the presence of active bleeding in the wound should be considered first. Whether the tracheal tube should be removed after surgery depends on the preoperative examination, the degree of infection and edema, and the adequacy of postoperative drainage. If there is massive edema and tissue induration on the wound surface of the floor of mouth, it is recommended to leave the tracheal tube in place and send the patient to the monitoring room for further observation and treatment.

The prognosis is often poor if the patient has a preoperative multi-space infection at the floor of the mouth, infection of a deep neck space, or infection involving the thoracic cavity and mediastinum. The patient must be admitted to the intensive care unit after surgery and treated with high-dose of systemic antibiotics. The tracheal tube must be left in place until the patient's systemic condition improves. In the process of extubation, an endotracheal tube changer shall be used to preserve the noninvasive intubation pathway and allow for immediate reintubation if necessary.

References

1. Zhiyuan Z, Bing S, Chenping Z. Oral and maxillofacial surgery. Shelton, CT: People's Medical Publishing House; 2020.
2. Miao W. Oral anesthesiology diagnosis and operation routine. Shelton, CT: People's Medical Publishing House; 2018.
3. Boyd Barry C, Sutter Steven J. Dexmedetomidine sedation for awake fiberoptic intubation of patients with difficult airways due to severe odontogenic cervicofacial infections. J Oral Maxillofac Surg. 2011;69:1608–12.
4. Wates E, Higginson J, Kichenaradjou A, McVeigh K. A severe deep neck odontogenic infection not prioritised by the emergency department triage system and National Early Warning Score. BMJ Case Rep. 2018;2018:bcr-2018-224634.
5. Doyle DJ, Hantzakos AG. Anesthetic Management of the Narrowed Airway. Otolaryngol Clin North Am. 2019;52(6):1127–39.

13 Anesthesia for Oral Maxillofacial and Neck Trauma

Shuang Cao

13.1 Introduction

The term trauma refers to physical damage to the body caused by mechanical, chemical, thermal, electrical, or other external forces beyond the body's capacity to withstand. The number of deaths due to traumatic injuries is as high as 5 million worldwide each year. According to the National Health Commission, the number of people who suffer from traumatic injuries such as traffic accidents, falls, and mechanical injuries in China is about 62 million each year, among which 700,000–800,000 die, making it the first cause of death for people under 45 years old.

The oral maxillofacial and neck areas are exposed parts of the human body, whether in peacetime or in wartime, are vulnerable to injuries. Although the oral and maxillofacial areas are different from those of the neck, they are the entrance of the digestive tract and the respiratory tract, and are anatomically and functionally related, which makes them have many commonalities in anesthesia management, especially airway management. This explains why this chapter discusses together the anesthesia management for patients who suffer from injuries in oral maxillofacial and neck areas together.

S. Cao (✉)
Department of Anesthesiology, Shanghai Ninth People's Hospital Affiliated to Shanghai Jiao Tong University School of Medicine, Shanghai, China

13.2 Oral Maxillofacial and Neck Trauma

The most common cause of maxillofacial and neck trauma is car accidents, followed by assaults, sports, falls, and war injuries. The mechanism of injury usually includes penetrating injuries, blunt contusions, blast injuries, and burns. The most common site of injury is the mandible, followed by the zygoma. The most frequently combined type of injury is extremity injury, followed by craniocerebral trauma, ocular trauma, and cervical spine injury. The most frequently occurring nerve injury is facial nerve injury.

13.2.1 Maxillary Fracture (Fig. 13.1)

1. *Le Fort I fracture.* The fracture line occurs on the low line of weakness and is a horizontal maxillary fracture, separating the maxillary pressure groove and hard palate from the rest of the maxilla. There are very few comorbidities, rarely life-threatening, and most patients are still able to open their mouths without signs of respiratory distress. Intubation requires consideration of loose teeth, bleeding, and difficulty with mask ventilation. Nasal intubation should be avoided if the fracture involves the nasal septum.

H. Jiang, M. Xia (eds.), *Anesthesia for Oral and Maxillofacial Surgery*,
https://doi.org/10.1007/978-981-19-7287-4_13

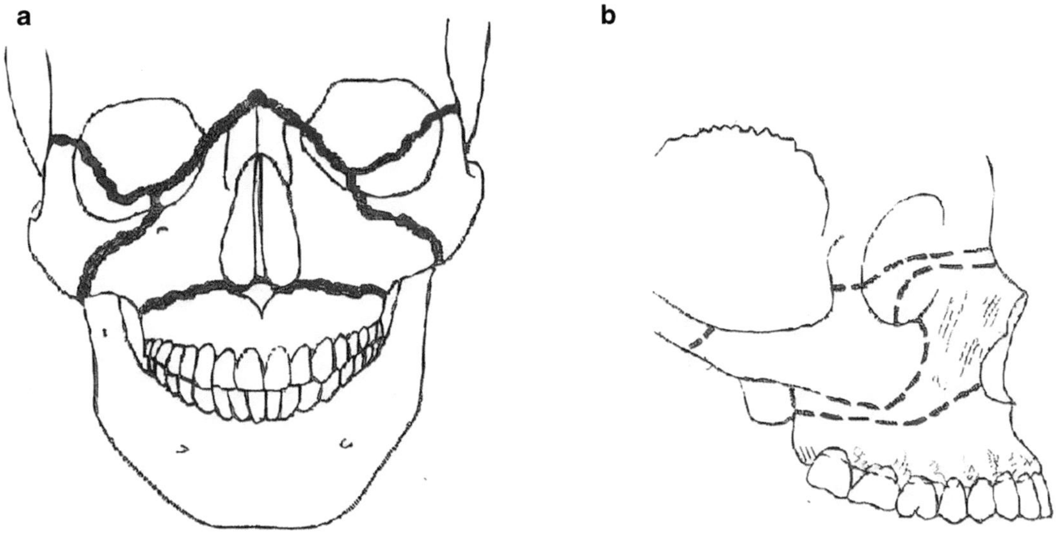

Fig. 13.1 The three types of maxillary fracture (**a**) frontal view, (**b**) profile view

2. *Le Fort II fracture.* The fracture line occurs on the median line of weakness and the entire fracture resembles the shape of a vertebral body when viewed from the front, hence it is also called by the name vertebral body fracture. This type of fracture often occur as a result of high-energy trauma and characterized by skull base fracture and cerebrospinal fluid leak. Considering that nasal bleeding and facial swelling will result in difficulty in mask ventilation and laryngoscopic exposure, or interference with fiberoptic bronchoscopic view, most fractures of this type can only be intubated through orotracheal tube, and nasal tracheal intubation is contraindicated.
3. *Le Fort III fracture.* Occurring in the high line of weakness, this is the most severe type of maxillary fracture. The middle 1/3 of the face is completely separated from the skull base by force (i.e., craniofacial separation). Patients often have severe compound injuries such as skull base fractures, and often have coma, aspiration, or other causes of airway obstruction. In addition, facial swelling, cerebrospinal fluid leakage, and nasal bleeding can cause difficult mask ventilation. Patients with this fracture type have an open connection between the skull base and the nasal cavity, and nasotracheal intubation is likely to be inserted directly into the skull, which can cause secondary intracranial infection, making nasotracheal intubation absolutely contraindicated. A direct tracheotomy is usually performed.

13.2.2 Temporomandibular Joint Injury

The temporomandibular joint (TMJ) consists of three parts: the temporal fossa, the mandibular condyle, and the articular disc. For anesthesiologists, the degree of mouth opening of the patient after an injury to the TMJ and its adjacent tissues is of greater concern. The TMJ injury often results in a limitation of the mouth opening, or even trismus. On the one hand, it may be directly due to injury to the joint itself, bone fragments embedded in the joint cavity, or occlusal hematoma, which is a mechanical cause of mouth opening limitation. On the other hand, it may be due to post-traumatic pain or reflex spasm of the occlusal muscles, i.e. non-mechanical causes of mouth opening restriction. Non-mechanical causes of mouth opening difficulties can be relieved by general anesthesia and muscle relaxants. In other words, a patient who has limited mouth opening can become able to open his or her mouth after receiving anesthesia. However, if the joint itself is damaged, i.e., mechanically, neither general anesthetics nor muscle relaxants can change gnathospasmus, and orotracheal intubation is not possible. If the TMJ is damaged for more than 2 weeks, the degree of limited mouth opening cannot be relieved by general anesthetics or muscle relaxants either due to fibrosis of the occlusal muscles.

13.2.3 Mandibular Fracture

The mandible is located in the lower part of the face and is horseshoe-shaped. It is the largest part of the individual bones of the maxillofacial region and is the facial bone most prone to fracture except for the nose. A mandibular fracture, especially a median chin fracture, can cause narrowing of the lingual bed and obstruction of the airway due to the pulling action of the hyoglossus, genioglossus, and mylohyoid, resulting in respiratory distress or even mechanical asphyxia, and although upright position can relieve this obstruction, one needs to be alert to the risk of aggravating cervical spine injury (Fig. 13.2).

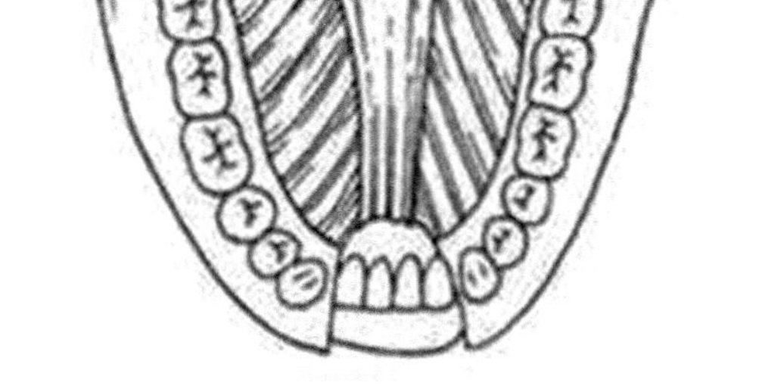

Fig. 13.2 The displacement of mandibular double fracture

With regard to the fracture of the mandible body, although significant tongue base retraction is not common, it can lead to a side displacement of the tongue base, with a left-sided fracture shifting the tongue base to the right and vice versa. This can also alter the normal anatomical relationship of the larynx. With a laryngoscope, the glottis may be perceived as "high" or even not visible at all. Restriction of mouth opening due to mandibular fractures may be due to mechanical obstruction (displaced condylar fracture fragments combined with zygomatic arch depression fractures) rather than pain or spasm, and therefore may not improve with the use of neuromuscular blocking agents during anesthesia and induction.

13.2.4 Neck Trauma

There are three types of neck trauma according to anatomical regions: region I is the clavicle to the cricoid cartilage. It is a high-risk zone which includes the large blood vessels at the entrance of the thoracic cavity, the lungs, the trachea, and the cervical esophagus. Cervical wounds may extend down into the interior of the thoracic cavity, resulting in massive bleeding, pneumothorax, shock, and ventilation difficulties that may require emergency thoracotomy. Therefore, adequate venous access, supplementation of blood products such as fresh plasma and cold precipitation, and invasive arterial pressure monitoring are required; region II is from the cricoid cartilage to the mandibular angle. Injuries in this region can be explored through a unilateral or transverse cervical incision, and hemostasis in this region is easier than in region I. The airway may be compressed by tissue rupture, edema, or hematoma; region III is from the mandibular angle all the way to the base of the skull. It is also a high-risk zone, where the surgery is complex and difficult. Preoperative angiography or computed tomography (CT) angiography can be helpful in planning anesthesia procedures.

The major clinical manifestations of severe neck trauma are given in Table 13.1. When assessing patients for severe neck trauma, the

Table 13.1 Major clinical manifestations of severe neck trauma

1. Active bleeding from the wound
2. Dysphagia, hoarseness, wheezing
3. Interruption of the trachea or larynx
4. Blood flow into the tracheobronchial tubes
5. Subcutaneous emphysema
6. Large or pulsating hematoma
7. Bleeding from the oropharynx
8. Cervical wound flap
9. Neurological deficits (spinal cord, brachial plexus)

wound should be examined for active external bleeding, dysphagia, wheezing, subcutaneous emphysema (possibly due to laryngeal or tracheal rupture), enlarged hematoma, open neck trauma, or neurologic deficits due to spinal cord or brachial plexus injury. Early death is associated with asphyxia or hypotensive shock due to airway compromise.

Any patient with a penetrating neck wound and airway injury should receive emergency airway management. Tracheal intubation should be performed by experienced personnel, and if tracheal intubation is unsuccessful, a surgical airway must be established. After securing the airway, the patient should undergo a formal neck exploration. Neck trauma should not be examined outside the operating room because of the risk of thrombus dislodgement and uncontrolled bleeding.

13.2.5 Laryngotracheal Injuries

The signs, symptoms, bronchoscopic findings, and CT images of laryngotracheal injuries are given in Table 13.2. The signs, symptoms, and severity of injury may not be directly proportional. Associated injuries include those in skull base, intracranial, neck, cervical medulla, esophagus, and pharynx. One quarter of all patients have injuries to the cervicothoracic vessels. Blunt injuries to the larynx usually involve the trachea. Some patients with blunt anterior cervical trauma initially have a normal airway but may develop progressive airway compromise over the next few hours due to laryngeal rupture, emphysema, and hematoma expansion. The patient should be adequately observed from the time of injury, including out-of-hospital transport and admission, and the need for intubation should be determined. If there is airway obstruction, wheezing, or trauma to the neck, sternum, or clavicle, direct injury resulting in tracheal compression should be suspected.

Table 13.2 Major manifestations of laryngotracheal injuries

Signs and symptoms	Subcutaneous emphysema, crepitus, air leakage, external bleeding and bruising, petechiae, hematoma, dyspnea, hypopnea, wheezing, cough, dysphonia, hoarseness, dysphagia, salivation, hemoptysis, tracheal displacement, nerve injury
Bronchoscopy findings	Laceration, edema, hematoma, vocal cord abnormality, airway compression, or distortion. Note: Tracheal injury may be external to the visible mucosa and evidence of injury may not be seen on fiberoptic bronchoscopy
CT images	Compression or deformation of the airway and surrounding structures, fractures, laceration, edema, hematoma, abnormal cavitation

Laryngotracheal separation is a special type of trauma. Tracheal intubation may make the separation more severe and turn airway narrowing into airway loss. In patients with airway rupture, it is important to allow tracheal intubation to pass through the area of injury without causing further damage or by using surgical methods to insert a tracheal tube around the injury and into the distal trachea.

13.3 Anesthetic Management of Oral Maxillofacial and Neck Trauma

Anesthetic management for oral maxillofacial and neck trauma also follows the principles of Advanced Trauma Life Support (ATLS): A—airway with spine control, B—breathing, C—circulation with hemorrhage control, and D—disability. If life-threatening injuries exist, priority should be given to treatment, and other treatments will be performed after the condition is stabilized.

13.3.1 Pre-anesthesia Assessment

13.3.1.1 Airway Assessment

Because oral maxillofacial and neck trauma usually disrupts the normal airway structures and difficult mask ventilation and intubation are common, airway assessment should be as comprehensive and rapid as possible. Airway obstruction due to facial edema or hematoma tends to develop rapidly and may aggravate with time, so the patient should be evaluated repeatedly within the first few hours. Methods of determination include: (1) the presence or absence of difficulty in conversation and vocalization: the clarity of consciousness and the patency of the airway are quickly determined by conversing with the patient. If the patient's answers are on-topic and clear, then the patient is considered to be conscious and the airway is patent. (2) Signs of airway obstruction: if the patient is confused, observe whether there is snoring, wheezing, three concave signs, abnormal breathing, cyanosis, and agitation; for abnormal respiratory rhythm, airway obstruction, or asphyxia, open the airway as soon as possible and give effective ventilation support. (3) Presence of foreign body aspiration: For comatose patients, foreign bodies in the oropharynx (such as sediment, tissue fragments, denture, secretions, or regurgitation of gastric contents) should be checked and removed in a timely manner. (4) Presence of cervical spine injury: For awake patients, if there is no neck pain, tenderness, or limitation of neck movement, it is suggested that there is no cervical spine injury. For unconscious patients or patients who lost consciousness immediately after the injury, or with neck pain, severe radiating pain, and any neurological signs and symptoms, it is indicative of combined underlying cervical instability, and should be treated accordingly as if it were accompanied by cervical fracture [1].

13.3.1.2 Assessment of Neurological Function

A rapid assessment of neurological function can be performed using the AVPU system, which includes four aspects: awake, verbal response, painful response, and unresponsive. The degree of wakefulness and orientation is clarified by asking the patient questions, and then limb mobility and pain response are checked. In addition, the Glasgow Coma Scale (GCS) (Table 13.3) can also be used to grade the injury: (1) 3–8 is severe brain injury; (2) 9–13 is moderate brain injury; (3) 14–15 is mild brain injury.

Cerebral nerve, spinal cord, and peripheral nervous system functions can be assessed by specific motor and sensory tests of the limbs in subsequent examinations.

13.3.1.3 Circulatory Assessment

Due to the abundant blood supply and arterial anastomotic branches in the oral and maxillofacial region, severe uncontrollable bleeding and even circulatory failure are pretty common in after injuries involving more than two-thirds of the maxillofacial region or the entire region In addition, massive bleeding sometimes forms blood accumulation in the sinus cavity (cranial cavity, maxillary sinus, etc.) or is swallowed by the patient into the gastrointestinal tract and ignored, so proper assessment should be made in a timely manner in order not to be delayed in rescue.

The patient's circulatory status can be initially determined by changes in heart rate, pulse, blood pressure, and peripheral tissue perfusion (SpO_2). When the patient shows symptoms such as tachy-

Table 13.3 Glasgow Coma Scale

Eye opening	Points	Verbal response	Points	Motor response	Points
Spontaneous	4	Oriented	5	Obeys commands	6
To speech	3	Confused	4	Localizes pain	5
To pain	2	Inappropriate	3	Withdraw to pain	4
No response	1	Incomprehensible	2	Abnormal flexion to pain (decorticate posturing)	3
		No response	1	Extension to pain (decerebrate posturing)	2
				No response	1

Table 13.4 Clinical grading and assessment of blood loss in injured patients

	Manifestations	Assessed blood loss
Grade I	Increased pulse rate, normal blood pressure, and respiration	Around 70% (>750 mL)
Grade II	Restlessness, pulse rate > 120/min, increased respiratory rate, decreased systolic blood pressure, decreased pulse pressure, capillary refill test >2 s, normal urine output	15–30% (750–1500 mL)
Grade III	Clinical symptoms are more severe than those of grade II, with altered mental status and oliguria	30–40% (1500–2000 mL)
Grade IV	Drowsiness, confusion, coma, systolic blood pressure < 50 mmHg, anuria	>40% (>2000 mL)

cardia, weak or even non-palpable peripheral pulse, low or undetectable blood pressure, pallor, and cold or cyanotic extremities, shock or hypovolemia should be considered, and the bleeding should be controlled first and blood volume should be replenished as soon as possible. It is also important to assess the mental status: patients in hemorrhagic shock start to be irritable, followed by drowsiness. Younger patients are highly compensated and can maintain a normal blood pressure even when bleeding reaches 40% of blood volume. This compensatory shock state may be diagnosed by a decreased pulse pressure difference, increased heart rate, pale complexion, and increased lactate levels and acid-base imbalance. Blood loss can usually be estimated based on the following clinical manifestations (Table 13.4).

13.3.1.4 Imaging and Laboratory Tests

1. Imaging examination

   Patients with oral, maxillofacial, and neck trauma are often combined with multi-system injuries. Imaging examinations can not only clarify the diagnosis of the injury but also provide comprehensive information about the airway and its surrounding structures. (a) X-ray plain radiograph: chest X-ray plain film can show whether there are rib fractures, pneumothorax, and hemothorax, etc. (b) CT scan: This includes continuous CT plain scans of the head, maxillofacial region, neck, chest, abdomen, and pelvis. Newer CT techniques allow for three-dimensional reconstruction of the maxillofacial, organ, and vascular systems. (c) Ultrasound: Ultrasound of the abdomen and chest can help di1agnose ascites, pneumothorax, pleural effusion, and pericardial tamponade. (d) Digital contrast angiography (DSA): can help diagnose the integrity of the vascular system. (e) Endoscopy: including bronchoscopy and esophagoscopy, which can assist in clarifying the integrity of the trachea and esophagus.

   The timing and prioritization of imaging examinations should be decided after weighing the pros and cons based on the patient's condition and the degree of cooperation. If the patient's vital signs are stable and cooperative, the examination is convenient and quick, and the anesthesiologist and surgeon can accompany the patient, then the examination can be performed immediately; on the contrary, if the condition may deteriorate at any time and the examination site is far away and time-consuming, it may be safer and more reliable to perform the examination after securing the airway.

2. Laboratory tests

   Laboratory tests mainly include routine blood tests (hemoglobin, hematocrit), arterial blood gas test (acid-base balance index), blood lactate level, serum electrolytes, and coagulation function. Because injured patients lose whole blood but replenish it with crystals and/or colloidal fluid, early decreasing values of hemoglobin and hematocrit do not reflect the actual bleeding volume. Arterial blood gases are the most important test to reflect the patient's acid-base balance and oxygenation status. Arterial or venous lactate levels are the most sensitive indicators for assessing hypoperfusion and shock status. Serum electrolytes and coagulation tests are important. Abnormal coagulation on admission can be one of the indicators of massive blood loss as well as severe hemorrhagic shock. In addition to the above laboratory tests, blood cross-matching are also required.

13.3.2 Intraoperative Management

13.3.2.1 Airway Management

Establishing an artificial airway and maintaining airway patency are the primary issues. Trauma of the maxillofacial and cervical region usually destroys the normal airway structure, and in addition, it is often combined with cervical spine injury and full stomach, making airway management difficult and challenging [2]. The basic requirement for airway management is the safety of tracheal intubation and positive pressure ventilation. Optional tracheal intubation devices include direct laryngoscope, video laryngoscope, fiberoptic bronchoscope, etc. Patients with difficult airways should be preserved to breathe spontaneously under local anesthesia, reasonable sedation, and removal of blood and tissue debris from the airway, if they can cooperate. Options are: tracheal intubation under surface tracheal anesthesia under conscious sedation, intubation under maintained spontaneous ventilation (inhalation induction with volatile anesthetics). If there is no difficult airway, rapid sequential induction is more appropriate for patients with severe trauma or organ damage, inability to cooperate well, or hemodynamic instability [3].

1. Airway management of trauma in different regions.
   (a) Maxillofacial trauma: Simple mandibular fracture has little effect on airway management. Although mandibular and zygomatic arch injuries can result in restricted mouth opening or even trismus, this condition can be resolved with muscle relaxants. However, bilateral mandibular fractures can sometimes affect the degree of direct laryngoscopic exposure. Condylar fracture fragments may limit the degree of mouth opening of the patient and require the appropriate intubation device depending on the situation. Airway injury in midface fractures may require surgical assistance to establish an airway or submandibular intubation. Nasal intubation via fiberoptic bronchoscopy and high-flow oxygen administration in the setting of skull base fractures increases the risk of intracranial infection and may be used if the fracture line is not over the midline and the CT imaging sieve is intact.
   (b) Neck trauma: Airway manipulation may increase bleeding and/or tissue edema. Airway swelling or bleeding makes intubation difficult, and agitation may exacerbate bleeding or tracheal rupture during tracheal intubation. Rapid induction intubation reduces the risk of hematoma expansion due to bucking and sudden movement but may worsen airway obstruction.
   (c) Laryngotracheal rupture: Conventional laryngoscopy is more dangerous when used in the setting of laryngotracheal injury. If the airway injury is large or involves the subglottis, surgical airway creation may be the best approach. In some patients, tracheal intubation can be performed through the airway rupture or using a fiberoptic bronchoscope distal to the rupture to preserve as much of the patient's spontaneous breathing as possible.
2. Reduce the risk of cervical spine injury.
   (a) In the emergency setting, the presence or absence of cervical spine injury in patients with oral maxillofacial neck injury is usually unknown, and a definitive diagnosis of cervical spine injury may take hours or even days. Until then, all patients should be treated as if they have an associated cervical spine injury, and the neck must be supported by a neck brace to limit neck motion to avoid serious complications such as quadriplegia due to aggravation of the underlying spinal cord injury. Current studies concluded that tracheal intubation with fiberscope under local anesthesia has

the least impact and safest effect on the patient's cervical displacement, while neurological function assessment can be performed after intubation. Adequate preoxygenation, removal of as much airway blood, secretions or vomit as possible, effective surface anesthesia, and obtaining the cooperation of the traumatized patient are essential for successful intubation. Light wand and video laryngoscopic intubation also cause less cervical movement and less cervical displacement with compression of the cricoid cartilage. Regardless of the technique of intubation, manual in-line stabilization (MILS) of the cervical spine is most important: with the assistant at the bedside, the hands are fixed on both sides of the neck and mastoid to the extent that only the mouth can be opened and the chin lifted, keeping the head in as neutral a position as possible to complete the tracheal intubation [4].

3. Reduction of reflux aspiration.
   (a) All injured patients are considered to be "full stomach," and maxillofacial bleeding, intoxication, obesity, and drug addiction can further increase the risk of aspiration. Rapid Sequence Intubation (RSI) is a clinically indicated technique for the induction of general anesthesia in patients with a full stomach or at risk for regurgitation and aspiration. The key points of RSI include adequate preoxygenation, rapid sequential injection of pre-calculated doses of propofol and succinylcholine, implementation of the Sellick maneuver (thumb and index finger pushing back on the cricoid cartilage to close the upper esophagus with a pressure of 10N before loss of consciousness and an increase to 30N after loss of consciousness), and avoidance of positive pressure ventilation until the tracheal tube is successfully intubated and the catheter sleeve is inflated.
   (b) Although rapid sequential induction can be used in most trauma patients, patients with severe oral and maxillofacial trauma often have difficulty with mask sealing, positive pressure mask ventilation may exacerbate facial fractures and airway compressions, and preoxygenation is often difficult to achieve.
   (c) Regarding medication for induction, opioids should be considered as they may result in bucking and aggravate airway trauma. Prolonged respiratory depression due to opioids can place the patient in the most dangerous situation if intubation fails and effective ventilation is not possible.
   (d) The Sellick maneuver is not indicated in patients with laryngotracheal neck injuries because of the potential for airway bleeding or displacement. H_2 receptor blockers such as cimetidine and prokinetic agents such as metoclopramide can also be given intravenously, but these drugs take 1–2 h to produce their effects, so attention needs to be paid to the time point of administration. Oral antacids are contraindicated because of the risk of potential esophageal damage.
4. Different methods of establishing an artificial airway.
   (a) Nasotracheal intubation: In maxillofacial surgery, anesthesiologists have to share the airway with surgeons. In neck surgery, anesthesiologists have to stay away from the airway for the convenience of the surgeon. Nasotracheal intubation is more conducive to exposing the operative field, but skull base fractures and nasal bone fractures are contraindications to nasotracheal intubation. Nasotracheal intubation can be accomplished with the aid of direct laryngoscopy in most patients, but when direct laryngoscopic exposure is difficult, fiberoptic bronchoscopy can be used instead. In some types of surgery, nasotracheal intubation can be combined with other intubation modalities, for example, in patients with multiple facial fractures, intraoperative nasotracheal intubation can be converted to orotracheal intubation, thus avoiding

invasive operations such as tracheostomy and submandibular intubation.

(b) Orotracheal intubation: Since maxillofacial surgery often requires the use of maxillary and mandibular teeth to establish a normal occlusal relationship during surgery, the use of transnasal tracheal intubation is more advantageous than transoral tracheal intubation in this group of patients. When transnasal tracheal intubation is difficult to perform, or in patients with simple neck trauma, transoral tracheal intubation can be chosen.

(c) Submental intubation: When multiple fractures of the maxillofacial region are combined with skull base fractures and nasal bone fractures, nasotracheal intubation is contraindicated, and submental tracheal intubation can be used. The specific procedure is as follows: after orotracheal intubation, a submental incision of about 2 cm in length is made (about 12 cm from the submental margin), and a curved vascular clamp is used to connect to the mucosal incision at the floor of the mouth through the subcutaneous, platysma, and mylohyoid muscle in turn, and the vascular clamp clamps the external mouth of the tracheal tube and draws it out of the open soft tissue channel to the submental incision, and the tracheal tube is secured to the skin with a #4 suture. Extraorally, the tracheal tube is connected to the anesthesia machine. Intraorally, the tracheal tube is located between the tongue and the inner wall of the mandible and can be moved freely to facilitate intraoral manipulation. After the operation, the sutures are cut and the tracheal tube is removed from the submental incision to return to orotracheal intubation. Submental intubation is a simple procedure and avoids the serious complications caused by tracheotomy. Although the damage is less than that of tracheotomy, it is also an invasive operation, and improper operation may cause bleeding, oral skin fistula, sublingual gland duct, and lingual nerve damage.

(d) Surgical airway: According to the current management process of difficult airway guidelines, supraglottic ventilation can be performed through a mask or laryngeal mask when tracheal intubation fails. If mask or laryngeal mask ventilation still fails to maintain oxygenation, a surgical airway needs to be established rapidly.

Cricothyrotomy is the easiest and fastest method of tracheotomy for patients who cannot be intubated due to pharyngeal or laryngeal obstruction. The procedure is as follows: make a transverse skin incision between the thyroid cartilage and the cricoid cartilage about 2–4 cm long, cut the cricothyroid membrane close to the cricoid cartilage, enlarge the incision with a curved vascular clamp, and insert a tracheal cannula or endotracheal tube. The operation should avoid damage to the cricoid cartilage to avoid causing postoperative laryngeal stenosis. The cricothyroid membrane is clearly positioned, so it is simpler and easier to complete than tracheotomy, but it causes great damage to the larynx. The tube should not be carried for too long after cricothyrotomy, and if the patient cannot be extubated within 24 h, conventional tracheotomy should be chosen.

Tracheotomy is usually performed at the second to fourth tracheal rings to incise the cervical trachea, which is deeper than the cricothyroid membrane and less clearly positioned than the cricothyroid membrane. Sometimes a larger incision is required, so it usually takes longer, and there is a greater risk of bleeding due to damage to the thyroid tissue. In these patients, if the penetrating foreign body transects or severely tears the trachea, an incision of the injured lower trachea is required. Incision by wound access is also possible but should be done in the operating room [5].

13.3.2.2 Circulation and Other System Management

1. Circulation management: The goal is to maintain hemodynamic stability. Arterial cannulation (radial artery preferred) facilitates real-time monitoring of arterial blood pres-

sure and facilitates blood sampling for arterial blood gas analysis and other laboratory tests. Central venous placement facilitates rapid volume expansion and administration of vasoactive drugs, and femoral venous placement is often preferred as central venous access in patients with oral, maxillofacial and neck trauma. Volume resuscitation is guided by a pulmonary artery catheter or noninvasive hemodynamic monitoring (e.g., beat-to-beat output variability). A catheter is left in place to monitor urine output to assess intravascular volume status. In addition, the effect of anesthetics on circulation should be considered. Dramatic fluctuations in hemodynamics occur with excessive doses of sedative-hypnotic drugs, which are particularly harmful in patients in hypovolemic shock.
2. Temperature management: Monitor core body temperature; warm fluids and blood; keep the patient's body covered and control the operating room temperature > 28 °C; use warm blankets.
3. Coagulation management: If there is excessive blood loss, the surgeons are suggested to stop the operation and perform hemostasis; monitor hematocrit, calcium ion, and coagulation; pay attention to calcium supplementation when high-dose citrate products are used; supplement plasma, platelets, cold precipitation, fibrinogen, and prothrombin complex according to clinical symptoms or coagulation tests.
4. Other systems: If accompanied by craniocerebral trauma, maintain cerebral perfusion pressure greater than 70 mmHg; monitor airway pressure and tidal volume. If not, tidal volume can be set at 5–6 mL/kg ideal body weight, maintain peak airway pressure + plateau pressure less than 30 mmH_2O, use proper positive end-expiratory pressure to maintain PaO_2 greater than 60 mmHg, hypercapnia is permitted; be alert to pneumothorax; measure urine volume; monitor peripheral arterial pulsation.

13.3.2.3 Maintenance of Anesthesia

Maintenance of anesthesia can be done by inhaled or intravenous anesthesia. If a tracheal injury is present, it is safer to use inhalational anesthetics alone with continued preservation of spontaneous breathing for surgical repair. Sevoflurane may be the inhalational anesthetic of choice. The surgeon should avoid neuromuscular blockade when intraoperative neurological assessment is required and, if necessary, reverse the neuromuscular blocking effects of vecuronium and rocuronium with sugammadex. Narcotic analgesics should be administered promptly once the airway has been established. Given that these patients are likely to require mechanical ventilation postoperatively, there is no need to be overly concerned about the delayed awakening associated with high-dose narcotic analgesics. Dexmedetomidine is a commonly used adjunctive drug that provides some sedation without significant risk of respiratory depression.

13.3.3 Postoperative Precautions

1. Precautions for extubation: In postoperative patients with maxillofacial and neck trauma, airway obstruction and ventilation difficulties are very likely to occur after extubation due to mucosal edema, soft tissue swelling, pain, restricted mouth opening, head and facial bandages, and neck fixation. In addition, the surgical operation site is adjacent to the airway, which often causes changes in the anatomical structure of the airway, and the residual blood and secretions in the oropharynx are not removed in time after the operation, which also causes airway obstruction. Therefore, the airway status and ventilation should be re-evaluated before extubation to clarify whether the postoperative airway condition has improved or worsened compared with the preoperative condition, and choose an optimal time for extubation to avoid putting the patient at high risk as much as possible [6].

   It is important to conduct individualized assessment according to the patient's own conditions, and strictly control the indications for extubation. It is worth noting that airway swelling and compression may be further aggravated postoperativey for patients with Le Fort III, so extubation should be delayed until normal anatomy is restored or edema subsides. Patients undergoing maxillary fixation should always have wire cutters or rubber band scissors at the bedside to prevent airway obstruction. The relatively low expansibility of the neck can lead to airway compression even with a small amount of bleeding and requires postoperative observation in the ICU for 12–24 h. When the tracheal tube covers the injury site, edema at the injury can obstruct the airway after extubation, and an air leak test should be performed before extubation. Resuscitation intubation and tracheotomy tools should be prepared before extubation, and a tube changer should be used if necessary. After extubation, oxygen inhalation and close monitoring shall be performed routinely, so as to detect and deal with airway obstruction, vomiting and aspiration, and inadequate ventilation in a timely manner.

2. Reasonable use of drugs to prevent postoperative nausea and vomiting is recommended.
3. Local anesthetics, NSAIDs, acetamino¬phen, and opioids may be used postoperatively to provide effective multimodal analgesia.
4. Intravenous dexamethasone to reduce tissue swelling.
5. Any patient with severe open trauma should receive antibiotic prophylaxis that works against gram-positive bacteria for at least 24 h after the injury.

References

1. Baijing LY. Airway management of maxillofacial and neck trauma patients. Int J Anesthesiol Resusc. 2018;39(1):53–7.
2. Krausz AA, El-naaj IA, Barak M. Maxillofacial trauma patient: coping with the difficult airway. World J Emerg Surg. 2009;4:21. https://doi.org/10.1186/1749-7922-4-21.
3. Barak M, Bahouth H, Leiser Y, et al. Airway management of the patient with maxillofacial trauma: review of the literature and suggested clinical approach. Biomed Res Int. 2015;2015:724032. https://doi.org/10.1155/2015/724032.
4. Jain U, Mccunn M, Smith CE, et al. Management of the traumatized airway. Anesthesiology. 2016;124(1):199–206. https://doi.org/10.1097/ALN.0000000000000903.
5. Kellman RM, Losquadro WD. Comprehensive airway management of patients with maxillofacial trauma. Craniomaxillofac Trauma Reconstr. 2008;1(1):39–47. https://doi.org/10.1055/s-0028-1098962.
6. Lovich-Sapola J, Johnson F, Smith CE. Anesthetic considerations for oral, maxillofacial, and neck trauma. Otolaryngol Clin North Am. 2019;52(6):1019–35. https://doi.org/10.1016/j.otc.2019.08.004.

14 Anesthesia for Pediatric Oral and Maxillofacial Surgery

Jingjie Li

14.1 Introduction

Neonates and infants, emergency surgery, and combined respiratory problems (supraglottic airway obstruction, unplanned extubation, difficult intubation) remain high risk factors causing the reported anesthesia-related complications. Airway and respiratory management remain a major factor in complications and death from pediatric anesthesia. At the same time, oral and maxillofacial surgery are prone to complications and adverse events, which makes the importance of accurate management in pediatric oral and maxillofacial surgery more important.

Since children are not just a small version of adults, pediatric anesthesiologists must understand and be familiar with the anatomical and physiological characteristics of pediatric patients, and choose the appropriate tools and equipment according to different ages and take appropriate management measures to ensure the safety of surgical anesthesia for children.

J. Li (✉)
Department of Anesthesiology, Shanghai Ninth People's Hospital Affiliated to Shanghai Jiao Tong University School of Medicine, Shanghai, China
e-mail: chenx1853@sh9hospital.org.cn

14.2 Anatomy and Physiology

14.2.1 Physiology in Children

On top of their protuberant abs, children have disproportionately large heads perched on their tiny necks, with cartilaginous ribs atop a wide thorax of immature cartilage. Furthermore, the tongue and tonsils are disproportionately large compared to neighboring anatomy. Also, they have small nasal passages and do not breathe through their mouths until they have reached around 5 months old [1, 2].

Pediatric airways have long been thought of as funnels made up of cartilaginous and other soft tissue structures in the neck. The airway anatomy of a child is different from that of an adult due to the long floppy epiglottis and anterior and cephalad larynx. With a shorter neck, a child's larynx sits at the level of C4 (fourth cervical vertebra), whereas it is much lower for adults at C6 (sixth cervical vertebra) [3]. Recent studies involving computed tomography scans of neonates and infants have challenged the notion that the pediatric airway is funnel-shaped. These studies suggest that the pediatric airway is an elliptical structure with the subglottic area being the narrowest part prominent between the subglottic region and the cricoid. Additionally, these studies revealed that the airway is wider anteroposteriorly and narrows in the transverse direction from the subglottic region to the cricoid. The older the

H. Jiang, M. Xia (eds.), *Anesthesia for Oral and Maxillofacial Surgery*,
https://doi.org/10.1007/978-981-19-7287-4_14

child, the more these airways start looking like the cone that was described previously. There are significant differences in the pulmonary anatomy and physiology of children compared with adults. In a previous study by the same group, the subglottic area was found to be the narrowest transversely, thus posing the greatest resistance to the passage of an endotracheal tube. The ribs of children are more horizontally arranged and are composed of a greater amount of cartilaginous tissue than those of adults. This increases the elasticity of their chest walls, making them more prone to collapse on inspiration, leaving them with a small residual lung volume on expiration [4]. People with this type of lung have smaller alveoli and fewer of them. Weaknesses in the intercostal muscles and diaphragmatic musculature occur. A child with rapid growth has an increased oxygen consumption, and their limited physiologic reserve makes them less able to tolerate hypoxemia. As a result, they desaturate more rapidly and have shorter apnea safety times. Children compensate for the reduced volume and reserve by increasing their respiratory rate. By varying the respiratory rate (tidal volume breaths per minute), minute ventilation can only be maintained. At any given level of activity, the respiratory rate is almost double that of an adult, demonstrating this factor.

It is common for children of school age to get upper respiratory tract infections (URIs). In children with URIs, airways reactivity increases, making them more vulnerable to respiratory complications under anesthesia [5]. Scientific literature on the topic provides a range of information. In terms of clinicians looking to answer a simple question, "Should we anesthetize a child with a recent mild-moderate upper respiratory infection?", it can sometimes be challenging to distill the data available. In most cases, the information is based on retrospective observational studies rather than case-controlled studies. It has been suggested that children with a mild URI may be safely anesthetized as many of the problems encountered are easily treated without long-lasting consequences. There is also a strong correlation between this topic and airway instrumentation—supraglottic airways or intubation are commonly employed in anesthetic techniques. Using a non-intubated airway and anxiolysis, is it safer to anesthetize a child with a mild URI rather than using a laryngeal mask airway as a recently performed prospective study showed? This scenario cannot be proven or disproven by any evidence.

14.2.2 Cardiovascular Anatomy and Physiology in Children

Children's left ventricles tend to be relatively non-complaining and fixed. The size of their hearts and arteries increases as they grow. Diastolic fill and, therefore, stroke volume are restricted by the limited mobility of the left side of the heart. A decrease in stroke volume indicates that the heart rate has to be increased to maintain cardiac output, since cardiac output depends on heart rate and stroke volume. Age and the size of an organ both increase systolic and diastolic pressure.

Younger patients experience a blunted reflex response to hypotension via tachycardia or vasoconstriction due to their immature autonomic nervous system. It is also possible to expect a decreased response to exogenous catecholamines. When their volume is lost, neonates and infants become hypotensive and are rarely tachycardic.

A true cardiac event is rarely the cause of cardiac arrest in otherwise healthy children. It almost always results from hypoxic insults affecting the lungs. In children, hypoxia and respiratory embarrassment cause bradycardia, hypotension, and, ultimately, asystole. An example of this is the sedated child with potential airway compromise in the OMS office.

Pediatricians should also pay attention to the renal and gastrointestinal systems. It takes about 2 years for a child to reach normal kidney function. Even older children undergoing anesthesia in the office require meticulous and appropriate fluid administration and dosing of medications [6].

14.2.3 Anatomical and Physiological Characteristics of Pediatric Airway

1. Head and Neck

   Infants have a large head and a short neck, and the neck muscles are underdeveloped, which makes them prone to upper airway obstruction, even if intravertebral anesthesia is administered, improper position can cause airway obstruction.
2. Nose

   Pediatric nostrils are narrow and are the main respiratory channel for children within 6 months of age. Secretions, mucosal edema, blood, or inappropriate masks lead to nasal obstruction and upper respiratory tract obstruction.
3. Tongue and Pharynx

   Pediatric patients have small mouth and tongue, their pharynx is relatively narrow and vertical, prone to hyperplasia and tonsillitis.
4. Larynx

   Larynx position of newborns and infants is higher, and their glottis is located in the cervical 3 to 4 level [7]. Therefore, during tracheal intubation, the anesthetist can press the larynx in order to expose the larynx. Infants are with long and hard epiglottis, which is of "U" shape and forward displacement, blocking the line of sight, causing difficulties in revealing the vocal folds. A straight laryngoscope blade is usually used to pick up the epiglottis to have easier glottic exposure. Because of the narrow funnel-shaped laryngeal cavity (the narrowest part is at the level of the cricoid cartilage, i.e., the subglottis area), the soft cartilage, and the tender vocal cords and mucous membranes in children, they are prone to laryngeal edema. When the tracheal tube encounters resistance through the vocal cords, excessive force should not be used, and the tracheal tube should be replaced with a thinner one to avoid damaging the trachea.
5. Trachea

   The total trachea length of the newborn is about 4–5 cm, and the inner diameter is 4–5 mm. The bifurcation of the trachea is located high in the third to fourth thoracic vertebrae in newborns (in adults, it is at the lower edge of the fifth thoracic vertebrae). The angles of the main bronchi and trachea are basically equal in children under 3 years of age, and the chances of entering the left or right main bronchi are similar when the endotracheal tube is inserted too deeply or when a foreign body enters compared to adults [8].
6. Lung

   The number of alveoli in newborns is only 8% of that in adults, and the surface area of alveoli per unit body weight is 1/3 of that in adults, but their metabolic rate is about twice that of adults, so the respiratory reserve of newborns is limited [9]. The lung interstitium is well developed, and the capillary and lymphatic tissue gap is wider than that of adults, resulting in less air and more blood, so it is easy to be infected and inflammation is easy to spread, causing interstitial inflammation, pulmonary atelectasis, and pneumonia. Due to the poor development of elastic tissue, lung expansion is not sufficient, prone to pulmonary atelectasis and emphysema; premature infants due to immature lung development, lung surface active substance production or release is insufficient, which can cause extensive alveolar atrophy and reduced lung compliance.
7. Thorax

   The pediatric thorax is relatively small and barrel-shaped, with thin bones and muscles, underdeveloped intercostal muscles, and horizontal ribs, so the thoracic expansion force is small during inspiration, and breathing mainly depends on the vertical movement of the diaphragm, which is easily affected by factors such as abdominal distension.
8. Mediastinum

   The pediatric mediastinum occupies a large space in the thoracic cavity, limiting the expansion of the lungs during inspiration, so the respiratory reserve capacity is poor. The tissue around the mediastinum is soft and loose, rich in elasticity, and when there is a large amount of fluid in the thoracic cavity, or when there occurs pneumothorax and pulmonary atelectasis, it is easy to cause displacement of the organs in the mediastinum (trachea, heart, and large blood vessels).

14.3 Airway Management Guidelines

14.3.1 Airway Devices and Their Usage

14.3.1.1 Mask

The ideal pediatric mask should have an air cushion seal that can cover the bridge of the nose, cheeks and chin, and different sizes should be available for selection. The amount of dead space of the mask should be minimal. Transparent masks are more suitable for pediatric applications. In order to make children easy to accept, the mask is often made with fragrance or coated with fragrance when used, or soaked by cherry, strawberry, or mint liquid before use.

1. Choose the Appropriate Mask
   (a) Avoid pressing the sub-chin triangle with finger, which causes airway obstruction, pressure on the neck vessels or stimulation of the carotid sinus.
   (b) Prevent damage to the eyes caused by the edge of the mask.
   (c) When resting the mask, the head can be positioned laterally to facilitate the maintenance of a clear airway and the outflow of oral secretions.

14.3.1.2 Oropharyngeal Airway

When there is difficulty in mask ventilation, an oropharyngeal airway can be applied. The distance from the corner of the mouth to the angle of the jaw or earlobe is the appropriate length of the oropharyngeal airway for children.

The child should avoid holding the breath, choking, increasing secretion, poor breathing, inducing cough or laryngospasm, or even hypoxia when the nasopharyngeal airway is placed too shallowly. Keep the airway open, oxygenate with mask, assist ventilation, if necessary, deepen inhalation anesthesia, and then place the oropharyngeal airway after the anesthesia reaches a certain depth with smooth breathing.

14.3.1.3 Nasopharyngeal Airway

Nasopharyngeal airway can be used to relieve airway obstruction because it opens the nasopharynx and allows airflow to pass between the tongue and the posterior pharyngeal wall.

1. Nasopharyngeal airway

   Choose a suitable nasopharyngeal airway according to the distance from the tip of the nose to the earlobe or choose a suitable size of tracheal tube (less than 1 mm than the tracheal intubation tube used). Apply lubricant before insertion, and be gentle when inserting.
2. Indications
   (a) More tolerable than oropharyngeal airway, used when the child is awakened from anesthesia but has partial airway obstruction or a long recovery time.
   (b) In certain children with obstructive airway diseases or postoperative airway obstruction.
   (c) Oxygen supply and/or inhalation of anesthetic gases during certain airway microscopies or dental anesthesia.
   (d) For use in children with loose teeth when placement of an oropharyngeal airway is at risk.
   (e) Can also be used in children with OSAS.
3. Contraindications

   Coagulation disorders, skull base fractures, pathological changes in the nose and nasopharynx.

14.3.1.4 Laryngoscope

1. A straight laryngoscope blade is suitable for neonates or small infants, it can reach the back of the pharynx over the epiglottis, pick up the epiglottis to expose the glottis.
2. For older children, a curved laryngoscope blade can be used, with the tip of the blade carefully pushed into the junction of the epiglottis and the tongue root, and the stem lifted vertically to reveal the larynx. Do not use the incisors as a fulcrum to cock the tip of the blade forward.

14.3.1.5 Tracheal Tube

The wall thickness of the tracheal tube made by different manufacturers is different, so the selection of catheter should also pay attention to the outside diameter (OD) of the catheter in addition to the internal diameter (ID) of the catheter.

1. The Selection of Tracheal Tube

   The most commonly used method is based on age, ID (cuffed tube) = age/4 + 4, ID (uncuffed tube) = age/4 + 4.5 [10]. Measurement method in clinical practice: (1) tracheal tube OD is equivalent to the thickness of the last joint of the little finger of a child and (2) tracheal tube OD is equivalent to the diameter of the external nostril of a child. One larger and one smaller tubes should be prepared separately for anesthesia.

   The dead space of the airway decreases significantly after tracheal intubation, while the resistance to airflow increases significantly, and the difference in ID between the connector and the tube causes turbulence and increases the resistance to airflow, so the maximum internal diameter of the tracheal tube is chosen as far as possible without causing damage.

   In some cases, such as head, neck or chest surgery and prone surgery, or in children with difficult or abnormal airways, the tracheal tube may be subjected to direct or indirect pressure and may be prone to kinking or crushing, and a special nylon or wire-reinforced tube should be used.

   When used for airway laser surgery, it is necessary to use the tracheal tube wrapped by appropriate materials or treated by graphite soaking to reduce flammability.
2. Cuffed Tracheal Tube

   It is most ideal to select an uncuffed tracheal tube that passes through the glottis and subglottic regions without resistance to the largest airway pressure up to 20 cmH_2O when there is air leakage. However, in practice to do so just right is not easy. It is agreed the use of a high-capacity, low-pressure airbag does not increase postoperative airway complications and produces no significant difference in postoperative laryngeal complications from an uncuffed tracheal tube. A cuffed tracheal tube is available for all pediatric patients (except for preterm infants).

   Advantages of cuffed tracheal tubes: (1) prevent aspiration; (2) implement low-flow controlled ventilation; (3) provide reliable carbon dioxide and ventilation monitoring; (4) reduce environmental pollution and waste of anesthetic drugs due to air leakage; (5) avoid the choice of too thick catheters to ensure good ventilation and reduce postoperative laryngeal complications; and (6) reduce repeated examinations and reduce the chance of tube changes, and the damage caused by cuffs may be much less than that caused by repeated intubation due to tube changes.

   An uncuffed tracheal tube is more suitable for children with major surgery, who require manual ventilation and are at high risk of regurgitation. However, it should be noted that: (1) the cuffed tracheal tube is thicker than the uncuffed tracheal tube (the outer diameter is about 0.5 mm thicker); (2) the pressure inside the cuff should not be too high, especially when using N_2O, and the airbag pressure should be monitored when possible; and (3) the airbag should be relaxed and carefully inflated regularly to prevent tracheal injury caused by compression if the tube is intubated for a long time.

   The depth of tracheal tube insertion can be through the mouth or through the nose: (1) the depth of insertion through the mouth is about age (years)/2 + 12 cm or ID × 3 cm; (2) the length of insertion through the nose is age (years)/2 + 14 cm or ID × 3 + 2 cm [10]. After the position of the tube is determined, consider cutting off the excess part according to the desired length. The catheter depth should be reconfirmed after positioning. For prolonged use of the endotracheal tube, an *X*-ray should be taken to confirm the position of the tube.

14.3.1.6 Tracheal Intubation and Extubation

1. Tracheal Intubation Method

   Orotracheal intubation is the most commonly used intubation method for pediatric clinical anesthesia. If the glottis is not exposed satisfactorily, the assistant or the operator should use the left pinky to gently press the cricothyroid cartilage from the front of the child's neck to displace the vocal incisors downward into the line of sight. The upper incisors should not be used as a fulcrum for laryngoscopic prying, for they can be damaged in this way. In addition, take care not to pinch the upper and lower lips between the teeth and the lens causing damage, especially for children in the period of tooth replacement to pay more attention to the protection of teeth.

The direct visual nasotracheal intubation method can be used for prone surgery, head and face surgery, cases where intraoperative transesophageal cardiac ultrasound is to be performed, cases requiring postoperative continuous mechanical ventilation, and major and prolonged surgery, where transnasal tracheal intubation can be performed to facilitate the fixation of the tracheal tube. Before intubation, check the patency of the child's nostrils and apply 0.5–1% ephedrine drops to constrict the nasal mucosal vessels. The prepared tracheal tube is soaked in hot saline to reduce possible nasal mucosal injury during intubation. After induction of anesthesia, the catheter is gently inserted through one nostril, and after passing through the posterior nasal orifice, the glottis is seen with the help of laryngoscope in plain view, and the tube is fed into the trachea with the assistance of intubation forceps.

2. Points of Attention for Tracheal Sphincter
   (a) Pediatric patients' oxygen reserve is small, and their ability to tolerate hypoxia is even worse, so intubation should be completed quickly.
   (b) Pediatric tracheal intubation should be operated gently, do not use violence to place the tube, otherwise it is very easy to cause tracheal injury and postoperative laryngeal edema.
   (c) Be sure to listen to the breath sounds of both lungs after intubation and observe the capnography to determine that the tracheal tube is placed correctly.
   (d) Before catheter fixation, hold the tracheal tube correctly to ensure that there is no change in the position of the tube.
   (e) Use a suitable support to prevent twisting of the tracheal tube. When nasal intubation is performed, care should be taken to avoid the catheter from compressing the nose.
3. Tracheal Extubation
   (a) The child must have the following conditions before extubation: (1) the effect of anesthetics has basically subsided, no residual effect of muscle relaxants and narcotic analgesics (except for those extubated under anesthesia); (2) the child has started to wake up, normalized spontaneous respiration, and independent body movement; infants and neonates should be extubated in the awake state; (3) cough and swallowing reflexes have returned to normal; (4) stable circulatory function and no hypothermia.
   (b) Operation: When preparing for extubation, the secretions in the trachea, nasal cavity, oral cavity, and throat should be suctioned first, and extubation should be performed when fully awake or at a certain depth of anesthesia. Newborns and infants should be extubated while awake. For children with recent upper respiratory tract infection, extubation under deep anesthesia is recommended. Adequate oxygen should be administered before extubation, and be prepared for reintubation. After extubation, a mask can be given to provide oxygen, and if necessary, secretions from the oropharynx should be suctioned, but repeated suction stimulation should be avoided. Place the child in the lateral position after extubation to help avoid or reduce the occurrence of vomiting, regurgitation, and aspiration.

14.3.1.7 Laryngeal Mask Airway (LMA)

LMA has become popular in pediatric anesthesia and can be used for airway management in general elective surgery, and also as an alternative to tracheal intubation after failure. Most pediatric LMAs are size 1–2.5.

1. LMA indications: (1) surgery without the risk of vomiting and reflux, and for short general anesthesia procedures on the body and extremities that do not require muscle relaxation; (2) in children with difficult airways, when intubation is difficult and LMA is used, LMA can also guide the completion of endotracheal intubation; (3) through the laryngeal mask, fiberoptic bronchoscopy can be performed for laser treatment of small tumors of the vocal cords, trachea or bronchus; (4) in children with unstable cervical spine, LMA can be used for the treatment of small tumors of the vocal cords and trachea; (5) LMA has advantages for infants and children with tracheal stenosis because the tracheal tube will further reduce the internal diameter of the narrowed trachea; (6) LMA can be placed during emergency resuscitation, and effective ventilation can be established quickly and timely resuscitation can be achieved if the operation is skilled.
2. LMA Placement Method

   The successful placement of LMA requires appropriate depth of anesthesia. The cuff of LMA should be emptied first, the back side should be coated with lubricant, the cuff should face forward toward the posterior pharyngeal wall (reverse method), and the mask should be placed along the axis of hard palate. The reverse method turns the position of LMA after the mask is placed in the mouth, straight to the lower part of the pharynx, and the air sac should cover the larynx, then inflate the air sac and connect the breathing circuit. After observing the activity of the skin bag or gently hand-controlling the inflated lung to see the thoracic movement and confirm the correct position, it is properly fixed with adhesive tape or bandage.
3. LMA Contraindications: (1) children with full stomach, gastrointestinal obstruction, high intra-abdominal pressure, and high risk of reflux and aspiration; (2) children with infection or other pathological changes in the throat; (3) children with respiratory bleeding; (4) children with oropharyngeal surgery; (5) children with difficulty in fixing the LMA position in lateral or prone position.
4. Note
   (a) The laryngeal mask should not be selected exactly according to the weight, but according to the development of the child, the appropriate size of the LMA should be selected with reference to the standard weight.
   (b) The LMA should be correctly placed. If the mask is placed too deeply or too shallowly in children, it will easily rotate and shift.
   (c) Maintain adequate depth of anesthesia. Although the stimulation of the LMA is much less than that of the tracheal tube, too shallow anesthesia, swallowing, coughing, etc. may lead to displacement of the mask, which may result in laryngospasm in severe cases.
   (d) Special attention should be paid to the resistance of the airway and ventilation during anesthesia. If the resistance is too high or the air leakage is serious, the position of the LMA should be adjusted in time, and if necessary, the laryngeal mask should be immediately disconnected for mask ventilation or changed to tracheal intubation.
   (e) Spontaneous breathing or controlled ventilation can be maintained during anesthesia, but it is safe to keep spontaneous breathing, closely observe whether the ventilation volume is sufficient, $PetCO_2$ monitoring is especially important, if the ventilation is controlled ventilation, close observation of ventilation, gastric distension and airway resistance is required, and the time should not be too long.

(f) At the end of surgery, the LMA can be removed after the protective reflexes are restored or under deep anesthesia.
(g) The disadvantages of the LMA include: (1) the airway seal is not as good as that of the endotracheal tube, and it cannot protect the airway when vomiting and regurgitation occur; (2) the possibility of gas leakage is increased during positive pressure ventilation; (3) the airway is not absolutely guaranteed to be open; (4) the pediatric LMA, especially the small-sized LMA, is prone to malposition.

14.3.2 Ventilation Devices and Ventilation Patterns

The ideal pediatric ventilation circuit should have these characteristics: light weight, small dead space of the device, low resistance whether it is without valve or low resistance valve, small gas volume inside the circuit, should minimize CO_2 repeated inhalation, respiratory work should be small to avoid respiratory muscle fatigue; its structure should form a small turbulence; easy to wet inhalation gas and exhaust gas; suitable for autonomous, assisted, or controlled ventilation.

14.3.2.1 Circulatory Circuit

The use of low flow and tightly closed-circuit anesthesia in pediatric anesthesia has become increasingly common in recent years. The circulatory circuit used in adults can be safely used in pediatric anesthesia after modification (reducing the inner diameter of the threaded tube and using a small respiratory airbag).

1. Advantages
   (a) Reduction of operating room contamination.
   (b) Reduction of water and heat loss in the pediatric patient.
   (c) Reduced waste of anesthetic gas, making tight circulation low-flow anesthesia possible.
   (d) The same standardized anesthesia equipment as adults, so that all anesthesiologists can be skilled in its use.
2. Resistance to Ventilation
   (a) In the circulatory loop, the resistance generated by the tubing and respirator is about 1/3 of the total resistance of the loop, and the valve accounts for 2/3, while the resistance generated by the tracheal tube is at least ten times that of the loop in infants and children, so the current information believes that the resistance generated by the loop is perfectly acceptable in pediatric patients [11].
   (b) Good performance of the anesthesia machine live valve resistance is small, in general, children over 1 year old whether in control or spontaneous breathing, the respiratory muscles have enough strength to open the live valve, while in newborns or infants, the strength of control ventilation is sufficient to open the live valve; while in spontaneous breathing, the strength of its respiratory muscles may not be sufficient to open the respiratory live valve, therefore, these children use the circulatory circuit during spontaneous breathing, especially in the anesthesia awake extubation period When spontaneous breathing resumes, the circuit can be replaced by a "T" tube series with no or low resistance to ventilation.

14.3.2.2 Anesthesia Machines and Ventilators

At present, most anesthesia machines can be used for pediatric patients, and there is no need to have an anesthesia machine dedicated to pediatric patients; even neonates can be anesthetized using a circulatory circuit, but it is necessary to understand their pressure and volume characteristics to change the clinical estimation of ventilation.

1. In addition to the safety devices that modern anesthesia machines should have, they should also have the following functions:
   (a) the ability to dilute the concentration of inhaled anesthetics with compressed air;
   (b) the ability to connect special pediatric anesthesia circuits (such as the Mapleson circuit), which is an important feature of pediatric anesthesia;

(c) a ventilator that precisely gives small tidal volumes, high respiratory rates and pressure control modes;
(d) anesthesia machines for small infants, preferably with the function of compensating compression volume function.

2. Adjustment of Main Working Parameters of Ventilator
   (a) Tidal volume and ventilation volume: tidal volume 10–15 ml/kg, minute ventilation volume 100–200 ml/kg. However, it is worth noting that in pediatric mechanical ventilation, it is necessary to compensate for the volume of gas compression in the anesthesia loop and the dead space volume caused by the expansion volume of the loop, therefore, the tidal volume given by the airbox is much larger than the actual tidal volume of the child, so the parameters shown in the airbox are meaningless. Judgment of the appropriateness of ventilation should be determined by auscultation of respiratory sounds, observation of the amplitude of thoracic undulation and in combination with $PETCO_2$ or $PaCO_2$.
   (b) Inspiratory pressure: peak inspiratory pressure is generally maintained at 12–20 cmH_2O, and the maximum should not exceed 30 cmH_2O.
   (c) Respiratory rate and inspiratory and expiratory time ratio: the respiratory rate is generally adjusted to 20–25 breaths/min, and the inspiratory and expiratory time ratio is 1:1.5, adjustable to 1:1 in neonates [11].
   (d) Fraction of inspired oxygen (FiO_2): adjusted according to the different conditions of the child, generally advocating a FiO_2 of 0.8–1.0 for no more than 6 h, a FiO_2 of 0.6–0.8 for no more than 12–24 h.
   (e) Constant-volume ventilator, generally used for children weighing 15 kg or more. Special attention should be paid to changes in airway pressure to avoid pressure injuries. It should be noted that the change in fresh air flow has an impact on the output tidal volume, which is greater for smaller children. Therefore, when setting the ventilator or changing the fresh air flow, the child's thoracic relief, breath sounds, and peak inspiratory pressure should be repeatedly approved.
   (f) The ventilation mode using constant-pressure ventilator is necessary for pediatric patients, and it is commonly used for children weighing less than 10 kg, especially for children with high airway resistance, to avoid air pressure injury. However, ventilation volume is often affected by changes in airway compliance, so constant attention should be paid to whether ventilation is insufficient or excessive. The output air volume of the fixed-pressure ventilator will not increase due to excessive fresh air flow, but when the fresh air flow is too small for the airbox compressor to reach the set peak pressure, the tidal volume will be insufficient.
3. Monitoring of Ventilation
   (a) The monitoring of tidal volume and ventilation volume is the most basic monitoring index, and changes in their values should be noted at any time during the operation, especially when the airway resistance changes.
   (b) During mechanical ventilation, monitoring of airway pressure is a necessary indicator, especially in the fixed-volume breathing mode, where detection of airway pressure can avoid air pressure injury.
   (c) The partial pressure of end-expiratory carbon dioxide ($PETCO_2$) is a real-time indicator of good ventilation and should be a routine monitoring item during pediatric tracheal intubation. The difference between $PETCO_2$ and $PaCO_2$ in neonates and preterm infants is large and $PaCO_2$ should be measured when necessary.
   (d) Pulse oximetry (SpO_2) reflects the oxygenation of the body. It is closely related to the concentration of inhaled oxygen, and indirectly reflects the ventilation.

14.3.3 Principles and Methods of Management of Pediatric Difficult Airway

14.3.3.1 Common Causes of Difficult Airway in Pediatric Patients

1. Anatomical deformities of the head, face, and airway: cerebrospinal bulge, small jaw deformity, severe congenital cleft lip and palate, congenital tracheal stenosis, esophageal tracheal fistula, etc.
2. Inflammatory conditions: epiglottitis, submaxillary abscess, peri-tonsillar abscess, laryngeal papilloma, etc.
3. Tumors: benign, malignant tumors of the tongue, nose, floor of the mouth, pharynx and trachea, and tumors of the neck and chest may also compress the airway.
4. Trauma or motor system diseases: such as maxillofacial trauma, scar contracture after burns, ankylosing spondylitis, temporomandibular joint lesions, cervical spinal dislocation, or fracture, etc.

14.3.3.2 Assessment of Pediatric Difficult Airway

1. Medical History
   (a) Any experience of difficult intubation, history of airway surgery.
   (b) Any abnormal sleep performance, such as restless sleep, sleeping position with elongated neck and head tilted back; any sleepwalking or micturition associated with airway obstruction; any snoring or sleep apnea syndrome.
   (c) Any history of prolonged feeding time, swallowing with choking or nausea, breathing difficulty or inability to tolerate exercise in children.
2. Physical Examination
   (a) Check for nasal obstruction, deviated nasal septum, protrusion or loosening of incisors, and check whether the chin, hyoid bone, turbinate, and trachea are centered.
   (b) Check the degree of mouth opening: if the distance between the upper and lower incisors is less than the width of the child's own two fingers when trying to open the mouth, the child may be accompanied by a difficult airway.
   (c) Check the degree of neck retroflexion: reduced atlanto-occipital mobility may result in poor exposure of the vocal folds during laryngoscopy.
   (d) The shape and size of the mandible and jawbone, check if there is a small jaw.
   (e) Examination of the oral cavity and tongue; infants and children are often uncooperative, so complete visualization of the isthmus and uvula is often difficult, and Mallampati scoring methods may not be applicable in the pediatric population to predict difficult tracheal intubation.
   (f) Laryngoscopy: Indirect laryngoscopy is useful to assess the size of the base of the tongue, the mobility of the epiglottis and the visualization of the larynx and the posterior nostril. Pediatric direct laryngoscopy is often difficult to perform preoperatively.

14.3.3.3 Tools and Methods for Establishing the Airway

1. Non-Acute Airway

   Management of non-acute airway should be minimally invasive.
   (a) Conventional direct laryngoscopy: Macintosh (curved) and Miller (straight) laryngoscopes.
   (b) Bullard laryngoscope and Upsher fiberoptic laryngoscope: allows indirect visualization of the voice box.
   (c) Visual laryngoscopes: such as ClideScope video waiting scopes. (3) Visual laryngoscopes: such as the ClideScope video waiting scope.
   (d) Tube core type: (1) rigid tube core; (2) insertion probe (Bougie).
   (e) Light wand.
   (f) Visible rigid cores: such as Shikani rigid fiberoptic tracheoscope, Levitan rigid fiberoptic tracheoscope, etc.
   (g) Laryngeal mask (LMA): classic laryngeal mask (LMA-Classical, LMA-Unique), double tube laryngeal mask (LMA-

ProSeal, LMA-Supreme), intubated laryngeal mask (LMA-Fastrach).
   (h) Flexible Fiberoptic Intubation.
   (i) Retrograde intubation: This method mainly involves the insertion of a guidewire through the cricothyroid membrane puncture, leading from the oral cavity through the vocal cords, and then the tracheal tube enters the trachea through the guidewire.
2. Acute airway: The purpose of dealing with acute airway is to save life.
   (a) Mask positive pressure ventilation: place an oropharyngeal or nasopharyngeal airway, and complete ventilation by two people if necessary.
   (b) Laryngeal mask: can be used for both non-acute and acute airways, and in emergency situations, the mask most familiar to the operator should be selected for placement.
   (c) Combined esophagotracheal tube (ET-Combitube).
   (d) Cricothyroid puncture placement: a method of subglottic airway opening that can be used in emergencies where the supraglottic route cannot establish an airway. When neither ventilation nor intubation is possible, cricothyrotomy or tracheotomy placement is the only life-saving method and should be performed decisively and quickly.

14.3.3.4 Pediatric Difficult Airway Management

1. Prepare the tools for airway management before anesthesia, check the anesthesia machine, ventilation circuit, mask, airway and laryngoscope, tracheal tube, intubation probe, laryngeal mask, etc. to ensure that they are readily available. Prepare a cart or box for "difficult airway" management, containing the above-mentioned airway management tools.
2. Preoperative anticholinergics should be used to reduce oropharyngeal secretions and laryngospasm; the child should not be overly sedated, and if necessary, a small dose of anxiolytics should be monitored; if there is no emergency fasting, H2 blockers and gastrostat should be given preoperatively.
3. Unlike adults, pediatric patients are generally uncooperative and almost always require general anesthesia and are not suitable for awake tracheal intubation. Inhalation anesthesia is often used for induction, sevoflurane is often preferred, intravenous anesthetics should be used with caution, inotropic drugs are prohibited, and spontaneous breathing is maintained. After reaching a certain depth of anesthesia, laryngoscopy and intubation are attempted. Ketamine, midazolam, etc. can also be used for proper sedation and good surface anesthesia and/or regional nerve block.
4. Expected Difficult Airway
   (a) Determine the presence of a difficult airway in the child before anesthesia, select the appropriate technique, and determine the preferred and alternative options for tracheal intubation. Try to use techniques and instruments that the anesthetist is familiar with, and minimally invasive methods are preferred.
   (b) Adequate mask oxygenation first, ensuring oxygenation during intubation, prompt mask-assisted oxygen ventilation when SpO_2 drops to 90%, and always actively seeking opportunities to provide assisted oxygenation.
   (c) Preserve spontaneous breathing as much as possible to prevent a predicted difficult airway from becoming an acute airway.
   (d) Direct intubation or fast induction intubation if the laryngoscope can see the glottis; if there are difficulties in glottic exposure, intubation probe or light rod technique, assisted by fiberoptic bronchoscopy, or video laryngoscopy or trial intubation laryngeal mask can be used.
   (e) When intubation is repeatedly unsuccessful for more than three times, postponing or abandoning anesthesia and surgery is also a necessary treatment to ensure the safety of the child. The patient should be handled again after experience summary and adequate preparation are made.

5. Unexpected Difficult Airway
    (a) Before the main general anesthesia induction drugs and inotropic drugs are given, a ventilation test should be routinely performed to test whether controlled ventilation can be implemented, and those who cannot control ventilation should not be blindly given inotropic drugs and subsequent general anesthetic drugs to prevent the occurrence of an acute airway.
    (b) For patients who can be ventilated but are difficult in glottic exposure and tracheal intubation, choose the above-mentioned tools for a non-acute airway. To fully ventilate and achieve optimal oxygenation before intubation, intubation time in principle is not more than 1 min, or pulse oximetry is not less than 92%, and when unsuccessful, to ventilate again to achieve optimal oxygenation, analyze the reasons, adjust the method or personnel, and then intubate again.
    (c) For ventilation difficulties encountered after induction of general anesthesia, help should be sought immediately by calling a superior or subordinate physician to assist.
    (d) Also try to solve the ventilation problem in the shortest possible time: mask positive pressure ventilation (using oropharyngeal or nasopharyngeal airway), place a laryngeal mask and ventilate. Consider waiting for the child to recover spontaneous breathing and wake up after improved ventilation.
    (e) Ensure that the child is ventilated using the tools and methods of the acute airway described above.
    (f) Consider waking up the child and canceling the procedure to ensure the patient's life safety, and decide on the anesthesia method after full discussion.
6. Cautions
    (a) Choose the technique with which the anesthetist is most familiar and experienced.
    (b) When intubation fails, avoid repeated operations by the same person using the same method. You should analyze it in time, change ideas and methods or change personnel and techniques, and learn to give up after repeated failures several times.
    (c) Ventilation and oxygenation are the main purpose, while being minimally invasive.

14.4 Pediatric Anesthesia Techniques

14.4.1 Premedication in the Pediatric Population: Alleviating Anxiety

In either adult or pediatric patients, the purpose of premedication is to reduce anxiety and prepare the patient for the next level of anesthesia by accepting a mask or intravenous (IV). Dental treatment for pediatric patients may be compromised by their lack of cooperation in dental procedures, including examinations and radiographs [12]. Induction and maintenance of anesthesia are now more challenging due to an increased sympathetic tone. Patient anxiety increases the risk of missed appointments by three times and requires more chair time and hand holding. A poor experience can negatively impact future experiences for the child and parents despite the best efforts of the anesthesia team. Therefore, premedication appears to be an appropriate measure not only to reduce anxiety to "show" for the appointment, but also to have a conscious, cooperative, and comfortable child so the team can proceed with the anesthetic and surgical plan.

Premedication can be administered via enteral (oral), parenteral (often intramuscular [IM]), and inhalational routes [6]. In spite of the fact that enteral administration is the least threatening and most convenient method of administering premedication, it has several disadvantages. The cooperation of children and parents is essential to the process. Many drugs are administered empirically and cannot be titrated properly. In addition to variable responses, oral premedication has an equally unpredictable recovery pattern. Treatment plans can be hindered on a busy procedure day due to the unpredictable and extended action times of medication. A variety of creative forms of oral premedication are available for children, such as syrups, popsicles, and lozenges. Children are less likely to tolerate nasal sprays. In addition to being rapidly absorbed, a premedication should also have a rapid onset of action with a high therapeutic index, and it should not delay recovery. A variety of medications can be used as premedications, such as benzodiazepines, histamine blockers, opioids, scopolamine, barbiturates, and alpha agonists (dexmedetomidine and clonidine).

Benzodiazepines are an ideal choice due to their ease of absorption and limited cardiovascular effects. Diazepam, triazolam, and midazolam are common drugs in this class used as premedication. The liquid form of midazolam is well tolerated by children. The three medications differ in some characteristics. Onset time: diazepam>triazolam>midazolam; duration of action: diazepam>tirazolam>midazolam.

Preoperative anxiety can be reduced with diazepam, which has been extensively studied in pediatrics for its efficacy and safety. It has proven to not delay discharge. Because of its effects on postural stability, administering it in the office is safer for very young patients. Oral midazolam has a rapid onset of action, short duration of action, leaves no active metabolites, and has the desirable effect of retrograde amnesia. This product is readily accepted by children since it comes in the form of pleasantly flavored syrups and popsicles. The recommended dose for premedication is 0.5–1.0 mg/kg with a 15–20-mg maximum dose. Such dose is anticipated to work for around half an hour. The oral dose decided should not affect heart rate, respiratory rate, or blood pressure significantly. Not providing any analgesic effects remains to be the major shortcoming of the drug. Moreover, adverse reaction such as dysphoria, blurred vision, and undesirable behavior may appear on 3–4% of children can who were administered midazolam. Like all other oral premedications, oral midazolam also may be difficult to titrate, may have unreliable absorption, and moderate failure rates. Unfortunately, other medications such as triazolam have not been well-studied in children.

Dexmedetomidine becomes widely accepted as a single agent sedative for MRI or simple procedures. Unlike benzodiazepines or propofol which is a GABA-mimetic drug, dexmedetomidine as an alpha2 agonist embraces the advantage of producing the sedation which mimics natural sleep, anxiolysis, analgesia, sympatholysis, with minimal respiratory depression. The present recommended dose of the agent for premedication is 3–4 mg/kg intranasal and 1–4 mg/kg dosing orally.

Ketamine is another agent used for oral premedication. The dose recommended is 6 mg/kg, which typically takes 20 min to onset and can provide up to 30 min of sedation.

14.4.2 Routes of Administering Anesthesia

14.4.2.1 Intramuscular Anesthesia Technique

Anesthetic administered through this route encompasses the advantage that the onset of anesthesia is predictable to some extent, even with the most uncooperative pediatric patient. Nevertheless, the onset of anesthetic relies on the drug used and the site of injection, and it may be an unpleasant experience for the cooperative children. Many drugs, including benzodiazepines, ketamine, and dexmedetomidine, have been used in the IM technique.

Ketamine appears to be the more common choice of OMS using this route of anesthetic administration. It is an effective analgesic and amnesic drug that is known to dissociate the cerebral and the limbic system, thereby disrupting the translation of visual, auditory, and pain stimuli. It provides what is known as dissociative anesthesia. At subanesthetic doses, it provides analgesia without respiratory depression and reduces the need for anesthetics. The recommended IM dose of ketamine is 3–4 mg/kg. Anesthesiologists often add benzodiazepines, such as midazolam and glycopyrrolate, to injected ketamine to enhance its action while reducing undesired side effects. Ketamine can cause increased salivation, heart rate, blood pressure, and intracranial pressure. However, it stimulates smooth muscle dilation, thereby reducing the risk of bronchospasm. It is important to note that ketamine is available in two concentrations, 50 mg/ml and 100 mg/ml. The higher concentration of ketamine is indicated for IM injections, which can minimize the volume of the injection site. In larger children, the use of a lower concentration of ketamine may result in an injection volume of more than 3 mL and therefore is not recommended for injection at only one site.

A phenomenon known as "emergent delirium" has been associated with ketamine use, making practitioners wary of this drug. Concurrent use of benzodiazepines or propofol may reduce the risk of ketamine-induced delirium. Risk factors for delirium when using ketamine include female gender, over 10 years old, underlying psychiatric disorder, IV route, high dose and excessive noise stimulation upon emergence.

The IM injection technique requires parents and practitioners to be prepared, particularly in uncooperative children. The preparation involves a quiet room with minimal stimulation and a schedule that provides sufficient time for the onset action of anesthetics. Once the child becomes cooperative, a monitor must be placed and should be kept in place until discharge. It may be helpful to have an alternative route of administration of the anesthetic or prepare readministering the IM route. Longer recovery times can be expected if higher IM doses are used preoperatively.

14.4.2.2 Intravenous Anesthetic Technique

The IV route remains the most predictable route of administration of anesthetic and resuscitation drugs. One of its advantages is the rapid onset and offset of medications. Whereas, it requires placement of a catheter in a peripheral vein, which can be challenging for pediatric patients. Appropriate equipment is indispensable for careful administration of medications and fluids. Preoperative calculation of drug doses for anesthesia and emergencies is necessary as well. Fortunately, many new technologies such as applications may help dose calculation while ensuring accuracy.

Drugs such as benzodiazepines, opioids, ketamine, and propofol are the primary agents used in pediatric intravenous anesthesia. A single drug or a combination of two or more drugs insures the smooth performance of the procedure by achieving desired goals of anxiety, amnesia, analgesia, immobilization, sedation, and hypnosis. The intravenous route provides safety, rapid onset and offset of action, and predictable recovery. It is recommended that the IV catheter be maintained until discharge and the recovery unit or ward needs to be equipped with IV/IO equipment to prevent premature loss of this vascular catheter.

The use of an infusion pump during longer procedures minimizes fluctuations in drug serum concentrations and guarantees a smoother intraoperative anesthetic course. Normally, the pump may assure improved cardiovascular and respiratory stability, less patient movement, and more quickly recovery as a result of less medication used.

Providing and training in the use of intranasal access devices is also advised to be included in facilities that choose to treat children. Placing IV in children is a challenging process requiring skill, especially when the prevalence of childhood obesity makes the task even more difficult. In cases where peripheral vascular access is difficult to obtain, the most reliable option is intraosseous (IO) access, especially in emergency situations [13].

14.4.2.3 Inhalational Anesthesia Technique

Since 1844, dentists have been familiar with the technique of inhaled anesthesia using nitrous oxide. Nitrous oxide has been shown to have a broad safety margin in the pediatric population with minimal side effects. It is rapid in induction and emergence, and is an effective analgesic. It is known to cause insignificant cardiovascular and respiratory changes. When added to a second inhaler, it promotes anesthesia through a second gas effect.

Inhalation techniques are much better tolerated and considered less invasive, and at the same time, result in almost no extra respiratory adverse events comparing with IV route [14]. Often, the mask is easily accepted by curious children, especially when a fruity smell is added and the unpleasant odor of the plastic mask is diminished. In most cases, anesthetic gas is delivered quickly and the onset of anesthesia is rapid. For uncooperative children, crying can actually be helpful. Because when they are crying, they take long, deep breaths that allow the lungs be filled with anesthetic.

Sevoflurane has become the inhalation agent of choice for most OMS offices. It is a halogenated ether with a rapid onset of action and predictable recovery. It has a sweet, slightly irritating fruity odor and is well accepted by pediatric patients. The gas itself does not irritate the airway compared with other options, and induction is characterized by a reduced incidence of breath-holding and laryngospasm. It has been proven to be safe for use with epinephrine local anesthesia. Standard ASA monitoring, including preoperative temperature measurement, is recommended when using inhaled agents. If sevoflurane is used for procedures exceeding 30 min, it is recommended that continuous invasive temperature monitoring to be adopted.

For cooperative pediatric patients, several minutes' preoxygenation prior to induction may achieve ideal effect. Sevoflurane can be used as a single inhalation agent or in combination with nitrous oxide. Gradual titration of the gas to achieve the effect is preferred. Once the patient is past the second stage of anesthesia, an IV and administering anesthetic drugs via that route should be started. At then, gas inhalation is stopped and the oxygen is maintained by mask or nasal cannula.

For uncooperative children, the single-breath technique is effective. Priming the circuit with 8% sevoflurane and preoxygenation is often impractical for a crying child. Crying promotes rapid inhalation of highly concentrated gas and induction is quickly finished. After induction, the IV may be administered, the gas discontinued, and the technique can be converted to total IV anesthesia.

Of all inhalational anesthetics, it is sensible to consider placing an IV. This is especially important if the patient is relatively small, obese or young, or in any case where the anesthesia provider feels that placing an IV may be a challenge, especially in the event of an unplanned event. The IV may never be used, but can provide a safeguard in the emergencies. It is best done when things are under control and before surgery begins, rather than in an emergency or mid-surgery.

Halothane gas is a trigger for malignant hyperthermia (MH). Potential family and personal medical histories regarding MH should be discussed with the patient and parents prior to planning inhalational anesthesia. Facilities using MH triggering agents are advised to be prepare for MH events, including stocking adequate amounts of dantrolene and practicing how to reconstitute it. Newer dantrolene products make this process less cumbersome, in addition to reducing the amount of dantrolene that needs to be stored.

14.4.3 Anesthesia for Pediatric Cleft Lip and Palate Surgery

Cleft lip and palate deformities, as the most common congenital malformations of the maxillofacial region, account for 2/3 of all facial malformations. While the worldwide prevalence of such deformities is about 1.5 per 1000 live births, the rate varies six-fold for cleft lip/palate and three-fold for cleft palate [15, 16]. Reports in Asian populations put overall rates around 1.76–1.81 per 1000, reflecting the higher prevalence in this region [17, 18]. Genetic and environmental factors are the main reasons causing congenital malformations of the maxillofacial region. Besides, clefts can be further divided into syndromic and nonsyndronic clefts. The syndromic clefts include chromosomal syndromes, teratogens, and uncategorized syndromes [19].

Specifically, cleft lip is a failure of fusion of the anterior nasal and maxillary processes, resulting in various degrees of clefting through the lip, alveolus, and nasal floor (incomplete clefts do not cross the nasal floor, whereas complete clefts imply a lack of connection between the floor and medial elements of the lip) [20]. There are two types of cleft palate, the hard and soft palate, which result from the failure to fuse the palatal shelf of the maxillary process [20]. In the embryonic developmental cycle, cleft palate occurs in stages IV to VIII. Depending on the location of the failure of fusion of the various facial processes, they appear at different times in the embryonic period, depending on the disturbance to development that occurs during the process [21].

Understanding the occurrence, development and characteristics of children with cleft lip and palate will help anesthesiologists properly implement anesthesia management, which in turn will ensure the smooth performance of the surgery.

14.4.3.1 Classification and Surgical Treatment of Cleft Lip and Palate

There are many ways to classify cleft lip and palate. Here is the classification based on the degree of cleft opening that is most commonly used in our clinic.

1. Unilateral Cleft Lip
   (a) Unilateral incomplete harelip/cleft lip: unilateral cleft of the lip that does not reach the nasal base.
   (b) Unilateral complete harelip/cleft lip: a cleft lip that runs through the upper lip to the nasal base.
2. Bilateral Cleft Lip
   (a) Bilateral incomplete harelip/cleft lip: bilateral cleft lip where neither cleft reaches the nasal base.
   (b) Bilateral complete harelip/cleft lip: bilateral cleft running through the upper lip to reach the nasal base.
   (c) Bilateral mixed harelip/cleft lip: one side of the upper lip is completely cleft and the other side is incompletely cleft.
3. Cleft soft palate: only the soft palate is cleft (no distinction between right and left cleft palate), which may be limited to the uvula.
4. Incomplete cleft palate: a complete cleft of the soft palate with a partial cleft hard palate (no distinction between right and left cleft palate) and a complete alveolar process.
5. Unilateral complete cleft palate: a complete split from the uvula to the incisive foramina, reaching to the alveolar ridge and attaching to the alveolar row.
6. Bilateral complete cleft palate: occurring simultaneously with bilateral cleft lip, a cleft exists in the premaxillary bone extending to the alveolar ridge, leading to the isolation of nasal septum, forehead and anterior lip part from the center.

Cleft lip and palate deformities not only damage children's appearance, but also affect the morphology and function of their maxillofacial organs. Also, cleft lip and palate repair surgery can affect the facial growth and development. Considering the positive and negative effects of all treatment measures, children with cleft lip and palate need sequential treatment which is a complex and lengthy systematic treatment method, requiring multidisciplinary, multifaceted treatment and observation in order to achieve or approach normal appearance, function, and psychological well-being of pediatric patients.

The treatment of cleft lip and palate consists of two phases, namely, phase I (initial) treatment and phase II treatment. Initial treatment, including cleft lip (palate) repair, initial correction of cleft lip secondary to nasal deformity and correction of incomplete palatopharyngeal closure, is usually completed before patients are 5–6 years old. Phase II treatment is usually scheduled after patients are 8 years old, including orthodontic treatment, alveolar cleft repair, and orthognathic surgery.

1. Phase I Cleft Lip and Palate Treatment

   The best time to repair initial cleft lip and cleft lip secondary to nasal deformity is within 3–6 months after the birth of pediatric patients. Prior to the surgical treatment, children should be taken good care to meet the weight requirements of the surgery. Bilateral cleft lip can be repaired either in one or two operation. The interval between two operations should be no less than 2–3 months.

The optimal surgery time for phase I treatment is when patients are 1–1.5 years old. The children's development and the presence of any systemic abnormalities also need to be evaluated before the procedure is performed.

The best time to correct palatopharyngeal insufficiency is between 5 years and 6 years of age. The main clinical manifestation of palatopharyngeal insufficiency is the high nasal voice that affects their speech.

2. Phase II Cleft Lip and Palate Treatment

   The best time to repair an alveolar cleft bone defect is from 9 years to 11 years of age, before the cuspids erupt in the cleft area. The remaining nasal and labial deformities should be rectified again after or at the same time as the alveolar cleft bone grafting [22].

   The best time to treat dental and maxillofacial malformations in children with cleft lip and palate is from 14 years to 16 years of age. Le Fort I osteotomy is most frequently used.

14.4.3.2 Characteristics of Anesthesia Management in Cleft Lip and Palate Surgery

Cleft lip and palate is one of the most common congenital malformations of the maxillofacial region, and the anesthesia management of cleft lip and palate surgery should take into account the characteristics of the disease, in addition to the traits of pediatric anesthesia and repeated anesthesia. Also, for cleft lip and palate caused by chromosomal aberrations and single gene mutations, attention needs to be paid to the altered physiological or pathological conditions ignited by the concomitant occurrence of multi-malformation.

1. Characteristics of Pediatric Airway

   The larynx of pediatric patients is normally anterolateral and cephalad. Their nasal cavity is relatively narrow. Their tongue is comparatively large, and their epiglottis is long and drooping. The short trachea and neck make the exposure of glottis difficult, which increases the difficulty of intubation as tracheal mucous membrane edema may occur. Infants and young children have short and narrow airway and because their respiratory system is not well developed, they have fewer alveoli and faster metabolism. Thus, mild laryngeal edema may cause serious ventilation disorders, increasing the resistance of the airway, affecting the oxygenation, and triggering hypoxemia.

   Moreover, the palate and maxillofacial area of pediatric patients are rich in blood flow; therefore, intraoperative and postoperative bleeding in the trachea may easily cause aspiration. Edema in the operative area after cleft palate surgery as well as filling of iodoform gauze and nostril plastic tubes for compression of hemorrhage may also affect the patency of the airway.

   Some pediatric patients who require orthognathic and orthodontic treatment may also have micrognathia, which is a potential factor of difficult airway. They are prone to upper airway obstruction which may be escalated when glossoptosis happens during induction of anesthesia. Therefore, such patients should be adequately evaluated prior to anesthesia.

2. Adverse Neurological Reflexes

   As the oral and maxillofacial area has abundant nerves and is sensitive to pain, the carotid sinus reflex may be induced under surgical stimulation. Furthermore, apnea, hypotension, bradycardia, and even cardiac arrest may occur. Therefore, it is necessary to closely monitor the changes in the vital signs to detect and prevent them in a timely manner.

3. Pediatric Anesthesia

   As mentioned above, pediatric patients have fewer alveoli and low lung compliance. During inspiration, their chest wall tends to collapse, resulting in lower residual lung air volume during exhalation. The reduced functional residual air volume limits the oxygen reserve during the hypoxic phase of intubation. As a result, infants and children are more susceptible to pulmonary atelectasis and hypoxemia.

In infancy, the left ventricle is underdeveloped and poorly compliant, and cardiac output is very sensitive to changes in heart rate.

Their low fat reserves and large body surface area make them prone to heat loss in the low-temperature environment of the operating room. Also, during surgery, operations such as exposure of wounds, infusion of intravenous fluids, and the influence of the anesthetic drugs on the thermoregulatory center, can exacerbate the loss of heat. Hypothermia may lead to delayed awakening, myocardial provocation, respiratory depression, and other adverse outcomes in pediatric patients. Their body temperature should be closely monitored in order to identify hypothermia and hyperthermia timely.

The incidence of perioperative complications may rise if pediatric patients suffer from upper respiratory tract infection 2 weeks prior to surgery, predisposing them to asthma, laryngospasm, hypoxemia, and pulmonary atelectasis. During extubation, laryngospasm should be prevented.

14.4.3.3 Anesthesia Techniques in Cleft Lip and Palate Surgery

General Anesthesia

1. Pre-anesthesia Visit and Preparation

   Usually, the anesthesiologist should visit patients and their families 1 day before surgery to review the entire hospital history of patients and make purposeful inquiries with their families. The focus should be on: (1) delivery history, whether pediatric patients have intrauterine distress, preterm delivery, forceps or birth injury; (2) history of congenital diseases, especially children with congenital heart disease and some newly diagnosed heart murmurs, and pediatric cardiologists should be consulted or an echocardiogram should be performed; (3) patients' feeding, nutritional, and growth status; (4) patients' sleep condition, including whether children can sleep peacefully or lie down, whether there is snoring or suffocating awake phenomenon; (5) recent upper respiratory tract infection history, which can increase the incidence of complications such as asthma, laryngospasm, hypoxemia, and atelectasis.

   Pediatric patients who have infectious diseases before surgery should rearrange the surgery when diseases are controlled. If the surgery is so urgent that cannot be delayed, preoperative administration of anticholinergic drugs and inhalation of humidified gas need to be considered. When to perform the surgery should refer to laboratory reports in which children should meet the requirements that white blood cells is below 10,000/L and hemoglobin is greater than 100 g/L. During the anesthesia visit, the anesthesiologist should briefly introduce the process of anesthesia, and explain the importance of preoperative fasting and abstinence so that they can cooperate and strictly observe the fasting time.

2. Premedication

   There are great disagreements on premedication for pediatric patients, and preoperative sedatives are usually omitted. However, when children are unable to control their emotions, giving sedatives is a reasonable choice. Anticholinergic agents such as atropine and valacyclovir hydrochloride can be routinely applied. The recommended injection time of these agents is half an hour before surgery, which can effectively reduce the incidence of bradycardia during induction of anesthesia, and at the same time, the accumulation of secretions can also be mitigated, so to prevent obstruction of small airways and airway tubes. Scopolamine should be used with caution in children.

3. Implementation of Anesthesia

   General anesthesia was administered either by intravenous induction or by inhalation induction, which has been introduced in previous text. Generally, for intravenous induction in pediatric patients, the order of administration is the same as in adults, with propofol followed by nondepolarizing inotropes. Inhalation induction can also be used if patients are unable to cooperate in opening the vein. An important step in the intubation process, whether awake or under general anesthesia, is the adjunctive application of endotracheal mucosal spray for surface anesthesia. The small internal diameter of the catheter used in this group of patients limits the use of fiberoptic laryngoscopes and blind tracheal intubation devices, because they will cause edema of the tender pharyngeal tissues and consequent adverse events.

4. Intraoperative Monitoring and Management

   Intraoperative monitoring in children is similar to that in adults, but with a slight difference: pediatric monitoring has a much smaller margin of error.

   (a) Respiratory Monitoring and Management

      The anesthesiologist can only monitor patients away from them because during surgery, the surgeon operates in front of the patients, making it challenging to manage patients perioperatively. Therefore, it is especially important to closely monitor the patient's breathing and to detect and treat abnormalities such as too deep intubation, twisting, folding, and dislodging of the tube and the connector in a timely manner. Before administering controlled ventilation, gas flow, tidal volume, and respiratory rate should be accurately set according to the child's weight, and the high and low limits of the airway pressure alarm should be adjusted. Oxygen saturation and carbon dioxide testing is particularly important in infants and children, and the pulse oximetry probe is preferentially placed in the right hand or earlobe for newborns. When the child weighs less than 10 kg, capnography values are often inaccurate, that there may be a false increase in inspiratory baseline CO_2 and a false decrease in expiratory peak CO_2.

   (b) Circulation Monitoring and Management

      Although the duration of cleft lip and palate repair surgery is not long, the monitoring and management of circulation should not be neglected. Intraoperative fluid intake and output should be recorded to accurately estimate the blood loss and supplement crystalloid and colloid fluids promptly. Autologous blood transfusion can be planned preoperatively. In pediatric patients, it is important to drain as much gas as possible from the pressure line and use small volume fluid flushes during the infusion to prevent air embolism, accidental heparinization, or fluid overload.

   (c) Temperature Monitoring and Management

      Pediatric patients' low fat reserves and large body surface area make them prone to heat loss in the low-temperature environment of the operating room. Also, during surgery, operations such as exposure of wounds, infusion of intravenous fluids, and the influence of the anesthetic drugs on the thermoregulatory center, can exacerbate the loss of heat. Hypothermia may lead to delayed awakening, myocardial provocation, respiratory depression, and other adverse outcomes in pediatric patients. Their body temperature should be closely monitored in order to identify hypothermia and hyperthermia timely.

   (d) Perioperative Fluid Infusion

      Because of the limited margin of error that pediatric patients can accept, more attention should be paid to their fluid management. Their fluid infusion should consider the fluids required for physiological maintenance, fasting losses and intraoperative losses. Fluids for physiological maintenance are calculated based on the 4:2:1 principle: 4 ml/(kg h) for the first 10 kg, 2 ml/(kg h) for the second 10 kg, and 1 ml/(kg h) for the remaining body weight. The fluid loss was calculated according to the fasting time. The amount of preoperative fasting and hourly fluid required were replenished by 50% in the first hour and 25% in each of the second and third hours. For intraoperative losses, it is worth noting that children have a small intravascular volume and rapid fluid infusion increases the risk of electrolyte disturbances.

5. Post-anesthesia Recovery

After cleft lip and palate surgery, patients' head and face are mostly fixed by bandage. The inappropriate extubation time may induce respiratory distress. Therefore, in order to ensure that they safely pass through the post-anesthesia recovery period, they should be sent to the post-anesthesia care unit (PACU) after surgery. The anesthesiologist in charge should hand over patients to the PACU physician. Necessary monitoring and documentation should also be maintained in the PACU, and children's consciousness, respiration, and pharyngeal reflexes should be closely observed.

In addition, the operation field should also be closely observed, especially whether there is blood oozing. If blood oozes from the wound, using small cotton swab to gently wipe blood away. The wound should be disinfected with 75% alcohol before changing the dressing. If the wound is bruised with blood, saline should be used to clean the wound in order to prevent infection. If the blood oozing is serious, it must be treated immediately. The priority is to distinguish the causes of blood oozing. For example, severe bleeding, blood drainage soaking the dressing, rapid swelling of the wound, negative pressure drainage tube pumping fresh blood or even abnormalities such as decreased blood pressure and increased pulse rate may be the results of active bleeding in the wound and the surgeon should be notified immediately to re-suture it. If excessive blood loss or shock symptoms occur, blood and fluid transfusion should be given promptly.

Furthermore, body temperature should be of particular interest during this period. Postoperative fever is generally a normal reaction if the temperature is not too high. However, if the temperature is >39 °C, the cause should be identified and corrected as early as possible. Treatment includes physical cooling, infusion of cool fluids or enema with chloral hydrate. Pediatric patients with hyperthermia are more likely to have dehydration and acid-base and electrolyte disturbances.

Pediatric patients should be extubated only when their swallowing and coughing reflexes have fully recovered, their respiratory and circulatory functions are stable, and no risk of airway obstruction exists. If their intubation lasts for too long, early administration of adrenal glucocorticoids can prevent laryngeal edema. Normally, cleft palate patients are more likely to have upper airway obstruction, and a nasal airway can be placed prior to extubation to reduce the incidence of airway problems. After they awake, clinicians should check whether they have laryngeal edema and wound bleeding. They could adopt a head-high position to mitigate edema 6–8 h after recovery from anesthesia. The monitoring of their vital signs should be continued to ensure the patency of their airway and provide oxygen if necessary. The hoarse of vocal cord caused by laryngeal edema due to general anesthesia intubation can be treated with symptomatic treatment (such as nebulized inhalation). If they snore or have glossocoma, immediate treatment should be provided. When suctioning, the suction tube should not touch the wound. Their families can enter the PACU to comfort and console the anxiety patients.

References

1. Physiology for Children. JAMA. 2014;311(17):1811. PMID: 24794384. https://doi.org/10.1001/jama.2013.279481.
2. Thornton PS, Stanley CA, De Leon DD, Harris D, Haymond MW, Hussain K, Levitsky LL, Murad MH, Rozance PJ, Simmons RA, Sperling MA, Weinstein DA, White NH, Wolfsdorf JI, Pediatric Endocrine Society. Recommendations from the Pediatric Endocrine Society for evaluation and management of persistent hypoglycemia in neonates, infants, and children. J Pediatr. 2015;167(2):238–45. Epub 2015 May 6. PMID: 25957977. https://doi.org/10.1016/j.jpeds.2015.03.057.

3. Prakash M, Johnny JC. Whats special in a child's larynx? J Pharm Bioallied Sci. 2015;7(Suppl 1):S55–8. https://doi.org/10.4103/0975-7406.155797.
4. Huelke DF. An overview of anatomical considerations of infants and children in the adult world of automobile safety design. Annu Proc Assoc Adv Automot Med. 1998;42:93–113. PMCID: PMC3400202.
5. Tait AR, Malviya S. Anesthesia for the child with an upper respiratory tract infection: still a dilemma? Anesth Analg. 2005;100(1):59–65. PMID: 15616052. https://doi.org/10.1213/01.ANE.0000139653.53618.91.
6. Krishnan DG. Anesthesia for the pediatric oral and maxillofacial surgery patient. Oral Maxillofac Surg Clin North Am. 2018;30(2):171–81. PMID: 29622311. https://doi.org/10.1016/j.coms.2018.02.002.
7. Hiller AS, Kracke A, Tschernig T, Kasper M, Kleemann WJ, Tröger HD, Pabst R. Comparison of the immunohistology of mucosa-associated lymphoid tissue in the larynx and lungs in cases of sudden infant death and controls. Int J Leg Med. 1997;110(6):316–22. PMID: 9387014. https://doi.org/10.1007/s004140050095.
8. Szpinda M, Daroszewski M, Woźniak A, Szpinda A, Mila-Kierzenkowska C. Tracheal dimensions in human fetuses: an anatomical, digital and statistical study. Surg Radiol Anat. 2012;34(4):317–23. Epub 2011 Oct 8. PMID: 21984196; PMCID: PMC3334485. https://doi.org/10.1007/s00276-011-0878-7.
9. Herring MJ, Putney LF, Wyatt G, Finkbeiner WE, Hyde DM. Growth of alveoli during postnatal development in humans based on stereological estimation. Am J Physiol Lung Cell Mol Physiol. 2014;307(4):L338–44. Epub 2014 Jun 6. PMID: 24907055; PMCID: PMC4137164. https://doi.org/10.1152/ajplung.00094.2014.
10. Anderson B, Bissonnette B. Pediatric anesthesia: basic principles, state of the art, future. Shelton, CT: People's Medical Pub; 2011.
11. Kamlin C, Davis PG. Long versus short inspiratory times in neonates receiving mechanical ventilation. Cochrane Database Syst Rev. 2004;2003(4):CD004503. PMID: 15495117; PMCID: PMC6885059. https://doi.org/10.1002/14651858.CD004503.pub2.
12. Campbell RL, Shetty NS, Shetty KS, Pope HL, Campbell JR. Pediatric dental surgery under general anesthesia: uncooperative children. Anesth Prog. 2018;65(4):225–30. PMID: 30715931; PMCID: PMC6318733 (Winter). https://doi.org/10.2344/anpr-65-03-04.
13. Dornhofer P, Kellar JZ. Intraosseous vascular access. In: StatPearls. Treasure Island, FL: StatPearls; 2022; PMID: 32119260.
14. Porter LL, Blaauwendraad SM, Pieters BM. Respiratory and hemodynamic perioperative adverse events in intravenous versus inhalational induction in pediatric anesthesia: a systematic review and meta-analysis. Paediatr Anaesth. 2020;30(8):859–66. https://doi.org/10.1111/pan.13904. Epub 2020 Jun 5. PMID: 32358815.
15. Little J, Cardy A, Munger RG. Tobacco smoking and oral clefts: a meta-analysis. Bull World Health Organ. 2004;82(3):213–8. Epub 2004 Apr 16. Pubmed PMID: 15112010.
16. Mossey PA, Shaw WC, Munger RG, Murray JC, Murthy J, Little J. Global oral health inequalities: challenges in the prevention and management of orofacial clefts and potential solutions. Adv Dent Res. 2011;23(2):247–58. Pubmed PMID: 21490237.
17. Kim S, Kim WJ, Oh C, Kim JC. Cleft lip and palate incidence among the live births in the republic of Korea. J Korean Med Sci. 2002;17(1):49–52. PubmedPMID: 11850588.
18. Wang W, Guan P, Xu W, Zhou B. Risk factors for oral clefts: a population-based case-control study in Shenyang, China. Paediatr Perinat Epidemiol. 2009;23(4):310–20. PubmedPMID: 19523078.
19. Murray JC. Gene/environment causes of cleft lip and/or palate. Clin Genet. 2002;61(4):248–56. PubmedPMID: 12030886.
20. Semer N. Practical plastic surgery for non surgeons. Philadelphia: Hanley& Belfus; 2001. p. 235–43.
21. Proffit W, Fields H, Sarver D. Contemporary orthodontics. 5th ed. Amsterdam: Elsevier Mosby; 2012.
22. Shaye D, Liu CC, Tollefson TT. Cleft lip and palate: an evidence-based review. Facial Plast Surg Clin North Am. 2015;23(3):357–72. Epub 2015 Jun 12. PMID: 26208773. https://doi.org/10.1016/j.fsc.2015.04.008.

Anesthesia for Oral and Maxillofacial Surgery in the Elderly

15

Jingjie Li

15.1 Introduction

In many developed countries, population aging has become a spreading issue, as a result, in these countries, the elderly population (defined as population with age ≥65 years) is the fastest growing segment of the population. Aging increases a person's probability of undergoing surgery and also increases perioperative morbidity, which has been reported to increase sharply in older adults after age 75 years.

Elderly patients are usually more sensitive to anesthetics, which means that in the anesthesia management for the elderly, fewer drugs are needed to achieve the desired clinical outcome, and the anesthetic effects are prolonged. The most important outcome and overall goal of perioperative care for the elderly population is to accelerate recovery and to avoid functional decline.

When managing anesthesia in elderly patients, it is important to keep in mind that aging involves a progressive loss of functional reserve in all organ systems to varying degrees. In addition, compensation for age-related changes is usually more adequate; however, significant limitations in physiologic reserve remain during periods of stress, such as the perioperative period.

15.2 Characteristics of Elderly Patients

15.2.1 Characteristics of Anesthesia Management

15.2.1.1 High Prevalence of Multiple Systemic Diseases

One of the characteristics of systemic diseases in the elderly is that a patient often has multiple systemic diseases [1, 2]. Anesthetic management of such elderly patients requires consideration of the interrelationship of multiple systemic diseases. Table 15.1 shows some common systemic diseases in the elderly.

15.2.1.2 Symptoms of Systemic Diseases May be Atypical

Because of the susceptibility of the elderly to a variety of systemic diseases, systemic diseases may alter each other's symptoms and their typical symptoms are often not as pronounced as in young and middle-aged patients. Examples include painless acute myocardial infarction (often seen in elderly women with diabetes) and infections without febrile symptoms, which may make diagnosis and management in anesthesia management difficult.

J. Li (✉)
Department of Anesthesiology, Shanghai Ninth People's Hospital Affiliated to Shanghai Jiao Tong University School of Medicine, Shanghai, China
e-mail: chenx1853@sh9hospital.org.cn

H. Jiang, M. Xia (eds.), *Anesthesia for Oral and Maxillofacial Surgery*,
https://doi.org/10.1007/978-981-19-7287-4_15

Table 15.1 Common systemic diseases in the elderly

1. Circulatory system	
	Hypertension, angina pectoris, myocardial infarction, heart valve disease, congestive heart failure
2. Respiratory system	
	Pneumonia, chronic obstructive pulmonary disease (COPD), asthma, tuberculosis
3. Cerebrovascular system	
	Cerebral infarction, cerebral hemorrhage, subarachnoid hemorrhage
4. Metabolic and endocrine system	
	Diabetes mellitus, lipid abnormalities, hypothyroidism, hyperthyroidism
5. Digestive system	
	Peptic ulcer, gastroesophageal reflux disease, pharmacogenic digestive system diseases
6. Mental and nervous system	
	Dementia, depression, Parkinson's disease
7. Bone, exercise system	
	Osteoporosis, rheumatoid arthritis
8. Blood, immune system	
	Anemia, multiple myeloma, myelodysplastic syndrome

15.2.1.3 Great Individual Differences

The function of most organs declines gradually with physiological aging. However, the age at which the function of these organs begins to decline and the state of decline varies from person to person. In addition, when pathological aging occurs, individual differences become even greater. Anesthesia should not be administered uniformly based solely on a mechanical assessment of age.

15.2.1.4 Common Dementia and Mild Cognitive Impairment

By 2012, it was estimated that one in seven patients aged 65 or older had dementia, and it is predicted that by 2025, one in five patients aged 65 or older will have dementia. Even if dementia does not develop, the elderly will experience an increased frequency of mild cognitive impairment and thus may experience difficulty in obtaining medical records. In addition, these patients may not follow preoperative management such as fasting and abstinence from food and drink very well.

15.2.1.5 Patients Often Take Multiple Medications at the Same Time

Older patients often have multiple systemic diseases and thus may be taking several to a dozen medications. In the management of these elderly patients, it is necessary to consider the interactions between the various medications they are taking and the anesthetics.

15.2.2 Anatomical and Physiological Characteristics

15.2.2.1 Circulatory System

1. Heart

   Although heart volume does not change with age, heart weight increases with age due to myocardial hypertrophy, increased fibrous and adipose tissue, and sclerotic changes in the mitral and aortic valves.

   The size of the heart increases slightly with age, especially the left ventricle. The thickness of the left ventricular wall increases mildly with age, and the left and right ventricular volumes tend to decrease, and the heart fills more slowly.

   In the conduction system, the number of pacing cells in the sinoatrial node decreases significantly from around age 60 to age 75 when the number of cells drops to 10% of that at age 20. Changes from the atrioventricular node to the atrioventricular bundle are less pronounced than in the sinoatrial node, and only slight changes occur in the more distal conduction bundles.

   Resting heart rates in the elderly are not much different from those of younger and middle-aged adults, but the maximum heart rate that can be achieved during exercise decreases with age. Left ventricular diastolic function is impaired due to decreased myocardial compliance and compensatory atrial hypercontraction. Consequently, in the presence of arrhythmias, such as atrial fibrillation, the single cardiac output is significantly reduced. Increased peripheral vascular resistance due to atherosclerosis increases afterload and systolic blood pressure [3].

The elderly heart is susceptible to heart failure because of its decreased reserve capacity against load.

2. Vascular system

Thickening and reduced stretch of the vessel walls of the aorta and middle arteries, and narrowing and reduced elasticity of the lumen of the small and fine arteries can be seen. The thickening of the arterial wall is more pronounced in the intima. Systolic blood pressure increases with age, but diastolic pressure decreases in the elderly, resulting in an increase in pulse pressure. Decreased sensitivity of the baroreceptor in the aorta and venous sinuses leads to decreased baroreceptor reflex function and predisposes to orthostatic hypotension, resulting in large diurnal variations in blood pressure.

In addition, changes in the connective tissue of the vessel wall can cause the aorta to thicken and stiffen. One result of such changes is an increase in blood pressure—as is the case in most elderly patients. At the same time, increased blood pressure leads to an increased burden on the heart, which can lead to thickening of the heart muscle (hypertrophy), while other arteries can thicken and stiffen as well.

15.2.2.2 Respiratory System

With humans' aging, respiratory muscle strength decreases, the trachea and the rib cartilage calcify, and the connective tissue between the alveolar epithelium and the capillaries of the lungs hardens. These changes cause a decrease in lung and thoracic compliance, an increase in closed volume, closed capacity, functional residual air volume, and a decrease in total lung volume. Closed capacity is about 10% of total lung volume at about age 20, but increases to about 30% at age 70. Exertional lung volumes, FEV1 and FEV1% decrease with age [4, 5].

In addition, there is a decrease in alveolar surface area, a decrease in pulmonary diffusing capacity, a decrease in arterial partial pressure of oxygen (PaO_2) due to an increase in physiological shunt, and an increase in the alveolar-arterial partial pressure of oxygen gradient (A-aDO_2).

As mentioned above, respiratory function in the elderly declines almost linearly with age.

Swallowing and cough reflexes are diminished, and aspiration pneumonia caused by occult aspiration (saliva flowing into the lungs during sleep) is common.

15.2.2.3 Autonomic Nervous System

The thermoregulatory function is decreased, and body temperature is susceptible to hypothermia during general anesthesia due to the ambient temperature of the operating room. The responsiveness of chemoreceptors is decreased, as is the heart rate reflex to hypercapnia and hypoxemia [6].

15.2.2.4 Liver

The number of hepatocytes decreases with age, as does cytochrome P-450 (CYP) activity in hepatocytes. Liver weight decreases to approximately 3/4–2/3 that of younger and middle-aged patients [7], and hepatic blood flow is reduced. These changes result in a reduction in hepatic drug metabolism. The frequency and severity of drug-induced liver injury increases in older patients taking multiple medications [8].

The presence of dyspnea, smoking, coughing, and wheezing can be assessed from the history. Valuable information regarding pulmonary function can be obtained by questioning the elderly patient concerning ability to climb stairs provided that other causes for stopping (e.g., claudication, degenerative osteoarthritis) can be excluded.

Patients with COPD should receive preventive therapy with mucolytic and broncho-dilating agents. Pulmonary infection should be well controlled before surgery. Chest physical therapy may decrease postoperative pulmonary complications.

15.2.2.5 Kidney

Renal atherosclerosis and vitelliform degeneration are the main causes of micro-atherosclerotic nephropathy, and tubular atrophy and glomerulosclerosis may also occur.

In renal cortical function, glomerular filtration rate (GFR), renal blood flow, renal plasma flow, and creatinine clearance are decreased. In renal medullary function, urine concentration and dilution are decreased. In renal tubular function, sodium storage is diminished and sodium excretion is increased. Renin-angiotensin-aldosterone production is also reduced [9, 10].

As with respiratory function, these functions decline linearly with age.

15.2.2.6 Metabolism and Endocrine

Numerous alterations in hormonal secretion occur with aging. In general, these tend toward the disintegration of the normal cyclic secretory patterns resulting in lower total circulating levels. In addition, declines in receptors and post-receptor function further decrease the ability of the hormonal orchestra to maintain coordinated function throughout the organism.

Basal metabolic rate decreases with age and is approximately 30% lower at age 80 than in youth and middle age.

There is little change in the synthesis or secretion of cortisol, ACTH, or T4, but the conversion of T4 to T3 is reduced, resulting in low levels of T3.

Blood levels of the adrenal androgens dehydroepiandrosterone (DHEA) and dehydroepiandrosterone sulfate (DHEA-S) decline linearly with age starting in the early 20s. In clinical practice, DHEA-S concentrations are measured in the blood, and high DHEA-S concentrations are considered a biomarker of longevity, as higher concentrations mean less cardiovascular disease and longer life expectancy [11].

Insulin secretion and glucose tolerance decrease with age, while hemoglobin Alc (HbAlc) increases.

15.2.2.7 Nervous System

With age, atherosclerosis of the cerebral blood vessels increases and cerebral blood flow decreases. The metabolic rate of the brain also decreases. The autoregulatory function of cerebral blood flow shifts to the hypertensive side compared to that of middle-aged and young adults. Therefore, the decrease in cerebral blood flow due to the decrease in blood pressure, as well as the decrease in pressure receptor reflexes, can easily cause upright hypotension and syncope.

Various changes in the transmission mechanisms of neurotransmitters such as dopamine, norepinephrine, monoamine neurotransmitters (e.g., 5-hydroxytryptamine), and acetylcholine can cause Parkinson's disease, depression, dementia, etc.

Brain function decreases after a certain age (which varies from person to person). Some areas of the brain in some populations decrease by up to 1% per year without any loss of function [12]. In other words, a loss of brain function is not a certain result of age-related changes. However, it is still possible for brain function to decline with age, in conjunction with numerous factors such as changes in brain chemicals (neurotransmitters), changes in the nerve cells themselves, toxic substances that accumulate in the brain over time, and genetic changes.

15.2.2.8 Blood, Body Fluid, and Immune System

Red blood cell count, hemoglobin level, and serum albumin level decrease with age. Total body water content decreases, especially intracellular water content, thus making it more susceptible to dehydration.

With age, the immune system becomes slower to respond. Aging decreases immune function and predisposes to reactivation of herpes viruses and tuberculosis, and the development of cancer is also associated with decreased immune function. Also, an autoimmune disease may develop. At the same time, the body heals more slowly with aging [13].

15.2.2.9 Sensory System

Aging raises the threshold of producing sensation, which means more stimulation is needed for the elderly to become aware of the sensation.

The latency to light reflex increases with age. Glaucoma, diabetic retinopathy, retinitis pigmentosa, age-related macular degeneration, and cataracts are the leading causes of blindness, and the occurrence of these diseases increases with age.

Hearing loss becomes more severe with age. Hearing in the high-frequency range decreases significantly, but the low-frequency range also decreases gradually [14].

15.2.3 Pharmacological Characteristics

Age alters both pharmacokinetic and pharmacodynamic aspects of anesthetic management, and these changes need to be considered when administering medication. The functional capacity of organs declines and coexisting diseases further contribute to this decline.

The elderly is more sensitive to anesthetic agents and generally require smaller doses for the same clinical effect, and drug action is usually prolonged (Table 15.2).

15.2.3.1 Pharmacokinetic Changes [17, 18]

Age-related pharmacokinetic changes lead to prolonged drug half-life and increased maximum blood concentration of drugs in the elderly. Pharmacokinetics is defined by the phases of drug absorption, drug distribution, drug metabolism, and drug excretion; it is also influenced by age-related changes in the following aspects.

1. Drug absorption

   Aging leads to a decrease in gastric acid secretion, an increase in gastric pH, a decrease in the rate of gastric emptying, a decrease in blood flow in the gastrointestinal tract, and a decrease in the area of the gastrointestinal tract to absorb drugs. These factors are thought to reduce the absorption of oral drugs and prolong their absorption time. However, in clinical practice, they do not affect the absorption of oral drugs to a great extent, except for iron and vitamins, and they do not change much compared to those in young and middle age.
2. Drug distribution

   In the elderly, there is a relative increase in the percentage of body fat due to a decrease in muscle tissue, and this trend is stronger in women. Fat-soluble drugs are more likely to accumulate in adipose tissue due to increased distribution and a longer duration of action.

   On the other hand, due to the low total body water content, the volume of distribution of water-soluble drugs decreases, and the increase in blood concentration at the beginning of drug administration very much enhances the efficacy of the drug.

   A decrease in serum albumin, the binding protein of the drug, leads to an increase in the plasma concentration of the unbound drug. Especially for drugs with high albumin binding, the number of unbound drugs increases, thus increasing the volume of distribution (the total volume of body fluid required when calculated from the measured plasma drug concentration after equilibration of the drug in the body) and tending to prolong the duration of action of the drug.
3. Drug metabolism

   Most drugs are metabolized primarily in the liver, and aging is associated with a decrease in the number of hepatocytes, a decrease in hepatic blood flow, and a decrease in the activity of cytochrome P-450 (CYP), an

Table 15.2 Clinical pharmacology of anesthetic agents in the elderly [15–17]

Drug	Brain sensitivity	Pharmacokinetics	Dose
Inhaled agents	↑		↓
Thiopental	→	Volume↓	↓
Etomidate	→	Volume↓	↓
Propofol	↑	Clearance↓	↓
Midazolam	↑	Clearance↓	↓
Morphine	↑	Clearance↓	↓
Remifentanil	↑	Clearance↓	↓
Atracurium	–	–	→
Cisatracurium	–	–	→

important drug-metabolizing enzyme in the liver. There were no significant differences in the activities of ethanol dehydrogenase, acetylation binding, and glycolysis compared to those in young and middle age.

Hepatic metabolism of drugs depends mainly on the activity of drug-metabolizing enzymes and hepatic blood flow; therefore, hepatic drug metabolism time is prolonged in the elderly.

4. Drug excretion

   Most drugs are excreted through the urine. Due to reduced renal blood flow and decreased glomerular filtration rate caused by aging, drug excretion is reduced and drug concentration in the blood increases. The degree of reduction in drug excretion correlates with a decrease in creatinine clearance. Reduced renal excretion, combined with reduced hepatic drug metabolism, is a major factor in altering pharmacokinetics in the elderly.

   Some drugs are excreted from the liver into the bile. In elderly patients with obstructive jaundice, drugs excreted through the bile are prohibited in principle.

15.2.3.2 Pharmacodynamic Changes [18]

Pharmacodynamics changes with age. Therefore, even if the blood concentration of the drug remains constant, age-related changes in responsiveness occur. The sensitivity of some receptors to which the drug binds may increase or decrease, while others remain unchanged. For example, beta-blockers are less effective because of the decreased sensitivity of beta-receptors, whereas benzodiazepines are more effective because of the increased sensitivity of benzodiazepine receptors. In addition, aging generally decreases tolerance to drug side effects and toxicity.

15.2.3.3 Drug Interactions

There are more than 50 CYPs, which are classified as CYP1A1, CYP1A2, CYP2B6, CYP3A4, etc. based on the homology of amino acid sequences. When a drug metabolized by a specific CYP is combined with a drug that inhibits the activity of the same CYP, the process of metabolism of the former drug by the CYP is inhibited and its effect is enhanced. For example, the melatonin receptor agonist ramelteon, which has been increasingly used as a sleeping pill for the elderly because it does not produce the same effects as amphetamines, is metabolized mainly by CYP1A2 and is therefore contraindicated in combination with the antidepressant fluvoxamine (a strong inhibitor of CYP1A2).

15.3 Anesthesia Practice in the Elderly

15.3.1 Preoperative Management

15.3.1.1 Preoperative Assessment

Special attention should be paid to diseases that increase with age when performing preoperative assessments (Table 15.1). In addition, the reserve capacity of the respiratory system, circulatory system, liver, kidneys, and other organs that may become problematic during general anesthesia should be assessed.

15.3.1.2 Preoperative Management Issues Specific to the Elderly

1. Dementia and mild cognitive impairment

   Dementia is the deprivation of once acquired intellectual functions for some reason, resulting in a significant decrease in daily or social/occupational functioning compared to previous levels due to memory impairment, as well as aphasia and apraxia, so that the patient is unable to maintain independence in daily life. A condition in which a patient has memory impairment but is still able to maintain independence in daily life is referred to as "mild cognitive impairment."

   There are three main types of dementia. Alzheimer's disease: senile plaques (beta-amyloid deposits) in the brain, neurogenic changes (aggregation and fibrosis of Tau proteins), neuronal degeneration and loss, and brain atrophy; dementia caused by infection: such as Creutzfeldt-Jakob disease; and reversible dementia: caused by hypothyroidism, normal pressure hydrocephalus, and chronic subdural hemorrhage.

Dementia and mild cognitive impairment make it difficult for patients to comply with preoperative management regimes, such as abstinence from food and drink, medical history taking, and obtaining informed consent for anesthesia. Dementia and mild cognitive impairment are also important risk factors for postoperative delirium.

2. Malnutrition

It is estimated that 10–20% of elderly patients are malnourished, and malnutrition is associated with prolonged hospitalization and postoperative complications.

Diseases and conditions specific to the elderly, such as dysphagia, dementia, depression, living alone, and being bedridden, are factors that contribute to malnutrition.

Nonsteroidal anti-inflammatory drugs and inosine drugs, which are often taken for long periods in the elderly, have side effects that cause anorexia, which can also cause malnutrition. Anthropometric measurements and blood tests are used as indicators to assess malnutrition (Table 15.3). The ideal weight ratio needs to be calculated by measuring height, but this may be difficult to achieve in bedridden elderly patients. The weight loss ratio can be assessed by measuring weight alone.

3. Apraxia

Apraxia is the loss of mental and physical functions due to rest, inactivity, or immobility. Elderly people are often bedridden, which is the main cause of apraxia. The various functional declines resulting from apraxia include cardiopulmonary, mental, and neurological (Table 15.4), and should be managed with full recognition that this is a contributing factor to difficulties in perioperative management.

4. Depressive disorders

It is estimated that 3–5% of elderly patients suffer from depressive disorders such as depression and depressive states, while the prevalence of depressive disorders is 10–15% among elderly patients seen in nonpsychiatric units [22]. Depressive disorders are a risk factor for postoperative delirium, which prolongs hospitalization and has a significant impact on postoperative quality of life. For patients on

Table 15.3 Malnutrition indicators [19–21]

Body measurement		
Ideal weight ratio (%) = current weight (kg)/ideal weight (kg) × 100% Ideal weight (kg) = height (m)^2 × 22		
1.1.	80–89%	Mild malnutrition
	70–79%	Medium malnutrition
	Lower than 70%	Serious malnutrition
Weight loss ratio (%)		
Duration	Obvious weight loss	Serious weight loss
1 week	Lower than 2%	Greater than 2%
1 month	Lower than 5%	Greater than 5%
3 months	Lower than 7.5%	Greater than 7.5%
6 months	Lower than 10%	Greater than 10%
Blood examination		
Item	Half-life (day)	Malnutrition standard (/dL)
Serum albumin	17–23	Lower than 3.5 g
Transferrin	7–10	Lower than 200 mg
Methotrexate	2–3	Lower than 17 mg
Retinol-binding protein	0.5	Lower than 3.0 mg

Serum albumin is the most widely used blood test as an indicator of malnutrition. Serum albumin has a relatively long half-life of 17–23 days, and it is important to note that nutritional interventions to improve a patient's nutritional status do not result in an immediate increase in albumin levels

Table 15.4 Changes brought by apraxia

Cardiopulmonary function	Decrease in beat volume, spirometry, and minute ventilation
Mental function	Decrease in cognitive ability, depression, anxiety
Joints	Decreased activity, degeneration, rickets
Bones	Reduced bone density, osteoporosis
Muscles	Reduced muscle strength, muscle atrophy
Digestive system	Reduced appetite, malnutrition

tricyclic antidepressants, please contact their primary care physician in advance to switch to other antidepressants, such as tetracyclic antidepressants, selective 5-hydroxytryptamine reuptake inhibitors, or 5-hydroxytryptamine-norepinephrine reuptake inhibitors.

15.3.1.3 Premedication

Elderly patients require lower doses of premedication. Opioid premedication is valuable only if the preoperative condition of the patient involves severe pain. Anticholinergics are not required since salivary gland atrophy is usually present. However, H_2 antagonists are useful, to reduce the risk of aspiration. Metoclopramide could also be used to promote gastric emptying, although the risk of extrapyramidal effects is higher in elderly patients [23].

The dose of premedication is lower in elderly patients. Patients should be premedicated with opioids only if severe pain is identified during the preoperative evaluation. Anticholinergics are not required because elderly patients usually have salivary gland atrophy. H_2 antagonists may reduce the risk of aspiration. Metoclopramide may also be used to facilitate gastric emptying, although in elderly patients there is also a higher risk of extrapyramidal effects.

Premedication with anxiolytics and tranquilizers may be used to reduce preoperative anxiety and insomnia. Medications that may be used for this purpose include benzodiazepines, cyclopentadienone, melatonin receptor agonists, and oxytocin receptor antagonists. In addition, the melatonin receptor agonist ramelteon and the appetite peptide receptor antagonist suvorexant are administered. Considering the increased sensitivity to these drugs with age, the doses administered should be lower than in young and middle-aged patients. Since many elderly patients are taking multiple psychotropic medications, their medications should be checked to ensure that there is no overlap with medications previously used by the patient.

Scopolamine, a belladonna drug, may cause delirium in the elderly and should not be used.

Narcotic analgesics may cause severe respiratory depression in the elderly, especially when used with sedatives, which are significantly more potent, and should be reduced and closely monitored for causing respiratory depression.

15.3.2 Intraoperative Management

15.3.2.1 Commonly Used Anesthetics

1. Inhaled anesthetics.

   The minimum alveolar concentration (MAC) of inhaled anesthetics decreases with age. The decrease in MAC with age can be calculated by [24]

   $$115\% - 0.6 \times \text{age}$$

   With the above formulation, it can be calculated that a 10-year increase in age results in a decrease of approximately 6% in MAC.

   As functional residual capacity increases with age, the absorption of inhaled anesthetics slows down and the induction time of inhaled anesthetics is prolonged. High concentrations of desflurane, sevoflurane, and isoflurane, which are volatile inhalants now widely used in Japan, tend to cause hypotension and reduced cardiac output; therefore, administration at high concentrations should be avoided.

2. Intravenous anesthetics

   The ED_{50} of intravenous anesthetics decreases with age. As with inhaled anesthetics, the degree to which ED_{50} decreases with age can be calculated by [25]

   $$115\% - 0.6 \times \text{age}$$

   The decrease is approximately 6% for every 10 years of age.

   At age 80, the ED_{50} decreases by approximately 30%.

   (a) Propofol

      In the elderly, both induction and maintenance doses should be reduced because of the tendency for hypotension due to vasodilation. In addition, if the infusion rate is too fast during induction of anesthesia, significant hypotension can occur, so the infusion rate should be slowed down. When using target-controlled infusion (TCI), the predicted blood levels should be reduced to 1/2–2/3 of those in younger and middle-aged patients.

Patients with liver disease should be cautioned that the duration of action may be prolonged.

(b) Barbiturates

Barbiturates have a high binding rate to serum albumin. In the elderly, serum albumin is lower, so unbound barbiturates are increased, resulting in increased volume of distribution and prolonged duration of action. Sensitivity to barbiturates also increases with age and therefore the dose should be reduced.

(c) Ketamine

Ketamine should not be used in patients with hypertension or ischemic heart disease because it increases blood pressure and heart rate by stimulating sympathetic nerves, and also increases cerebral blood flow, cerebral metabolic rate, and intracranial pressure.

3. Analgesic anesthetics

(a) Remifentanil

In the elderly, it has stronger respiratory depression function at lower doses and causes heart rate and blood pressure to fall as in young and middle-aged patients. The initial and maintenance doses should be reduced to 1/3–1/2 the dose in young and middle-aged patients.

(b) Fentanyl

The incidence of respiratory depression is higher than in young and middle-aged patients. The dose should be reduced.

(c) Muscle relaxants

It is generally accepted that the pharmacodynamics of muscle relaxants show little change due to aging. In terms of pharmacokinetics, non-depolarized muscle relaxants are metabolized by the liver or excreted by the kidneys, resulting in a prolonged duration of action. Succinylcholine, a depolarized muscle relaxant, is degraded in plasma by butyrylcholinesterase and has no prolonged duration of action.

Rocuronium and vecuronium are the most widely used non-depolarized muscle relaxants and are indicated in elderly patients because of their minimal circulatory effects and because their muscle-relaxing effects are rapidly antagonized by the γ-cyclodextrin derivative sugammadex, and are thus indicated in the elderly.

15.3.2.2 Practice of General Anesthesia

1. Induction of anesthesia

The sunken cheeks in elderly patients due to edentulous jaws or multiple missing teeth may make it difficult for them to put on the mask. Gauze can be inserted into the mouth to make the patient's cheeks fuller and able to fit the mask. To prevent the gauze from falling into the airway, it is best to use gauze with a gripping handle.

Before induction of anesthesia, adequate oxygenation should be given through high concentration oxygen inhalation. The choice of inhalational anesthetics, intravenous anesthetics, or a combination of both for induction should be based on the preoperative evaluation. Inhaled anesthetics should be administered at low concentrations, gradually increasing the inhalation concentration, and intravenous anesthetics should be administered slowly. High concentrations of inhaled anesthetics and rapid administration of intravenous anesthetics may result in severe circulatory depression and significant hypotension.

2. Tracheal intubation

The height of the larynx relative to the cervical spine decreases with age. Therefore, it is often easier to expose the larynx with a laryngoscope in elderly patients than in young and middle-aged patients. On the other hand, it should be noted that due to the resorption of the alveolar bone caused by periodontal disease, the remaining teeth are often unstable and may fall out when exposing the larynx. In addition, older patients have a high incidence of rheumatoid arthritis and may have difficulty with tracheal intubation due to reduced mobility of the cervical spine. Tracheal intubation using video laryngoscopy or fiber optic bronchoscope should be considered for such patients.

Close care should be taken to prevent respiratory depression when using midazolam or propofol for conscious tracheal intubation in elderly patients under sedation. In addition, because elderly patients are prone to elevated blood pressure during awake intubation, continuous intravenous antihypertensive drugs such as calcium antagonists or nitroglycerin are often used during tracheal intubation.

3. Maintenance of anesthesia

   Inhaled anesthetics, intravenous anesthetics, narcotic analgesics, muscle relaxants, and other drugs used to maintain anesthesia should not be overdosed in elderly patients.

   Compared to young and middle-aged patients, the elderly are more prone to circulatory changes during the maintenance of anesthesia and therefore often require the use of elevating and hypotensive medications. Care should be taken not to overdose on these medications.

   Respiratory management is usually achieved through respiratory regulation, as the respiratory depressant effects of the drugs used tend to be enhanced in the elderly. Due to reduced pulmonary-thoracic compliance in the elderly, positive pressures tend to be higher in the elderly than in young and middle-aged patients during respiratory regulation of inspiration. Care should be taken to avoid excessive positive pressures and to reduce the mean airway pressure during the combined time of inspiration and expiration so that expiration time is adequate and venous return is not reduced.

4. Awakening and extubation

   Elderly patients are prone to elevated blood pressure and tachycardia during awakening and extubation. When antihypertensive drugs or β-blockers are used, overdose should be avoided. To antagonize the muscle-relaxing effects of the non-depolarized muscle relaxants rocuronium and vecuronium, the γ-cyclodextrin derivative sugammadex is better than the anticholinesterase drugs neostigmine and edrophonium chloride in combination with atropine because it has less circulatory changes and is more suitable for the elderly.

15.3.3 Postoperative Management

The most common postoperative complications in elderly patients are pulmonary complications, such as pneumonia and atelectasis, and central nervous system disorders, such as postoperative delirium and postoperative cognitive impairment.

15.3.3.1 Postoperative Pulmonary Complications

Risk factors for postoperative pulmonary complications include postoperative transnasal insertion of a gastric tube, excessive preoperative sputum, chronic obstructive pulmonary disease (COPD), and smoking. Aging reduces the reflexes of the pharynx and, together with decreased swallowing function, increases the risk of aspiration and predisposes to pulmonary complications related to aspiration.

15.3.3.2 Postoperative Delirium [26, 27]

Postoperative delirium is a temporary loss of brain function resulting in abnormal psychomotor confusion. In the context of this confusion, concentration, attention, memory, judgment, and the ability to perceive orientation are impaired. The diagnostic criteria for delirium are based on DSM-5 criteria (Table 15.5).

Postoperative delirium, which occurs after anesthesia or surgery, is one of the most important perioperative management problems commonly seen in the elderly. The onset of postoperative delirium is usually 1–3 days after surgery. Delirium can lead to life-threatening behaviors, such as self-extraction of tracheal

Table 15.5 Diagnostic criteria for delirium

A	Abnormalities in attention (i.e., decreased orientation, ability to focus, maintain, and shift attention) and impaired awareness (decreased ability to perceive the environment in which they are located)
B	Abnormalities occur over a short period (usually hours to days), with changes compared to consistent levels of attention and cognitive ability, and changes in single-day severity
C	Often associated with cognitive impairment (e.g., memory loss, confusion, abnormalities in language, visuospatial cognition, perception)
D	The abnormalities mentioned in A and C are difficult to distinguish from other pre-existing neurocognitive disorders, and generally do not occur in states with low levels of consciousness (e.g., in a drowsy state)
E	Abnormalities caused by other diseases, poisoning, or withdrawal of a substance (i.e., abuse of drugs or medical supplies), or exposure to toxic substances, or by physiological changes brought on by multiple diseases, as evidenced by medical records, physical examinations, and clinical findings, with clear evidence

tubes intravenous fluid catheters, which can prolong postoperative recovery and lead to delayed bed departure and resumption of treatment.

Postoperative delirium in Alzheimer's patients can easily be misinterpreted as a worsening of dementia or resistance or refusal to treatment or medical personnel. Although delirium shares the same broad cognitive impairment as dementia, delirium differs from dementia in its rapid onset, the presence of diurnal variation in symptoms, lack of attention and concentration on the surroundings, and disturbed sleep rhythms.

There are three types of delirium: hyperactive, in which the patient has an agitated psychomotor state, is emotionally unstable, irritable, and refuses to cooperate with medical treatment; hypoactive, in which the patient has a diminished psychomotor state with a tendency toward inactivity and drowsiness, similar to coma; and mixed, in which the patient has a psychomotor state with a mixture of symptoms from the two previous types. The onset of the hyperactive type of postoperative delirium is relatively easy to detect, whereas the onset of the hypoactive type of postoperative delirium may be detected later and may even be missed. This may be one of the reasons for the large variation in the incidence of postoperative delirium between reports. Postoperative delirium has been reported to occur in 5–15% of all anesthetized patients, especially after cardiac and femoral fracture repair procedures, but also in a small number of patients after head and neck tumor surgery.

It has been suggested that the pathogenesis of delirium involves neurological hyperactivity, such as neurological hyperfunction of dopamine, norepinephrine, and glutamate, and neurological abnormalities of 5-hydroxytryptamine and γ-aminobutyric acid (GABA) in the cerebral cortex, limbic system, and upper brainstem, areas that are profoundly associated with cognition, memory, emotion, and sleep-wake cycles. Microhemorrhages in the brain caused by surgery have also been reported to be associated with postoperative delirium.

Risk factors for the development of postoperative delirium have been reported to include age over 70, dementia, depression, insomnia, postoperative pain, electrolyte abnormalities, and the use of anticholinergic drugs and benzodiazepines.

To prevent postoperative delirium, it is important to recognize and address the risk factors, as well as to improve the environment. Management of intraoperative hypotension and postoperative pain is important for patients with a high likelihood of delirium. The use of scopolamine (an anticholinergic drug) in premedication is a risk factor for delirium and thus should not be used in elderly patients.

The environment should be improved by adjusting daytime and nighttime lighting, adjusting monitor volume, organizing medical equipment, using familiar household items, and allowing family members to visit and accompany the patient.

The first choice in treating postoperative delirium is to find and eliminate the cause, i.e., correct hypoxia, eliminate postoperative pain, correct dehydration, and electrolytes, and discontinue the causative medications. Dissuasion of the patient is not effective and often exacerbates the symptoms. Wearing glasses, hearing aids, and moderate lighting may also help, as delirium can be exacerbated when the senses are suppressed. If the cause of delirium has not been eliminated, or if it is caused by multiple causes, pharmacologic treatment should be administered. Treatment of postoperative delirium includes butalbital drugs, such as haloperidol, atypical antipsychotics, such as risperidone, and antidepressants, such as trazodone. Benzodiazepines are not usually used because they can exacerbate delirium. However, if delirium is thought to be caused by the discontinuation of a benzodiazepine, it may be combined with an antipsychotic. Cholinesterase inhibitors should be used if the cause of delirium is known to be caused by anticholinergic drugs or drugs with anticholinergic effects. Dexmedetomidine and ramelteon may also reduce the incidence of postoperative delirium in elderly patients.

15.3.3.3 Postoperative Cognitive Impairment [28, 29]

Postoperative cognitive impairment refers to cortical dysfunction, such as language, movement, perception, memory, attention, executive function, and social adaptation, that occurs after surgery. It is one of the most common postoperative central nervous system disorders in the elderly, along with postoperative delirium. Postoperative cognitive dysfunction occurs with high frequency after cardiac surgery, but even after general anesthesia for noncardiac surgery, the disorder has been reported in approximately 25% of elderly patients at 1 week postoperatively and in approximately 10% at 3 months postoperatively.

It is generally believed that the disease has multiple causes, including the spread of inflammatory responses to the brain during surgery, microemboli, genetic predisposition, and age-related organic changes in the brain. Risk factors for the development of the disease include advanced age, prior history of cerebrovascular disease, alcohol abuse, preoperative cognitive impairment, postoperative infection, and respiratory complications.

Although postoperative delirium and postoperative cognitive impairment are generally considered to be distinct conditions, it has also been suggested that postoperative delirium may be an early symptom of postoperative cognitive impairment.

15.4 Conclusion

Elderly patients are susceptible to the stress of trauma, hospitalization, surgery, and anesthesia in ways that are only partly understood. Accordingly, minimizing perioperative risk in elderly patients requires thoughtful preoperative assessment of organ function and reserve, meticulous intraoperative management of coexisting disorders, and vigilant postoperative pain control [23].

References

1. Gheorghiade M, De Luca L, Fonarow GC, Filippatos G, Metra M, Francis GS. Pathophysiologic targets in the early phase of acute heart failure syndromes. Am J Cardiol. 2005;96(6A):11G–7G. PMID: 16196154. https://doi.org/10.1016/j.amjcard.2005.07.016.
2. Hutnik CM, Nichols BD. Cataracts in systemic diseases and syndromes. Curr Opin Ophthalmol. 1999;10(1):22–8. PMID: 10387315. https://doi.org/10.1097/00055735-199902000-00005.
3. Cardiovascular Considerations in the Older Patient. Physiopedia. 2022. https://www.physio-pedia.com/index.php?title=Cardiovascular_Considerations_in_the_Older_Patient&oldid=300043. Accessed 19 May 2022.
4. Lee J, Kang T, Yeo Y, Han D. The change of lung capacity in elderly women caused by life span. J Phys Ther Sci. 2017;29(4):658–61. Epub 2017 Apr 20. PMID: 28533605; PMCID: PMC5430268. https://doi.org/10.1589/jpts.29.658.
5. Mimae T, Miyata Y, Kumada T, Handa Y, Tsutani Y, Okada M. Interstitial pneumonia and advanced age negatively influence postoperative pulmonary function. Interact Cardiovasc Thorac Surg. 2022;34(5):753–9. PMID: 35137092; PMCID: PMC9070519. https://doi.org/10.1093/icvts/ivac014.
6. Choi W, Mizukami K. The effect of whole body vibration by sonic waves on mood, the autonomic nervous system, and brain function in elderly. Nihon Ronen Igakkai Zasshi. 2020;57(4):441–9. PMID: 33268629 (Japanese). https://doi.org/10.3143/geriatrics.57.441.
7. Katayama M, Yamazumi K, Kino K, Tsuru M, Fukazawa T, Shimada H. Changes in the liver weight in the elderly. Nihon Ronen Igakkai Zasshi. 1990;27(5):584–8. PMID: 2263016 (Japanese). https://doi.org/10.3143/geriatrics.27.584.

8. Pedraza L, Laosa O, Rodríguez-Mañas L, Gutiérrez-Romero DF, Frías J, Carnicero JA, Ramírez E. Drug induced liver injury in geriatric patients detected by a two-hospital prospective pharmacovigilance program: a comprehensive analysis using the Roussel Uclaf Causality Assessment Method. Front Pharmacol. 2021;11:600255. PMID: 33613279; PMCID: PMC7892439. https://doi.org/10.3389/fphar.2020.600255.
9. Euans DW. Renal function in the elderly. Am Fam Physician. 1988;38(3):147–50. PMID: 3046266.
10. Alehagen U, Aaseth J, Alexander J, Brismar K, Larsson A. Selenium and coenzyme Q10 supplementation improves renal function in elderly deficient in selenium: observational results and results from a subgroup analysis of a prospective randomised double-blind placebo-controlled trial. Nutrients. 2020;12(12):3780. PMID: 33317156; PMCID: PMC7764721. https://doi.org/10.3390/nu12123780.
11. Veronese N, De Rui M, Bolzetta F, Zambon S, Corti MC, Baggio G, Toffanello ED, Crepaldi G, Perissinotto E, Manzato E, Sergi G. Serum dehydroepiandrosterone sulfate and incident depression in the elderly: the Pro.V.A. study. Am J Geriatr Psychiatry. 2015;23(8):863–71. Epub 2014 Nov 6. PMID: 25537161. https://doi.org/10.1016/j.jagp.2014.10.009.
12. Ageing and the Brain. Physiopedia. 2022. https://www.physio-pedia.com/index.php?title=Ageing_and_the_Brain&oldid=293202. Accessed 19 May 2022.
13. Fuentes E, Fuentes M, Alarcón M, Palomo I. Immune system dysfunction in the elderly. An Acad Bras Cienc. 2017;89(1):285–99. PMID: 28423084. https://doi.org/10.1590/0001-3765201720160487.
14. Ianiszewski A, Fuente A, Gagné JP. Association between the right ear advantage in dichotic listening and interaural differences in sensory processing at lower levels of the auditory system in older adults. Ear Hear. 2021;42(5):1381–96. PMID: 33974783. https://doi.org/10.1097/AUD.0000000000001039.
15. Mei X, Zheng HL, Li C, Ma X, Zheng H, Marcantonio E, Xie Z, Shen Y. The effects of propofol and sevoflurane on postoperative delirium in older patients: a randomized clinical trial study. J Alzheimers Dis. 2020;76(4):1627–36. PMID: 32651322; PMCID: PMC7844419. https://doi.org/10.3233/JAD-200322.
16. Zhang Y, Shan GJ, Zhang YX, Cao SJ, Zhu SN, Li HJ, Ma D, Wang DX, First Study of Perioperative Organ Protection (SPOP1) Investigators. Propofol compared with sevoflurane general anaesthesia is associated with decreased delayed neurocognitive recovery in older adults. Br J Anaesth. 2018;121(3):595–604. Epub 2018 Jul 27. PMID: 30115258. https://doi.org/10.1016/j.bja.2018.05.059.
17. Davis PJ, Cook DR. Clinical pharmacokinetics of the newer intravenous anaesthetic agents. Clin Pharmacokinet. 1986;11(1):18–35. PMID: 3512140. https://doi.org/10.2165/00003088-198611010-00002.
18. Andres TM, McGrane T, McEvoy MD, Allen BFS. Geriatric Pharmacology: an update. Anesthesiol Clin. 2019;37(3):475–92. Epub 2019 Jun 19. PMID: 31337479. https://doi.org/10.1016/j.anclin.2019.04.007.
19. Peterson CM, Thomas DM, Blackburn GL, Heymsfield SB. Universal equation for estimating ideal body weight and body weight at any BMI. Am J Clin Nutr. 2016;103(5):1197–203. Epub 2016 Mar 30. Erratum in: Am J Clin Nutr. 2017 Mar; 105(3):772. PMID: 27030535; PMCID: PMC4841935. https://doi.org/10.3945/ajcn.115.121178.
20. Appelbaum N, Clarke J. Ideal body weight calculations: fit for purpose in modern anaesthesia? Eur J Anaesthesiol. 2021;38(12):1211–4. PMID: 33876785. https://doi.org/10.1097/EJA.0000000000001515.
21. Benoist S, Brouquet A. Nutritional assessment and screening for malnutrition. J Visc Surg. 2015;152(Suppl 1):S3–7. PMID: 26315577. https://doi.org/10.1016/S1878-7886(15)30003-5.
22. Wilkinson P, Ruane C, Tempest K. Depression in older adults. BMJ. 2018;363:k4922. PMID: 30487197. https://doi.org/10.1136/bmj.k4922.
23. Kanonidou Z, Karystianou G. Anesthesia for the elderly. Hippokratia. 2007;11(40):175–7.
24. Lobo SA, Ojeda J, Dua A, et al. Minimum alveolar concentration. In: StatPearls. Treasure Island, FL: StatPearls; 2022. https://www.ncbi.nlm.nih.gov/books/NBK532974/.
25. Dimmitt S, Stampfer H, Martin JH. When less is more—efficacy with less toxicity at the ED50. Br J Clin Pharmacol. 2017;83(7):1365–8. Epub 2017 Apr 6. PMID: 28387051; PMCID: PMC5465328. https://doi.org/10.1111/bcp.13281.
26. Inouye SK, Westendorp RG, Saczynski JS. Delirium in elderly people. Lancet. 2014;383(9920):911–22. Epub 2013 Aug 28. PMID: 23992774; PMCID: PMC4120864. https://doi.org/10.1016/S0140-6736(13)60688-1.
27. Hshieh TT, Inouye SK, Oh ES. Delirium in the elderly. Clin Geriatr Med. 2020;36(2):183–99. PMID: 32222295. https://doi.org/10.1016/j.cger.2019.11.001.
28. Kotekar N, Shenkar A, Nagaraj R. Postoperative cognitive dysfunction - current preventive strategies. Clin Interv Aging. 2018;13:2267–73. PMID: 30519008; PMCID: PMC6233864. https://doi.org/10.2147/CIA.S133896.
29. Lin X, Chen Y, Zhang P, Chen G, Zhou Y, Yu X. The potential mechanism of postoperative cognitive dysfunction in older people. Exp Gerontol. 2020;130:110791. https://doi.org/10.1016/j.exger.2019.110791. Epub 2019 Nov 23. PMID: 31765741.

Anesthesia for Oral and Maxillofacial Head and Neck Tumor

16

Yu Sun and Ming Xia

16.1 Introduction

Oral and maxillofacial tumors are a major part of head and neck tumors and so far surgery remains to be the main treatment for oral and maxillofacial tumors, which makes up the major part of the comprehensive and sequential treatment. Among all types of tumors, the oral and maxillofacial tumors occur at a relatively high rate, especially in India and Southeast Asia, with a large patient population. According to American Cancer Society (ACS), oropharyngeal tumors ranked ninth among all malignant tumors. According to the statistics in 2004, oropharyngeal tumors accounted for 2.1% of all tumors, and in 2007, this percentage increased to 2.4%. The analysis of inpatient cases of oral and maxillofacial surgery in our center (Shanghai Ninth People's Hospital) from 1954–2006 showed that the surgical amount of tumor surgery accounting for about 37% of the composition of oral and maxillofacial surgery, and more than 99% of them were performed under general anesthesia with tracheal intubation [1]. Therefore, we are supposed to focus on anesthesia for oral and maxillofacial tumors, which is going to be further discussed in this chapter.

From the epidemiological survey, the occurrence of oral and maxillofacial tumors is related to dental health and addiction to tobacco and alcohol, etc. Among the tumor patients, the elderly account for a larger proportion, and the ratio of male to female is about 1.48:1 [2]. Tumors are generally considered to be either benign or malignant. Benign tumors may be locally invasive but do not metastasize to distant sites. Malignant tumors are not only locally invasive but also have the potential to metastasize to other sites in the body. According to this survey, the ratio of benign to malignant oral and maxillofacial tumors is 1:1, and the common benign tumors are mixed tumors of parotid gland, ameloblastoma, maxillofacial angioma, etc. Cancer is most common in malignant tumors while sarcoma is rather rare. According to the site of lesion, the cancers can be divided into cheilocarcinoma, gingival carcinoma, tongue cancer, buccal carcinoma, carcinoma of mouth floor, etc., which involve all anatomical parts of the maxillofacial and intraoral areas.

From the perspective of anesthesiology, oral and maxillofacial tumors have the following characteristics: (1) the incidence of airway difficulties is very high in patients with maxillofacial tumors, and airway management during the whole perioperative period shall be rather tricky;

Y. Sun · M. Xia (✉)
Department of Anesthesiology, Shanghai Ninth People's Hospital Affiliated to Shanghai Jiao Tong University School of Medicine, Shanghai, China
e-mail: xiaming1980@xzhmu.edu.cn

H. Jiang, M. Xia (eds.), *Anesthesia for Oral and Maxillofacial Surgery*,
https://doi.org/10.1007/978-981-19-7287-4_16

(2) many patients with maxillofacial tumors are elderly, addicted to smoking or drinking, dystrophic or with certain comorbidities. Furthermore, considering the impact of preoperative radiotherapy on the body's immunity, detailed preoperative risk assessment and treatment are crucial (3) Radical surgery of maxillofacial malignant tumors can lead to large trauma and bleeding; meanwhile it is relatively difficult to stop bleeding, and hence reducing surgical bleeding providing corresponding blood protection measures should be considered for anesthetists (4) Similarly, due to the large trauma, it is often necessary to perform a repair of free tissue flap defect; thus it usually takes long for surgeries and long surgical management; smooth anesthesia and stable internal environment are significant to reduce postoperative complications and improve prognosis; (5) many of the blood vessels and nerves in the head and face are connected to the cranium, so it is important to be aware of brain protection during anesthesia.

16.2 Oral and Maxillofacial Head and Neck Tumor and Airway

The relationship between the airway and tumor of oral and maxillofacial head and neck is inseparable. First of all, the tumor may occupy the airway space or deform the airway by applying external compression, so that the airflow in and out of the airway can be affected, resulting in complete or incomplete airway obstruction, and in such cases, relieving the obstruction is the first task. Secondly, most of the maxillofacial head and neck tumors require intubation to ensure effective ventilation, while the specific anatomical location for tumors to grow adds difficulty to airway operations such as mask ventilation, laryngeal mask ventilation, endotracheal intubation and extubation. Furthermore, the surgical operation is in the vicinity of the airway, and a section of the endotracheal tube may be exposed to the surgical view. As a shared place for both anesthetists and surgeons, the airway has to be well managed by anesthetist with the premise of not influencing the surgical operations.

16.2.1 The Tumor and Airway Obstruction

A tumor is a solid or semi-solid mass within bone or soft tissue that is made of cells that are different than cells usually found in that location. In addition to tumors of the same type as other parts of the body, there are also facial tumors that only occur in the maxillofacial region, such as odontogenic tumor and salivary gland tumor. The naming of the tumors is mostly based on their anatomic regions. From the aspect of anatomic structures, the oral and maxillofacial region can be divided into collar surfaces and oral cavity. The former includes facial soft tissues and maxillofacial bones, such as maxilla, mandible, zygoma, temporomandibular joint, salivary glands, etc.; the latter includes teeth, alveoli, lips, cheeks, tongue, palate, pharynx, etc. There are several types of soft tissue tumors which may be found on the lips, cheeks, tongue, mouth floor (under the tongue), and gums. Maxillofacial tumors, especially intraoral carcinomas, can lead to different degrees of airway obstruction. For patients with airway obstruction, their tolerance to surgery and hypoxia must be assessed preoperatively.

16.2.2 Tumors and Their Influence on Airway Management

16.2.2.1 Lip Tumors

Common ones are hemangioma and lip cancer, which usually do not affect the degree of mouth opening, but if the tumor is huge or invades the intraoral tissues, it can affect the placement of laryngoscope. Hemangioma tumors are usually soft and have a certain degree of mobility, so the tumor can be pulled aside to expose the laryngoscope for endotracheal intubation. In contrast, lip cancer has a small range of movement and is prone to frictional bleeding, so adequate prior evaluation is required.

16.2.2.2 Buccal Cancer Tumor

Because it grows on the lateral side of the mouth, it usually does not obstruct the passage of anesthesia catheter, and there is no restriction of mouth opening in the early stage. However, when the tumor invades the buccal muscle and masticatory muscle, mouth opening restriction gradually appears, and the influence of mouth opening on laryngoscopic exposure should be fully considered at this time.

16.2.2.3 Gingival Tumor

Gingival cancer is mostly of ulcerative type, easy to bleed, and invades the alveolar bone at an early stage, resulting in loosening of teeth and possible loss of teeth. Before laryngoscopic exposure, whether the teeth are missing or loose should be checked, and rubbing the tumor surface should be avoided during operation. Upper gingival cancer may invade the nasal cavity, thus the ipsilateral nasotracheal intubation should be avoided; when gingival cancer invades the posterior molar area and pterygoid muscle, difficulty in opening the mouth may occur.

16.2.2.4 Tumor of Palate

Large tumors in the anterior part of the palate can lead to facial deformation and cause difficulties in oxygen delivery by mask confinement. The hard palate tumor often bulges toward the nasal cavity and one side of the nasal tract is easily invaded, depending on the size of surgical resection and intubation through the contralateral nostril. For patients who require total maxillectomy, nasotracheal intubation is more appropriate. Inadvertent nasotracheal intubation during maxillectomy has been reported. Soft palate cancer is more malignant and often involves the pterygopalatine fossa, and patients have clinical manifestations of restricted mouth opening.

16.2.2.5 Tongue Tumor

Tongue cancer usually refers to the cancer of the front two-thirds of the tongue body, while the tumor at the root of the back one-third of the tongue belongs to the category of oropharyngeal cancer. When tongue cancer invades the pharyngeal-palatal arch, patients will have difficulty in opening their mouth. Huge tumors in the ventral part of the tongue can sometimes occupy the entire oral cavity. Tongue cancer may invade the tongue root and pharyngeal wall backward, and laryngoscope should be avoided to damage the tumor body when intubating. In case of tumor with ulcerated surface or hemangioma of the tongue, it is more likely to bleed after injury, so special attention should be paid when using laryngoscope.

16.2.2.6 Tumors of the Floor of the Mouth and Oropharynx

Cancer of the floor of the mouth is most common in the anterior floor of the mouth, which occurs on both sides of the tongue ligament. The tumor invades the gingiva and the lingual plate of the mandible, then spreads backward to the posterior floor of the mouth and invades the floor muscles to the deeper level, resulting in limited tongue movement and fixation in the mouth, which is an important factor leading to difficult intubation. The oropharyngeal area is not large in scope, and the tumor is easy to invade the surrounding area, which can easily cause obstruction and can be followed by sleep apnea syndrome. Therefore, it is necessary to discuss carefully with the surgeon before surgery and make a proper assessment with the help of imaging data. If the tumor is found to be very close to the epiglottis or the vocal cords, the trachea may interfere with the operation, and there are also problems such as difficulty in breathing after extubation, so preoperative tracheotomy may be considered.

16.2.2.7 Maxillary Sinus Cancer

Maxillary sinus cancer is one of the most common cancers in the nasal cavity and paranasal sinuses. When it invades the temporomandibular joint, it can cause restriction of mouth opening. When the tumor spreads to the infraorbital plate, total maxillary osteotomy is often required, and it is not suitable for nasotracheal intubation.

16.2.2.8 Tumor of the Parotid Area

Generally, it does not affect the degree of mouth opening, and there is no obvious obstruction to the catheter path, so it is usually possible to choose fast induction of bright vision intubation. However, some malignant tumors of the parotid gland with large local infiltration and involvement of the buccal muscle may cause restriction of mouth opening, and some tumors with large tumors may also hinder the administration of oxygen by mask pressure.

16.2.2.9 Tumor of Chin and Neck

Tumors in the chin and neck can affect the mobility of the head and neck to the extent that laryngoscopic exposure is difficult, which needs to be evaluated before surgery. On the other hand, if the tumor is huge, it may squeeze and displace the vocal cord to the opposite side, making intubation difficult. Hygroma of the chin and neck is a type of neck tumor commonly seen in young children and is a type of lymphangioma. Large hygromas can invade the pharynx, vocal cords, and trachea, resulting in respiratory distress.

16.2.3 Impact of Prior Treatment on Airway Management

Preoperative radiotherapy makes anesthesia more difficult: (1) local tissues have radiation reactions after radiotherapy, which are more rigid, less mobile, and prone to bleeding, making anesthesia and intubation more difficult; (2) radiotherapy may decrease platelets and increase the risk of bleeding, reducing the patient's tolerance for surgical anesthesia.

The trauma and scarring of previous surgery, changes in local anatomy caused by tissue reconstruction, and the scarring of the anterior neck after the previous tracheotomy can have a great impact on the upcoming anesthesia and intubation, and the incidence of difficult intubation is significantly higher. In such patients, awake intubation should be chosen whenever possible, and the same side of the nasal cavity as during the previous surgery should be chosen for intubation. In patients with total bilateral mandibular resection and exposed floor of the mouth, such patients can be directly tracheotomized.

16.3 Oral and Maxillofacial Head and Neck Tumor Surgery and Bleeding

16.3.1 Blood Transfusion for Oral and Maxillofacial Tumor Surgery

The blood supply of oral and maxillofacial head and neck is rich, and it is relatively difficult to stop bleeding, especially for radical surgery of malignant tumor, resection of primary foci, combined craniomaxillofacial enlargement resection and corresponding osteotomy process; the blood loss in surgery is often difficult to control. In recent years, with the improvement of overall medical level, the rate of early detection and diagnosis of tumors has increased; the improvement of surgical techniques, the shortening of operation time, and the use of hemodilution techniques and controlled hypotension techniques have greatly reduced intraoperative bleeding.

Factors related to the amount of intraoperative blood transfusion include: (1) the site of surgery. Surgical bleeding is often greatest in the maxilla or midface, such as when advanced maxillary sinus carcinoma invades the base of the middle cranial recess or the pterygopalatine fossa, the surgery requires the removal of the entire maxilla, the bone plate of the middle cranial recess and the facial lesion, and the bleeding is very large; (2) tumors of high malignancy, with extensive resection, a large defect area needs to be covered and there is relatively more bleeding; surgeries in which the adjacent flap can repair the defect lead to less bleeding than surgeries requiring free tissue; (3) the nature of the tumor. The bleeding and transfusion volume of neurofibroma surgery in the maxillofacial area is higher; (4) the blood transfusion volume is often higher for long surgery, which is of course related to the complexity and difficulty of the surgery; (5) the physiological condition of the patient before surgery. Patients with preoperative anemia also require a larger perioperative transfusion volume. Patients with a history of preoperative hypertension and poorly controlled blood pressure are prone to show intraoperative hemodynamic fluctuations, which then lead to increased bleeding and transfusion volume [3].

16.3.2 Blood Transfusion-Related Problems

There are a large number of reports arguing the relationship between allogeneic blood transfusion and tumor recurrence. The current consensus is that transfusion-mediated immunosuppression may be mediated by leukocytes in blood products, so try to transfuse blood products with leukocytes removed. In addition, transfusion of allogeneic blood has been associated with postoperative infections. Blood transfusions can cause the spread of infectious diseases, including hepatitis and acquired immunodeficiency syndrome (AIDS). Adverse effects of blood transfusion also include hemolysis, febrile reactions, and dilutional coagulation disorders, electrolyte disturbances, hypothermia, and microthrombus input after massive transfusion. Therefore, on the basis of safeguarding the oxygen supply of patients and maintaining effective circulating blood volume, various measures are utilized to reduce unnecessary allogeneic blood transfusion.

16.3.3 Measures to Reduce Blood Transfusion

16.3.3.1 Controlled Hypotension

The application of controlled hypotension in maxillofacial tumor surgery is conducive to the reduction of tissue bleeding during resection of primary foci and provides a dry surgical field, which makes the tissue anatomy easy to identify and is also suitable for certain delicate operations such as vascular anastomosis in the process of tumor repair, so the application of controlled hypotension in oral and maxillofacial surgery is very common at present.

Controlled hypotension has its prerequisite. It presupposes adequate blood volume so as not to damage the tissues and organs. The usual practice is to use plasma substitutes such as hydroxyethyl starch and gelatin for volume expansion immediately after induction to ensure adequate circulating blood volume while also playing a hemodilution role.

Controlled hypotension is limited. The safe limit is to not affect the blood perfusion and oxygen supply of the tissues and organs, and the magnitude of pressure reduction is not less than 50 mmHg, or the time to drop below 50 mmHg is not more than 15–30 min. From the practical point of view, because the whole tumor surgery time is relatively long, it is only necessary to implement strict controlled hypotension during the steps with more bleeding such as osteotomy and tumor resection, while during the microscopic operations such as vascular anastomosis, the blood pressure can be controlled slightly below the base, and the pressure should be restored immediately after the end of vascular anastomosis, which helps the blood supply of the graft on the one hand, and helps the surgeon to judge and stop the bleeding on the other hand.

The implementation of controlled hypotension: (1) can achieve the purpose of hypotension by deepening anesthesia with inhalation anesthetics; (2) application of hypotensive drugs, commonly used such as vasodilators (sodium nitroprusside, nitroglycerin, etc.), calcium channel blockers (Perdipine, etc.), adrenal receptor blockers (Esmolol, Labetalol, etc.). In controlled hypotension, the surgical site can be kept as high as possible above the rest of the body so that the blood pressure in the surgical field can be minimized without affecting perfusion to other sites. Invasive arterial monitoring is necessary during the process of lowering blood pressure.

16.3.3.2 Strict Blood Transfusion Indications

The importance of blood to the body lies in its ability to carry oxygen, maintain effective circulating volume, and maintain normal coagulation mechanisms. The normal organism has a certain compensatory capacity for blood loss and anemia.

For acute blood loss during surgery, the first thing to assess is the circulating volume, and improving the circulating volume can be done by supplementing colloids and crystals according to the actual situation of the patient. Some new plasma substitutes such as hydroxyethyl starch and gelatin have emerged, which are not only effective in expanding the volume, but also have a long maintenance time with few side effects, so for cases where the percentage of blood loss is less than 15%, blood transfusion is usually not given, and only crystals and colloids are supplemented. When the percentage of blood loss rises to 15–30%, blood transfusion can still be withheld for patients with good cardiopulmonary reserve and when surgery no longer causes continued bleeding. Blood transfusion is only considered when the percentage of blood loss is greater than 30%.

Another indicator that determines whether to transfuse or not is hemoglobin. There are advocates of open transfusion, i.e., transfusion is started when hemoglobin is below 10 g/dL, and there are also advocates of restrictive transfusion, i.e., transfusion is started only when hemoglobin reaches 7 g/dL or less [3]. However, the fact is that there is no uniform critical transfusion point for all patients in clinical practice. Clinical judgment and patient's vital signs indicators such as blood pressure, pulse rate, urine volume, and capillary filling are crucial for the need of blood transfusion. Hemoglobin greater than 10 g/dL is not transfused; below 7 g/dL, transfusion of concentrated red blood cells is considered; between 7 and 10 g/dL, comprehensive consideration can be made according to the patient's cardiovascular status, age, oxygenation, and whether bleeding is still continuing.

16.3.3.3 Autologous Transfusion Techniques

There are three major types of autologous transfusion techniques in common use: preoperative autologous blood collection techniques, acute normovolemic or hypervolemic hemodilution techniques, and intraoperative blood recovery techniques.

Preoperative autologous blood collection technique. This technique is used in maxillofacial tumor surgery and generally requires autologous blood donors with basal hemoglobin of not less than 11 g/dL and no serious cardiopulmonary disease. Patients have 800–1000 mL of autologous blood collected in batches over a period of 2–4 weeks prior to surgery and stored in a blood bank for use during surgery. This technique can also be combined with the application of erythropoietin to achieve maximum blood conservation [4]. The disadvantage of this technique is the need to wait 2–4 weeks before the surgery can be scheduled, and the other concern is the anemia caused by preoperative blood collection.

Acute hemodilution technique. Moderate hemodilution reduces the loss of red blood cells in the same amount of blood loss and unblocks the microcirculation, which facilitates the survival of the graft. Acute high-volume hemodilution, which involves supplementation with a colloid equivalent to 20% of one's own blood volume after induction of anesthesia, has the advantage of being easier to perform and does not lead to waste, but it is less effective than isovolemic hemodilution in saving blood and can result in cardiovascular accidents due to circulatory overload if not properly manipulated.

Due to the nature of the tumor and the need for intraoral manipulation, it is generally not recommended. Unlike intraoral tumors, neurofibromas and hemangiomas in the oral and maxillofacial head and neck are benign tumors and are not operated in the oral cavity. The application of intraoperative blood recovery techniques can significantly reduce the transfusion of allogeneic blood and avoid the adverse effects of massive transfusion of allogeneic blood. The use of intraoperative autologous blood recovery techniques for neurofibroma and hemangioma surgery has now become routine.

16.4 Pre-anesthesia Visit and Preparation

Preoperative preparation is divided into several aspects, such as medical history, physical examination, laboratory and imaging tests, consultation and conversation.

16.4.1 Medical History Information

16.4.1.1 History Related to Airway Obstruction

A detailed history can determine the severity of airway obstruction. In addition to asking whether the patient has snoring, shortness of breath, or dyspnea, it is also necessary to ask whether there is nocturnal shortness of breath and awakening. The presence of nocturnal symptoms often indicates an escalation in the degree of obstruction. In the severe stage of obstruction there is often also an impairment of gas exchange, and even difficulty with coughing occurs. Atelectasis and lung infections can further worsen the condition. Other symptoms suggestive of airway obstruction include changes in voice, choking sensation after exercise, abnormal swallowing, and patients complaining of uncontrollable secretions from the nose and mouth.

16.4.1.2 History Related to Vital Organ Function

There is a great correlation between age, addiction to tobacco and alcohol, and the development of oral and maxillofacial head and neck tumors. Therefore, there are many patients with comorbid chronic diseases such as chronic obstructive pulmonary disease, bronchitis, hypertension, coronary heart disease, diabetes mellitus, alcoholic cirrhosis and other chronic diseases in the patient population, and whether these comorbidities are properly controlled before surgery is related to the risk of surgery, postoperative complications, and mortality. Patients with comorbidities are evaluated and treated aggressively preoperatively, such as controlling hypertension, using bronchodilators to increase lung capacity, controlling respiratory infections, controlling cardiac arrhythmias, controlling blood sugar, placing temporary pacemakers preoperatively for patients with severe conduction block, nutritional support therapy, and correcting anemia and electrolyte disturbances. Since tumor surgery is a surgery of limited duration, early surgery after appropriate adjustment and balancing the conflict between surgical risk and surgical treatment are important elements of preoperative evaluation.

16.4.1.3 Preoperative Radiotherapy History

Preoperative radiotherapy to the head and neck region can lead to abnormal airway anatomy, tissue edema and swelling, peri-airway tissue fibrosis, and local movement restriction. It is particularly important to examine the degree of tissue stiffness under the chin and between the hyoid bones, and swelling and fibrosis in this area largely affect laryngoscopic exposure. Acute inflammatory-like side effects that occur after radiotherapy include epidermolysis bullosa and oral mucositis, and patients with oral mucositis are more likely to develop infection and bleeding during airway manipulation. Radiotherapy to the parotid region can present with oral dryness, while intraoral radiotherapy can also affect the dentition, and there is a correlation between dental health and difficult cannulation.

16.4.1.4 History of Preoperative Chemotherapy

Preoperative chemotherapy is also very common. The common chemotherapeutic drugs amino-methotrexate and paclitaxel have significant myelosuppressive effects and can cause thrombocytopenia and also neutropenic fever; bleomycin can cause pulmonary fibrosis; cisplatin has nephrotoxicity; paclitaxel and carboplatin can reduce the diffusion rate of carbon monoxide by 20% with long-term use (>5 months); cisplatin and doxorubicin also have central nervous system toxicity; amino-methotrexate has digestive system toxicity, manifested as stomatitis, diarrhea, weight loss, electrolyte imbalance, etc. For chemotherapy patients, preoperative assessment of organ function, blood and electrolyte tests are very important.

16.4.1.5 Preoperative Medication History and Previous Surgical History

Tumor patients may use opioids preoperatively due to pain and other reasons, and may show signs of cognitive dysfunction such as delirium, excessive sedation, and drowsiness. For patients presenting with psychiatric problems, it is necessary to identify the presence of metabolic disease, infection, and hypoxia, or overdose with other psychotropic drugs, or brain metastases. The number of previous surgeries and the time of the most recent surgery, the history of airway difficulties during previous anesthesia, the history of previous blood transfusion, and whether a tracheotomy has been performed in the past can help in the selection of the anesthetic plan and the preparation before anesthesia.

16.4.2 Preoperative Physical Examination

16.4.2.1 Nutritional Status

Malnutrition can be defined as 10% or more below the standard weight. In 25% of patients with oral and maxillofacial head and neck tumors, there is some degree of malnutrition. Malnutrition may be related to factors such as reduced mouth opening, painful swallowing and aspiration due to tumor, and may also be due to tumor anorexia, decreased mastication function, and tooth alveolar invasion. In addition, nausea and vomiting after radiotherapy and mucosal inflammation can also aggravate malnutrition. Patients with malnutrition need further examination of total lymph count, albumin, prealbumin, and other indicators.

16.4.2.2 Intubation Conditions

Visual examination. Some tumors can be directly observed, such as lip cancer, tumors of hard palate, gum cancer, tongue and abdomen tumors, skin cancer of scalp and face and neck, and hemangioma of maxillofacial region. The size, location, fragility of the tumor, and whether it is easy to bleed and fall off need to be recorded. Some tumors can cause localized elevation of the maxillofacial region, such as huge masses in the parotid area and lymphoedema, which are evaluated to see if they interfere with mask pressurized oxygen delivery. Some hemangiomas invade the anterior cervical region, and it is necessary to know whether tracheotomy and emergency ventilation are feasible. Patients need to be recorded for loose or absent teeth, small jaws, short neck, and swelling in the anterior cervical region. Patients with previous surgical history should be observed for the effect of surgical scars and skin flaps on intubation, and the presence of tracheotomy scars in the neck should be recorded.

Mouth opening and tongue extension. When the tumor invades the masticatory muscle and temporomandibular joint, it often leads to mouth opening restriction. Mouth opening refers to the distance between upper and lower incisors at maximum mouth opening. The normal value should be greater than or equal to 3 cm (two fingers); when it is less than 3 cm, there is a possibility of difficult intubation. Patients with tongue root mass or radiotherapy are often associated with difficulty in tongue extension, and difficulty in tongue extension also suggests the need for awake intubation.

Temporomandibular distance. It is the distance between the notch of the thyroid cartilage and the chin prominence of the mandible when the patient's head is tilted back to its maximum. If the nail-chin spacing is greater than or equal to 6.5 cm, there is no difficulty in intubation; between 6 cm and 6.5 cm, there is difficulty in intubation, but appropriate position adjustment such as in the sniffing position can be intubated with laryngoscopic exposure, so this patient needs to be further checked for comfort in the sniffing position; less than 6 cm (three fingers), there is difficulty in intubation with laryngoscope.

Neck flexion and extension. Neck tumors, lymph node metastases, and side effects of radiotherapy can all affect neck mobility. Neck flexion and extension refers to the range of movement from maximum flexion to extension of the patient's neck. The normal value is greater than 90° and up to 35° from neutral to maximum posterior elevation; less than 80°, there is difficulty in intubation. Cervical joint extension can be measured by taking lateral radiographs, CT, and MRI.

Mallampati test. The Mallampati test is performed with the patient sitting upright, facing the examiner, and forcefully opening the mouth and extending the tongue to the maximum. The examiner grades the pharyngeal structures according to their visibility: grade I, the soft palate, pharyngopalatine arch, and uvula are visible; grade II, the soft palate, pharyngopalatine arch, and uvula are partially covered by the tongue root; grade III, only the soft palate is visible; grade IV, the soft palate is not visible.

Palpation of the anterior cervical region. It can help to understand whether the trachea is displaced or not. In patients with huge thyroid tumors or tumors after multiple surgeries, the trachea may be displaced to one side. Anterior cervical palpation is also useful for understanding whether there is difficulty in cricothyroid puncture.

16.4.3 Laboratory and Imaging Examinations

For elderly tumor patients with more comorbidities, preoperative blood, urine routine, blood clotting time, liver and kidney function, blood glucose, electrolytes, and other laboratory tests are performed to exclude preoperative anemia and occult liver and kidney insufficiency due to radiotherapy and tumor medication. In patients with airway obstruction, blood gas analysis helps to understand the presence of hypoxia and hypercapnia. A 12-lead electrocardiogram and chest radiograph are also mandatory, and a chest radiograph is useful for the presence of pulmonary metastases. Cardiac function and echocardiography are also required in patients with cardiac disease, and pulmonary function is required in patients with respiratory insufficiency.

Frontal and lateral X-rays of the head and neck and CT and MRI scans are important to evaluate difficult airways. On the X-ray projection measurement chart, patients with too long mandibular hyoid spacing and too short distance from the posterior nasal crest to the posterior pharyngeal wall are prone to difficult intubation; abnormalities in craniofacial angles and lines (such as the length of the anterior skull base, the angle of the maxilla and mandible in relation to the skull base, and the angle of the maxilla and mandible in relation to each other) can also cause difficult intubation due to changes in the volume of the nasopharyngeal and oropharyngeal airways; with the help of CT and MRI, we can understand the extent of tumor invasion and whether there is airway stenosis; the simulated endoscope constructed by CT three-dimensional conformation can visually simulate the path of intubation, so as to judge whether there is intubation difficulty.

16.4.4 Preoperative Case Discussion and Family Talk

The treatment of head and neck tumor requires the collaboration between multiple departments and a medical team. Preoperative discussion with surgeon and otolaryngologist may include: (1) The scope of tumor invasion. Whether it has invaded the skull or the orbit or sinuses with corresponding physiological changes, and cases invading the nasal cavity may be contraindications for nasotracheal intubation. If it is a mass adjacent to the vocal cords, it is also needed to ask the ENT physician to perform nasal endoscopy and tracheoscopy. Blind intubation may cause aggravation of obstruction as well as tumor dislodgement and implantation. (2) In case of hemangioma, it is necessary to distinguish capillary type or cavernous hemangioma, because the latter will rapidly engorge and swell when the position is changed, such as when the head is lowered. When the patient holds his breath or coughs, the tumor will also swell rapidly and obstruct the airway due to obstructed reflux of the mass. Any factors that cause obstruction of reflux of the hemangioma should be avoided during intubation. (3) The plan of surgery. Preoperatively, the surgeon should be informed of the surgical plan, and the intraoperative bleeding volume, operating time, and the choice of arterial and venous puncture sites should be predicted according to the surgical plan. (4) Previous treatment. The time of the last surgery and the extent of the damage, the number of radiotherapy sessions, and whether there is a response to radiotherapy, especially the last intubation, are extremely important for the airway assessment. (5) Whether a tracheotomy and admission to the intensive care unit are required postoperatively.

As far as anesthesia is concerned, most patients need to be intubated awake, so a detailed explanation should be given to the patient before surgery about the necessity of awake intubation and intubation steps to obtain the patient's cooperation in the intubation process, and patients who need to be intubated or tracheotomized after surgery should also be informed before surgery.

16.4.5 Preoperative Medication and Fasting

Preoperative medication includes sedative, analgesic, and anticholinergic drugs. How to administer medication depends on the degree of airway obstruction. Patients without significant airway obstruction can be given medication as usual. Considering that benzodiazepines and opioids may cause respiratory depression, and anticholinergic drugs may dry up airway secretions and aggravate airway narrowing, preoperative medications may be waived in patients with severe preoperative airway obstruction. Preoperative fasting was performed as usual.

16.5 Induction of Anesthesia and Intraoperative Management

General anesthesia with endotracheal intubation is chosen for most oral maxillofacial head and neck tumor surgeries. Since this type of surgery is time-consuming and involves intraoral manipulation, supraglottic devices such as laryngeal masks are not suitable and are limited to emergency ventilation in case of failed intubation.

16.5.1 Induction Phase of Anesthesia

16.5.1.1 Pre-induction Preparation

Lower limb vein placement is usually chosen in oral and maxillofacial head and neck surgery. For patients undergoing digital subtraction angiography (DSA), anterolateral femoral flap, or peroneal muscle flap repair, venous puncture should be avoided in the lower extremity where the donor area is located. The connection of the monitor, including the placement of the electrocardiogram electrodes, should be considered whether it will interfere with the surgical operation and should be avoided if possible. The patient is again informed of the next anesthetic procedures, especially the awake intubation, to gain the patient's trust and cooperation and to avoid unnecessary stress. As the internal jugular vein is usually within the surgical area, the femoral vein is usually chosen for the puncture of the central vein. For patients who are to undergo central venous pressure monitoring, subclavian vein puncture is feasible. Similarly, arterial puncture is more commonly chosen for the dorsalis pedis artery [5, 6].

RAE catheters are most frequently used in maxillofacial surgery, with the exposed proximal end of the orotracheal tube curved downward and the exposed proximal end of the nasotracheal tube curved upward, facilitating both fixation and surgical manipulation. The wire thread reinforced catheter does not deform after bending and is used in surgery where the head position is frequently changed to avoid catheter collapse.

Prepare laryngoscope, intubation forceps, mask, core, ventilator, dental pad, connecting tube, and other devices in terms of intubation appliances. For patients with suspicious airways, prepare as many different types of appliances as possible, such as cushion pillows, various laryngeal lenses such as Macintosh and Miller, laryngeal masks, blind tracheal intubation devices, visual laryngoscopes, fiberoptic bronchoscopes, etc., depending on the needs and expertise of the operator.

16.5.1.2 Intubation Plan

Developing an intubation plan for maxillofacial tumor anesthesia is never a simple task. It is necessary to be familiar with the process of difficult airway management, and to have alternative plans and remedial measures immediately after the first plan fails.

Selection of intubation route. The intubation routes are: (1) endotracheal intubation through the nose; (2) endotracheal intubation through the mouth; (3) tracheotomy insertion of catheter. It is mainly determined by the location of the tumor and the surgical plan. The most commonly used is the nasotracheal tube, which has the advantages of better fixation of the nasal cannula and easy intraoperative management; better tolerance and suitable for postoperative retention of the tracheal tube; close to the posterior wall of the pharyngeal cavity and less interference with surgery. It is customary to choose the nostril on the opposite side of the tumor lesion for intubation. Before intubation, it is important to know whether the nasal cavity on the operating side is patent and to routinely prepare the nasal cavity. When the patient's nasal cavity is invaded by the tumor, or patients with long-term radiotherapy for nasopharyngeal cancer and malignant tumors of the palate and maxillary sinus requiring total maxillary osteotomy, orotracheal intubation is usually chosen. In patients with partial maxillary resection, nasotracheal intubation contralateral to the lesion does not usually interfere with the procedure, and transnasal endotracheal intubation is still widely chosen. Preoperative tracheotomy may be chosen in three cases: (1) when orotracheal or nasotracheal intubation is not possible; (2) when tracheal tube inevitably has to interfere with the surgical operation; and (3) when prophylactic tracheotomy is to be performed postoperatively and preoperative intubation is difficult. Unless the patient has obvious laryngeal stenosis or supraglottic obstruction, tracheal intubation is still the mainstay of general tumor surgery.

The choice of induction method. There are three common methods: (1) Fast induction intubation, i.e., placing the catheter after the muscle relaxation has completely taken effect. This is mainly suitable for patients without airway difficulties, such as mixed tumors of the parotid gland and some early tumors of the lip, cheek, and ventral surface of tongue. (2) Intubation or tracheotomy under conscious sedation and surface anesthesia, which is mainly suitable for patients who are suspected of having airway problems but can cooperate, and can be guided by videolaryngoscopy, light stick guidance, or trans-fiber bronchoscopy to guide intubation. After completion of the operation, the catheter position is confirmed to be correct, and then drug-induced sleep is induced. (3) Slow induction intubation with preserved voluntary breathing is suitable for patients with suspected airway difficulties who are uncooperative, such as pediatric patients, and the main methods are ketamine induction and inhalation anesthesia induction. Attention needs to be paid to the reduced tolerance of the elderly to drug-induced respiratory circulation, the induction pushing speed should be slow, and the circulation should be kept as stable as possible.

Remedies after failed intubation. Remedies after failed intubation include emergency ventilation techniques such as cricothyrotomy and transtracheal jet ventilation (TTJV) in hypoxic state and other airway control routes such as laryngeal mask ventilation and tracheotomy in nonemergency situations.

16.5.1.3 Difficult Airway Management [7–9]

First of all, we should distinguish which type of airway difficulty the difficult airway belongs to, whether it is mask ventilation or catheter insertion, whether it is the patient's inability to cooperate or tracheotomy difficulty. For uncooperative patients, such as pediatric patients, intubation can be induced while preserving spontaneous breathing, and ketamine or inhalation anesthesia induction is the more common method. For cooperative adult patients, awake intubation is undoubtedly the best option. The awake patient has sufficient muscle tone to keep the airway open, and muscle tension makes the tissues easily recognizable. The presence of protective reflexes in the awake patient reduces the risk of aspiration.

The term "awake" does not mean that no anesthetic drugs are used, but rather: (1) appropriate sedative and analgesic drugs; (2) complete surface anesthesia; and (3) local nerve block, through the appropriate medication to avoid choking, laryngospasm, etc., to make the intubation smoother.

Commonly used sedative and analgesic drugs include fentanyl, midazolam, etc. The application of midazolam can also enable the patient to obtain good paracrine amnesia and avoid adverse recall.

Endotracheal injection of local anesthetics and local anesthetic spray by cricothyroid puncture can reduce the stress of airway and is very useful in awake intubation. The specific operation is as follows: (1) inject 3–4 mL of 2% lidocaine through the cricothyroid puncture, and ask the patient to cough so that the local anesthetic can be evenly distributed; (2) spray the dorsum of the tongue, soft palate, and pharynx with 7% lidocaine spray (trade name Xylocaine); you can also gently lift the root of the tongue after placing the laryngeal lens, ask the patient to inhale deeply, and aim the spray at the epiglottis and supraglottis area.

The main methods of intubation in the awake state are fiberoptic bronchoscopy-guided intubation or video laryngoscopic intubation, both of which require perfect surface anesthesia and appropriate sedation and analgesia. Fiberoptic bronchoscopy is considered to be the first choice for difficult tracheal intubation, allowing for transnasal or transoral manipulation and visualization of some structures of the airway with less irritation and a high success rate. However, it cannot be used in the presence of significant bleeding and secretions in the pharynx, and the operator's technical inexperience will affect its success rate.

16.5.1.4 Intubation Complications

Common complications of intubation include throat pain, hoarseness, and dental injury. Complications such as pharyngeal mucosal laceration or perforation, subluxation of the arytenoid cartilage, vocal cord paralysis, and laryngeal nerve injury are rare. Throat pain or hoarseness usually improves within 72 h.

Complications of nasotracheal intubation include massive nasal bleeding, entry of the catheter into the retropharyngeal space during intubation, and removal of the turbinates during intubation, mostly due to pre-existing deformities or lesions of the nasal cavity and rough handling. In patients with massive nasal bleeding, a catheter should be left in place to act as a pressure hemostat. Try to clear the blood from the oronasal cavity and try to intubate from the other nostril. Avoid rough handling, and proper lubrication and softening of the tracheal tube can play a preventive role.

16.5.2 Anesthesia Maintenance Stage

Tumor surgery, especially malignant tumor surgery, should take into account the two main characteristics of remote operation and prolonged surgery in the anesthesia maintenance stage.

16.5.2.1 Operation on Distance

In oral and maxillofacial head and neck tumor surgery, the operation in the mouth or moving the head will cause the catheter to shift, which may cause the catheter to slip out or enter into one side of the bronchus during the surgery. On the other hand, since the tracheal tube passes through the surgical area, it is often covered by the surgical towel and the displacement and folding of the catheter is usually not easily detected; therefore, the fixation of the catheter is very important. Generally, the nasal catheter is easier to fix than the oral catheter, and the RAE catheter facilitates airway management. The catheter can also be secured to the nasal septum or the corner of the mouth with sutures or to the skin with a surgical patch. The air sac of the tracheal tube should also be checked for air leakage before the start of surgery to prevent the flow of large amounts of bloody secretions into the airway during surgery in the mouth.

Since the surgeon occupies the head end of the patient and the anesthesia machine needs to be positioned away from the head and connected to the tracheal tube by a long threaded tube, it may be necessary to extend the tubing for additional length, choosing a lightweight threaded tube to avoid pulling the endotracheal tube out by gravity. Check each connection for a tight fit. Monitor closely intraoperatively to prevent loosening of the connections. Monitoring of end-expiratory carbon dioxide partial pressure ($PetCO_2$), pressure-flow loop, and airway pressure can help identify problems in the respiratory circuit early.

16.5.2.2 Prolonged Surgery

Protection of the organism. Since oral and maxillofacial head and neck tumor surgery is usually long, attention should be paid to the protection of the organism: (1) Eye protection. In maxillofacial surgery, surgical suction and antiseptic drops can easily lead to eye damage. Apply foam antimicrobial eye ointment and sterile tape to the upper and lower eyelids before surgery, and remind the physician to avoid pressing the eyeball or pulling the eye contents during the surgical operation, which can reduce the risk of eye injury and blindness. (2) Protection of the nose. Excessive upward pulling of the catheter or overweight of the articulating tube will compress the nasal flange, and prolonged compression and nasal ischemia will lead to local skin necrosis and scar formation. (3) Protection of peripheral nerves. The surgical bed is too narrow and leads to intraoperative upper limb sagging or pressure, which can easily cause ulnar nerve injury, especially in obese patients; the upper limb is too abducted, or the pad liner is not placed in prone position, which can cause brachial plexus nerve injury. Therefore, it is necessary to confirm whether the position is appropriate before cutting the skin. (4) Protection of skin and mucosa. In the same position for a long time, care should be taken to avoid excessive pressure on certain gravity areas and to disperse the area under stress as much as possible. The electrodes and lead wires should not pass through the pressurized area [10].

Hypothermia. Intraoperative hypothermia can lead to impaired platelet function and reduced coagulation factor activity, resulting in increased surgical blood loss; hypothermia can reduce enzyme activity, resulting in delayed awakening; on the other hand, hypothermia is an important factor leading to free flap graft failure.

Intraoperative monitoring of body temperature is usually required, and rectal temperature can be monitored continuously. Methods to prevent hypothermia include: increasing the ambient temperature of the operating room, using an adjustable temperature insulation blanket, and using an infusion warmer for large amounts of fluid input.

Drug accumulation. In order to avoid drug accumulation, intraoperative methods can be adopted: (1) intraoperative use of static inhalation compound anesthesia, reduce the amount of a single drug; (2) choose a strong controllable, short duration, nonhepatic and renal metabolism of drugs such as inhalation anesthetics, propofol, remifentanil, atracurium, and other new anesthetics; (3) according to the need for surgical stimulation to adjust the dose of drugs; (4) intraoperative use of the push pump constant rate of drug delivery. The push pump administration can also reduce the fluctuation of blood oxygen concentration and make the anesthesia smoother.

Fluid management. The bleeding from the maxillofacial area can flow to the neck and occipital area and be absorbed by the mattress and surgical towel, etc. These hidden blood losses can easily lead to underestimation of bleeding and insufficient volume replenishment. On the other hand, patients are mostly elderly patients with more combined cardiovascular diseases, and excessive fluid rehydration can lead to cardiovascular overload and heart pump failure, so a more precise fluid management pattern needs to be maintained. Traditional methods, such as monitoring of invasive blood pressure, central venous pressure, and other hemodynamic indicators, help to guide rehydration, while hourly urine volume recording can indirectly reflect tissue perfusion. Goal-directed fluid therapy (GDFT) refers to individualized rehydration therapy by monitoring hemodynamic indices to determine the body's fluid needs. Studies have shown that intraoperative individualized GDFT can provide greater benefit for medium- to high-risk patients. Due to the limitations of oral and maxillofacial head and neck surgical sites, Flotrac/Vigileo or LiDCOTM rapid devices are often used clinically to monitor SVV, PPV, and other indicators to optimize volume management of the body, which can significantly improve patient prognosis and shorten the hospital stay.

16.6 Postoperative Management

16.6.1 Extubation

Factors affecting postoperative airway management strategy include: (1) whether postoperative anatomical changes in the nasal and pharyngeal cavities and large free tissue flap repair obstruct the upper airway, and whether edema of the soft tissues surrounding the resected lesion affects airway patency; (2) injury to the lingual nerve, vagus nerve, and one side of the phrenic nerve during surgery can lead to decreased swallowing reflex, elevation of the ipsilateral diaphragm, and decreased ventilation; (3) prolonged anesthetic drug accumulation, postoperative infection, potential bleeding hematoma in the operating area, and the patient's preoperative pulmonary function are also factors that cannot be ignored.

Postoperative extubation must be done with caution. The requirements for extubation in oral and maxillofacial tumor surgery include: (1) the patient is clearly conscious, the EEG dual-frequency index monitoring meets the requirements, there is no delirium and irritability, and protective reflexes such as coughing are well recovered; (2) muscle tone is completely restored, and there is no residual effect of inotropic drugs; (3) pulse oxygen saturation can reach the preoperative level when breathing air; (4) hemodynamic stability; (5) salivation at the corners of the mouth significantly less than before, and not much secretion during intra-catheter suction.

Extubation can be performed after the patient is fully awakened or 24–48 h after surgery. The special nature of oncologic surgery makes delayed extubation very common, and it is safer for cases with significant postoperative local swelling, suspected bleeding, or where the surgical site may affect breathing. Before extubation, aspirate the secretions from the mouth and nose, and place a gastric tube to remove the gastric contents. Check again for localized blood leakage or poor drainage, and check if the dressing is affecting breathing, then release the air bag and gently remove the catheter. For patients who originally had a difficult airway, place a guide tube such as a Cook AEC before withdrawing the tube, and then slowly withdraw the catheter to the vocal opening, stop and observe the respiratory situation, if there is nothing special continue to withdraw outward until it is completely withdrawn, while continuing to leave the catheter in place for 10–20 min, in order to be able to quickly redirect the insertion of the tracheal tube in case of emergency. Such patients also need to have a tracheotomy device routinely available at the bedside. After extubation, patients should still be given close respiratory monitoring, including SpO_2, heart rate, respiratory rate, etc. Patients should be alerted to hypoventilation when they appear irritable, delirious, or drowsy, and blood gas tests should be performed if necessary. Patients with obvious posterior tongue drop may have a nasopharyngeal airway placed, or the tongue may be pulled out and fixed outside the mouth after suturing.

16.6.2 Prophylactic Tracheotomy and Indwelling Tracheal Tube

There are some procedures that require prophylactic tracheotomy in the postoperative period, such as: (1) procedures involving supraglottic tissues such as the tongue root, pharyngeal cavity, and larynx, where the postoperative pharyngeal cavity wall loses support and the airway tends to collapse; (2) simultaneous bilateral cervical lymph node dissection, where there can be significant postoperative laryngeal edema; (3) extensive joint resection with mandibular osteotomy beyond the midline; (4) large intraoral free tissue flaps; and (5) patients with preoperative respiratory insufficiency. The purpose of selective tracheotomy is to secure the patency of the airway, and then after 5–7 days when the swelling subsides, block the tube and finally remove the tracheotomy tube. However, postoperative prophylactic tracheotomy also carries certain risks and complications, such as the risk of hypoxia if the local tissue collapses after the tracheal tube is withdrawn from the airway and the tracheotomy tube cannot be delivered in time. Therefore, it is important that the withdrawal process be slow, stopping when the distal end of the tracheal tube reaches the top of the fistula and then completely withdrawing when the tracheotomy tube is delivered into the trachea without error. Tracheotomy also increases the risk of lung infection. The inability to speak after tracheotomy can affect the patient's psychological recovery. Complications associated with tracheotomy include obstruction of the tracheotomy cannula, tracheoesophageal fistula, and post-tracheotomy tracheal stenosis (mostly seen in pediatric patients). Airway patency can also be effectively maintained by leaving a catheter in place for 1–2 days, reducing the rate of postoperative tracheotomy. It has been clinically found that leaving a tracheal tube in place for 24–48 h after surgery does not increase the incidence of intubation-related complications and can significantly shorten the length of hospital stay. The following should be noted when leaving the tracheal tube in place: (1) choose transnasal intubation as much as possible because patients tolerate transnasal tracheal tube better and it is easy to fix and manage; (2) give appropriate sedation and analgesia to avoid excessive swallowing to increase the friction between the tube and airway and the occurrence of laryngeal edema; (3) strengthen the care of the tracheal tube to avoid partial blockage of the tube, which causes hypoventilation. The sleeve should be deflated intermittently to avoid prolonged compression of the tracheal wall; (4) for patients requiring long-term ventilator therapy, tracheotomy should still be selected.

16.6.3 Postoperative Airway Management

Whether the tracheal tube is left in place or tracheotomy is performed, postoperative airway care is very crucial: (1) The airway should be cleared frequently to avoid secretions obstructing the airway or remaining near the exit of the tube, causing obstructed ventilation and hypoxia. Aspiration should be performed aseptically, and the duration of aspiration should not be too long; (2) Air and oxygen enter the lower airway directly through the catheter, which tends to dry the lower airway and increases the chance of lower airway infection, so airway nebulization and antibiotics should be given, and the accumulated sputum should be cleared by chest physiotherapy such as patting the back; (3) Low-flow oxygen should be given to meet the balance of oxygen supply and demand of the body; (4) The formation of tracheotomy sinus tract takes about 5 days, and if the tracheotomy cannula is to be replaced within 5 days, try to use Cook AEC or suction tube; (5) for the tracheotomy cannula or indwelling catheter placed, choose a high-capacity and low-pressure sleeve, and adjust the balloon pressure frequently to avoid local ischemic necrosis [11, 12].

16.6.4 Postoperative Monitoring Management

Due to the high number of elderly patients, combined cardiovascular, chronic obstructive pulmonary disease, and diabetes mellitus among tumor patients, and the special requirements of postoperative airway care, postoperative treatment in intensive care unit is often required. Routine postoperative monitoring of pulse oxygen saturation, blood pressure, central venous pressure, electrocardiogram, electrolytes, and blood gases can help detect some problems early, such as airway obstruction, hypoxia, hypoventilation, hypercapnia, hypotension, hypertension, arrhythmia, and myocardial ischemia, and provide timely and symptomatic treatment.

Postoperative head braking, prevention of vascular tip distortion, and flap observation are also important for patients undergoing free tissue flap repair, including bleeding, hematoma, poor flap blood supply, and poor local drainage, and early detection can help to remedy the situation in a timely manner.

16.7 Anesthesia for Common Types of Maxillofacial Tumor Surgeries

16.7.1 Surgery of Giant Neurofibroma of Maxillofacial Area

Giant neurofibroma in the head and neck of oral and maxillofacial region is less common nowadays. Such surgery takes a long time and the bleeding volume can be as much as thousands of milliliters. Controlled hypotension and autologous blood transfusion techniques can be used in anesthesia, as well as with local hypothermia to cause local vasoconstriction. The surgical technique of performing segmental suturing of the tumor prior to tumor removal also helps to reduce blood loss. The intraoperative management is mainly about the judgment of blood loss and fluid management. Due to the coverage of the head and facial dressing, blood flow to the back of the occiput and other factors can cause errors in the judgment of blood loss, which can be compensated by strengthening hemodynamic monitoring, and such patients need to perform invasive arterial and central venous pressure monitoring and leave the catheter in place. After massive transfusion of blood and fluids, it is necessary to prevent complications such as hypothermia, water-electrolyte disorders, and abnormal coagulation function.

16.7.2 Mental and Cervical Hygroma Surgery

Hygromas of the chin and neck are benign lymph-vessel tumors that are giant and are often combined with tracheal displacement and even difficulty in breathing, and usually occur in young children. Since young children cannot cooperate, endotracheal intubation is difficult. Ketamine can be given for induction by intramuscular injection or inhalation gas induction, preserving spontaneous breathing, supplemented with adequate surface anesthesia. Dyspnea during induction is usually related to the position of the head. Breathing difficulties are usually relieved if the patient's head is turned to the affected side. Considering that the catheter may have to be left in place for 1–2 days after surgery, nasotracheal intubation is usually chosen. The normal holding forceps are too large for operation in the pediatric oral cavity, so long forceps can be prepared to replace the holding forceps. Once artificial respiratory access is established, anesthesia is often smooth, tumor envelope boundaries are obvious, and bleeding is usually under control. Postoperatively, due to local tissue swelling, an indwelling tracheal tube under proper sedation and hormone and antibiotic treatment is required.

16.7.3 Cervical Lymphatic Dissection and Combined Maxillo-Cervical Radical Surgery

The most common metastatic route of oral and maxillofacial head and neck malignant tumors is through lymph nodes. Therefore, in addition to resection of the primary foci, the surgical treatment should also include cervical lymph node dissection according to the different stages and grades of the tumor, including radical and functional cervical lymph node dissection, or unilateral or bilateral cervical lymph node dissection. Cervical lymph node dissection and resection of the primary site at the same time is called combined radical treatment.

In radical cervical lymph node dissection, the sternocleidomastoid muscle, internal and external jugular veins, and associated lymph nodes must be removed. The matters that need to be noted during surgical anesthesia are: (1) when large vessels in the neck are injured, the bleeding volume is very large, and a large orifice intravenous channel must be left in place before surgery; (2) during the process of dissection, try to maintain smooth anesthesia, and beware of air embolism, whose initial symptom is a sudden drop in partial pressure of carbon dioxide at the end of expiration; (3) surgery when stimulating the carotid sinus, unexpected sinus bradycardia may occur, which can be prevented by giving 1% lidocaine local block, or stopping the operation immediately after sinus bradycardia occurs and giving atropine symptomatic treatment; (4) after internal jugular vein removal, the head and facial venous reflux is impaired, so the edema of the head and neck is very obvious, especially in patients who have bilateral cervical lymph node dissection at the same time; after bilateral internal jugular vein removal, the collateral circulation of vertebral veins cannot be established rapidly within a short period of time. Intraoperative head elevation, avoiding excessive intravenous rehydration, giving hormones, mannitol and other methods can relieve the symptoms of edema, and can also apply cryogenic techniques or appropriate cranial protection measures, and postoperatively also keep the head elevated, hormone therapy, leaving the endotracheal tube to keep respiratory ventilation, and considering tracheotomy in patients with bilateral cervical lymph node dissection; (5) damage to the right stellate ganglion and right cervical autonomic nerve during right cervical lymph node dissection will lead to prolonged QT interval and lower ventricular fibrillation threshold, especially when there is electrolyte disturbance at the same time, and it is necessary to strengthen perioperative monitoring.

16.7.4 Expanded Craniofacial Radical Surgery

In the past, malignant tumors in some parts of the head and face were considered incurable, but after craniofacial radical surgery, the 5-year survival rate of patients is significantly improved. If the tumor is involved in the orbit, the entire orbital contents should be removed, and if the tumor is involved in the dura mater, the local dura mater and brain tissue should be separated and removed together. Because of the deep location of these tumors and the involvement of intracranial blood vessels and nerves, the surgery is quite complicated and the risk of surgical anesthesia is also very high.

This kind of surgery has the characteristics of both oral surgery and neurosurgery: (1) because of combined intracranial and extracranial radical treatment, the trauma is very large, and the defect is also large after resection of the primary foci, which usually requires free tissue flap repair or even tandem flap repair, so the operation time is very long, which can be more than 10 h; (2) because of the large trauma, deep location, and the difficulty of hemostasis, the intraoperative bleeding is very large, especially for some malignant tumors such as the malignant tumor of maxillary sinus. The osteotomy of the maxilla is required, and the bleeding is very rapid in a short period of time. Appropriate controlled hypotension during osteotomy can reduce blood loss and make the surgical field clearer. For patients with heavy bleeding, intraoperative hemodynamic monitoring is necessary; (3) shallow hypothermia can be taken during surgery to reduce cerebral metabolism, and other cerebral protective measures include avoiding hyperglycemia, maintaining normal levels of partial pressure of end-expiratory carbon dioxide, moderate hemodilution, reducing blood viscosity, and improving cerebral blood flow; (4) for some patients monitoring of intracranial pressure is required.

16.7.5 Free Tissue Flap Surgery

After tumor resection, especially radical surgery, there are often large tissue defects. One-stage tissue reconstruction is performed to cover the trauma on the one hand, and for cosmetic reasons on the other hand, which is important to improve the inferiority complex of tumor patients and improve the quality of survival. Small traumas can be solved by skin grafting and local flap transfer, while large defects must be covered by free tissue flaps, and myocutaneous flaps have better shape effect and anti-infection ability than normal skin grafts.

Common free tissue flaps include soft tissue flaps, such as forearm flap, pectoralis major flap, latissimus dorsi flap, anterolateral femoral flap, etc.; there are also bony muscle flaps, such as peroneal muscle flap, iliac muscle flap, etc. The site and size of the tissue defect determine which flap should be used. During flap grafting, the flap undergoes two ischemic periods. The primary ischemic period starts from the time the flap is free and disconnected until after vascular anastomosis and reperfusion, which is usually around 60–90 mins, and the length of the ischemic period depends on the surgeon. Ischemia is followed by anaerobic cellular metabolism within the flap, which is quickly followed by a decrease in pH, lactate accumulation, increased calcium ion concentration, and accumulation of inflammatory mediators. The secondary ischemic phase occurs after small vessel anastomosis, and hypoperfusion is the main cause, which is more harmful than primary ischemia and can easily lead to flap death; with proper anesthetic techniques, ischemic damage in this phase can be interfered with.

The causes of flap graft failure are factors of anastomotic arteries or veins, such as anastomotic fistula, arterial spasm, and vascular embolism; and factors causing edema within the flap tissue such as improper operation, too long primary ischemic period, too much crystal supplementation, and no lymphatic reflux in the flap. From the physiological point of view, the main method to reduce the flap failure rate is to improve the blood supply and reflux of the flap. According to the Poiseuille formula, blood flow is proportional to the pressure difference between the two ends of the tissue, proportional to the fourth power of the vascular radius, and inversely proportional to blood viscosity. Increasing perfusion pressure, dilating vessels, and decreasing blood viscosity increase blood flow and increase flap survival, which are the three main points of free flap anesthesia. Balanced anesthesia, good analgesia, and normal body temperature contribute to vasodilation, while mild high-volume hemodilution contributes to increased perfusion pressure and decreased viscosity.

Good perfusion pressure is achieved by proper depth of anesthesia and fluid management. Usually, ascending agents are not used because most of them cause vasoconstriction. Small doses of dobutamine, appropriate fluid replacement, maintenance of central venous pressure at a level 2 cmH_2O above basal, and maintenance of urine output of 1 mL/(kg h) to 2 mL/(kg h) can be tried as indicators of satisfactory microcirculatory perfusion.

Mild controlled hypotension, good analgesia, and avoidance of vasoconstrictive drugs can maintain vasodilation and adequate blood flow. In case of vasospasm, topical medications such as papaverine hydrochloride and lidocaine can be given to release the spasm. A decrease in body temperature is an important factor in vasoconstriction, so normal body temperature must be maintained during the perioperative period. During temperature monitoring, core and peripheral body temperatures can be monitored simultaneously, and a difference of less than 2° between them indicates satisfactory tissue perfusion.

The reduction of blood viscosity is achieved by hemodilution. Dilution is usually achieved until the red blood cell pressure volume is around 30%. Further dilution reduces the oxygen supply to the flap tissue.

In addition to the survival of the flap, the requirement of small vessel anastomosis should be considered. The microsurgery operation is delicate and requires absolutely smooth anesthesia throughout, avoiding too deep or too shallow anesthesia.

16.7.6 Carotid Body Aneurysm Surgery

This surgery may involve severing or blocking the common carotid artery, and there may be a large amount of bleeding when separating the adhesions, which is a potential threat to the blood supply to the brain. The patient's ability of collateral circulation should be tested before surgery. A simple method is to compress the affected common carotid artery for half an hour; if there are no symptoms such as sensory vertigo, it indicates that the compensation is sound and the prognosis of surgery is better. There are chemoreceptors around the aneurysm, and aneurysm pulling will cause a drop in blood pressure and slowing of the heartbeat. The use of local anesthesia can reduce the reflexes of the carotid body. There are different opinions on controlled hypotension. Proponents believe that controlled full hypotension helps to reduce the risk of intraoperative hemorrhage, while opponents believe that hypotension leads to decreased cerebral perfusion, causing brain damage and increasing complications of cerebral ischemia such as postoperative hemiplegia. Our clinical experience is that controlled hypotension should be given moderately during stripping and dividing the tumor adhesions with more bleeding, while therapeutic hypertension should be given during surgical clamp closure, ligation, and resection of the common carotid artery to help maintain cerebral perfusion and avoid local cerebral ischemia due to insufficient perfusion of the collateral circulation in the hypotensive state.

References

1. Zhu Y. Anesthesia of modern oral and maxillofacial surgery. Jinan: Shandong Science and Technology Press; 2001.
2. Xinliang Z, Yinming Z, Boluan C. Modern anesthesiology. 3rd ed. Beijing: People's Medical Publishing House; 2003.
3. Chenping Z. Challenges in the treatment of oral and maxillofacial tumor. J Oral Maxillofac Surg. 2020;30(01):1–4.
4. Rongqiang J, Lin H. Experience of airway management in difficult anesthesia for oral and maxillofacial surgical oncology. Dept Oral Med Electr Mag. 2015;2(03):44–5.
5. Qiang Z, Pan H, Guocheng J, Xinming L, He W. Anesthesia for combined radical surgery of oral and maxillofacial malignancies in elderly patients. West China J Stomatol. 2000;05:353–4.
6. Zhifeng C, Hong J, Yang Y. Anesthesia of maxillofacial tumor surgery with free flap reconstruction. Perioper Saf Qual Assur. 2019;3(05):258–62.
7. Rohit J, Orla L. Anaesthesia for head and neck cancer surgery. Curr Anaesth Crit Care. 2009;20(1):28–32.
8. Robert G, Krohner DO. Anesthetic consideration and techniques for oral and maxillofacial surgery. Int Anesthesiol Clin. 2003;41(3):67–89.
9. Mishra S, Bhatnagar S, Jha RR, et al. Airway management of patients undergoing oral cancer surgery: a retrospective study. Eur J Anaesthesiol. 2005;22(12):510–4.
10. Yonghai S, Yuhuan S, Zonggang C. Enhanced recovery after surgery (ERAS) for patients with head and neck neoplasms. China J Oral Maxillofac Surg. 2019;17(02):186–9.
11. Jane Q, Omer L. Anaesthesia for reconstructive surgery. Intensive Care Med. 2009;10(1):26–31.
12. Zhang Z, Qiu W. Craniofacial resection of advanced oral and maxillofacial malignant tumors. Chin Med J. 2003;116(1):134–7.

Anesthesia for Orthognathic Surgery

17

Rong Hu

17.1 Introduction

Orthognathic surgery is a discipline that focuses on the study and treatment of bony dental and maxillofacial deformities, with the treatment goal of achieving functional and aesthetic recovery and maintenance. It integrates new theories, techniques, and progress in oral and maxillofacial surgery, orthodontics, aesthetics, psychology, anatomy, physiology, speech pathology, and anesthesia, and uses modern surgery in combination with orthodontic treatment to correct bony dental and maxillofacial deformities, in order to obtain the best results in terms of morphology, function, and aesthetics.

17.2 The Scope of Orthognathic and Maxillofacial Deformities and Orthognathic Surgery

17.2.1 Oral and Maxillofacial Deformities

Oral and maxillofacial deformities are defined as abnormalities in the size and shape of the jaws due to abnormal growth and development of the jaws, abnormal relationships between the upper and lower jaws and other bones of the skull and face, and consequent abnormalities in the dental and jaw relationships and function of the oro-mandibular system, often appearing as jaws and face abnormalities. For patients with oral and maxillofacial deformities, mild jaw deformities such as malocclusion, dental disorders, crowding, mild protrusion or recession can be corrected by simple orthodontic or adolescent orthopedic treatment, while moderate to severe jaw deformities need to be treated by a combination of orthognathic surgery and orthodontic correction.

17.2.1.1 Etiology

The etiology of oral and maxillofacial malformations includes congenital, acquired, and functional factors.

1. Congenital Factors

   These include genetic factors or abnormalities in embryonic development, the latter of which can be caused by abnormalities in the mother's internal environment during fetal development. For example, malnutrition during pregnancy, endocrine disorders, and the effects of teratogenic drugs can cause disorders of embryonic development, attachment, or fusion, which in turn can lead to malformations of the oral and maxillofacial system.

R. Hu (✉)
Department of Anesthesiology, Shanghai Ninth People's Hospital Affiliated to Shanghai Jiao Tong University School of Medicine, Shanghai, China
e-mail: hur1152@sh9hospital.org.cn

H. Jiang, M. Xia (eds.), *Anesthesia for Oral and Maxillofacial Surgery*,
https://doi.org/10.1007/978-981-19-7287-4_17

2. Acquired Factors

    Acute or chronic diseases, including growth spurts, such as acute rash disease, tuberculosis, and poliomyelitis, can cause dental and maxillofacial deformities, mainly of the lower jaw. Excessive secretion of growth hormones can lead to macromandibular disorders, etc. In addition, bad habits in childhood, including finger sucking and pencil biting, can cause anterior protrusion of the upper front teeth and, in severe cases, recession of the jaw. Injuries to the jaw and face during adolescence and childhood such as jaw fractures and temporomandibular joint injuries, as well as infectious diseases may bring facial deformities.
3. Functional Factors

    These include abnormalities in jaw development due to abnormalities in sucking, chewing, and breathing functions.
4. Bad Oral Habits [1, 2]

    Long-term maintenance of bad oral habits may affect the normal growth and development of the jaw and face, and is one of the main causes of malocclusion. These bad habits mainly include finger sucking, tongue spitting, lower lip biting, and lateral chewing.

17.2.1.2 Characteristics of Oral and Maxillofacial Region

The blood supply to the upper and lower jaws is multiple and very rich, with the maxilla being richer than the mandible. At present, orthognathic surgery is basically performed intraorally. The deep and complex anatomy of the site, and the fact that many operations cannot be performed under direct vision make some operations prone to bleeding and difficult to stop, especially when the maxillofacial artery is injured, which can lead to acute hemorrhage and even threaten life.

17.2.1.3 Examination

When examining a patient with a dental or maxillofacial malformation in preparation for subsequent diagnosis and treatment, the anesthetists need to be aware of a number of special circumstances. For example, if there are other pathologies associated with dento-maxillofacial deformities, including temporomandibular disorders, maxillofacial tumors, maxillofacial trauma, apnea syndrome, systemic diseases, etc., the anesthetists need to assess the patient's airway conditions, whether there are potential difficulties with mask ventilation or intubation, and the functions of the patient's organs in order to adequately prepare the patient for the subsequent operations. The patient's mental health issues due to dental and maxillofacial deformities also need to be understood, which may influence the patient's subsequent ability to cooperate with the anesthetic and postoperative recovery [3].

17.2.1.4 Classifications

Dental and maxillofacial malformations are classified as congenital, developmental, and acquired malformations according to their etiology. However, classifying them by the direction of the deformity is convenient for the choice of treatment methods. Under this classification, they have sagittal, vertical, left-right transverse, and asymmetrical deformities.

17.2.1.5 Treatment

Orthodontic techniques are routinely used to treat patients with malocclusion but whose skeletal relationships are normal. For malocclusion patients with mild to moderate abnormal skeletal, treatment is carried out using dental substitution and growth control. For patients with moderate to severe malocclusion, combined orthognathic-orthodontic treatment is the ideal solution if orthodontic masking treatment fails to correct the deformity or achieve aesthetic stability of the face.

17.2.2 Orthognathic Surgery

Orthognathic surgery consists mainly of maxillary osteotomies and mandibular osteotomies. Common maxillary osteotomies include Le Fort fractures, which are classified according to the course and location of the fracture line. These include Le Fort I osteotomy, Le Fort II osteotomy, Le Fort III osteotomy, and maxillary anterior osteotomy. Common mandibular osteotomies include sagittal split ramus osteotomy, osteotomy of mandibular body, vertical mandibular osteotomy, anterior segmental maxillary osteotomy, and genioplasty, of which sagittal split ramus osteotomy is the most common.

17.3 Anesthetic Management Features

Orthognathic surgery is a surgical operation to restore the position of the upper and lower jaws through osteotomy, debridement, bone grafting, movement and fixation to correct dental and maxillofacial deformities. Nowadays, orthognathic surgery is basically performed through an intraoral approach, which is deep, complex in anatomy, and many operations cannot be performed under direct vision, which may easily damage the maxillary and mandibular vessels. In addition, patients with moderate to severe orthognathic malformations may suffer from genetic, embryonic developmental abnormalities or developmental infections, trauma, and other factors that lead to jaw hypoplasia, jaw recession, temporomandibular joint damage, obstructive sleep apnea syndrome, and consequent cardiopulmonary abnormalities or systemic dysplasia, making the surgical anesthetic management of patients with orthognathic malformations unique [4].

17.3.1 Difficult Airway Management

Some patients with dental and maxillofacial malformations present with varying degrees of airway obstruction due to mandibular hypoplasia, mandibular retrusion, snoring, and even suffocating during sleep. In such patients, in addition to routine airway assessment, airway ventilation conditions can be comprehensively assessed by means of respiratory sleep monitoring and 3D airway reconstruction if necessary. For patients with suspected difficult tracheal intubation or even difficult mask ventilation, the anesthetist must formulate a comprehensive perioperative airway management plan and use sedative and analgesic drugs carefully according to their airway conditions before induction of anesthesia to ensure the patient's safety [5].

17.3.2 Tracheal Intubation Route Selection

The appropriate route of tracheal intubation is chosen according to the needs of the different surgical operations. For procedures involving the skull base, orbit, nose, maxilla and maxillary sinus, transoral tracheal intubation is preferred. Transnasal tracheal intubation is preferred for procedures involving the parotid region, the mandible, and the oral cavity. For special procedures with large craniomaxillofacial range, the route of tracheal intubation should be chosen in consultation with the orthognathic surgeon, taking into account various factors such as the operation of the surgical area and the need for postoperative recovery.

17.3.3 Remote Management

The area around the head of the orthognathic patient is occupied by the surgeon for performing surgery, forcing the anesthetist to manage away from that area, which is extremely detrimental to intraoperative monitoring of the airway. When the orthognathic surgeon is operating intraorally, there is a risk of endoleaks, blood, and foreign bodies entering the airway, making it more difficult to manage. In order to safely perform this "remote management" of the airway, endotracheal intubation is always used for general anesthesia, and a leak-proof endotracheal tube with a cuff is used to secure the airway, and perioperative mechanical ventilation is used to ensure adequate gas exchange while the patient is anesthetized. The anesthetist should monitor the vital signs and detect and manage any gliding, twisting, or folding of the tracheal tube during the operation.

17.3.4 Intraoperative Blood Loss

Due to the rich blood supply to the maxillofacial area, the difficulty in stopping bleeding, and the vasodilating effect of the anesthetic drugs, the intraoperative blood loss might increase during surgery. Orthognathic surgery is delicate and complex, with more blood loss from the surgical wound and a relatively long operative time. In surgeries such as maxillary Le Fort I and Le Fort II osteotomies, sagittal split ramus osteotomy, and vertical ramus osteotomy, severe blood loss can also occur due to bleeding from bone sections and soft tissue incisions, and difficulties in hemostasis. For these procedures, intraoperative hemodynamics monitoring should be strengthened to accurately estimate intraoperative blood loss and provide timely volume replacement. For procedures where significant intraoperative blood loss is expected, chemoprotective measures such as acute hemodilution and autologous blood collection can be given preoperatively, and controlled hypotensive techniques can be used intraoperatively to reduce blood loss. For procedures where large intraoperative blood loss is expected or where craniotomy is being considered, hypothermic anesthesia may also be administered to increase the tolerance of the patient's tissues and organs to ischemia and hypoxia.

17.3.5 Adverse Nerve Reflex

The oral and maxillofacial nerves are rich and nociceptive, and stimulation by surgical operations can easily cause oculo-cardiac vagal reflexes and carotid sinus reflexes, which can result in a decreased heart rate and blood pressure, or even cardiac arrest. Therefore, it is necessary to maintain the appropriate depth of anesthesia during the perioperative period, continuously monitor changes in the patient's vital signs, and detect and manage abnormalities in a timely manner.

17.4 Anesthesia Methods

17.4.1 General Anesthesia

17.4.1.1 Preanesthetic Evaluation and Preparation

1. Medical History and Physical Examination

   The anesthetist should have a thorough understanding of the patient's condition and physiological function prior to anesthesia and assess patient's tolerance of surgical anesthesia: querying history of the patient's admission and systemic medical history of general anesthesia and major surgeries, including cardiovascular disease, diabetes, liver, kidney, and thyroid function. In children and adolescents, a history of allergy to anesthetic drugs, family history of malignant hyperthermia, and pseudocholinesterase deficiency should also be sought; the prevention of serious systemic complications due to anesthetic-induced malignant hyperthermia and impaired succinylcholine metabolism due to pseudocholinesterase deficiency should be actively pursued to prevent respiratory muscle paralysis and delayed emergence.

   In patients undergoing maxillofacial surgery, pre-anesthetic the presence or absence of difficult tracheal intubation and difficult mask ventilation can help to reduce the risk of airway complications in patients during the perioperative period. Although there are many assessment tools available to predict a difficult airway, no assured prediction method exists. Age > 55 years old, beard, edentulousness, body mass index >26 kg/m^2, and snoring are considered to be independent risk factors for difficult mask ventilation [6]. Mouth opening <3 cm, modified Mallampati classification grade III ~ IV, restricted mandibular protrusion, short thyromental distance (<6 cm), and Cormack-Lehane laryngoscopic view grading system III ~ IV are considered to be at risk for potentially difficult tracheal intubation [7].

   In addition to airway assessment, pre-anesthesia should focus on assessing the functional status of vital organs, including the presence of hypertension, whether ECG findings suggest arrhythmias, myocardial ischemia, and ventricular hypertrophy, and the assessment of heart function. If the patient is suspected of cardiopulmonary disorders, further investigations such as ECG exercise tests, echocardiography, pulmonary function, and arterial blood gas analysis measurements should be performed. In addition, blood glucose and urinary ketones should be measured before anesthesia to determine the patient's tolerance to carbohydrates, and liver and kidney function should be measured to assess the degree of impairment. After a thorough assessment of the patient's physiological status, the anesthetist should work with the orthognathic surgeon to develop an appropriate treatment plan to improve anesthesia quality.

2. Psychological Assessment and Preparation

    Patients may experience a range of complex psychological changes during the onset and progression of the disease and throughout the consultation and treatment process. Patients who have already undergone surgery may experience extreme pessimism, stress, and fear when they know they are going to undergo surgery again. For elderly patients, they may be overly concerned about the progression of their disease and health condition, which may lead to anxiety and depression. Adequate communication with patients during the pre-anesthetic visit will enable anesthetists to understand and cooperate with medical treatments such as management during the emergence period and postoperative admission to the surgical intensive care (SICU) with a tube, as well as help to accurately understand and assess the patient's psychological status and prevent adverse psychological activities.

3. Premedication

    For patients with suspected difficult airways, sedative, hypnotic, and analgesic drugs are usually prohibited or used with caution before surgery. Intramuscular anticholinergic drugs, such as atropine 0.01 mg/kg–0.03 mg/kg, long tocopherol 0.5–1 mg, or scopolamine 0.005 mg/kg–0.01 mg/kg, can be given 0.5 h before surgery to relieve the patient's anxiety and pain, reduce glandular secretion, inhibit the occurrence of adverse cardiovascular reflexes, etc. Antihistamines and antacids can be considered 1–2 h before elective surgery. In patients of advanced age, with severe respiratory problems, significant airway obstruction, or increased intracranial pressure, pre-anesthetic medication may not be given for safety reasons.

17.4.2 Implementation of Anesthesia

17.4.2.1 Anesthesia Induction

Induction of anesthesia should be implemented with the principle of guaranteeing patient's safety, stability, and comfort and the method of induction should be selected according to the patient's characteristics and the availability of anesthetic equipment, drugs, and techniques.

1. Induction with Spontaneous Breathing

    This means that tracheal intubation is performed after induction by intravenous administration of sedatives, analgesics, hypnotics, inotropes, or inhaled anesthetics. This induction method should be used when the patient's general condition is good, no difficult mask ventilation and intubation is predicted, the anesthetic equipment is well established, and an experienced anesthetist is present.

2. Induction without Spontaneous Breathing

    This refers to the induction of anesthesia in which the patient's spontaneous ventilation is maintained. Prior to induction, appropriate amounts of sedatives and analgesics may be administered intravenously to facilitate surface anesthesia of the pharynx and endotracheal mucosa. Tracheal intubation may be performed using tools such as videolaryngoscopy, light wands, fiberoptical bronchoscope, or blind tracheal intubation devices while preserving voluntary breathing [8]. This induction method is usually used in patients whose pre-anesthetic airway assessment reveals the possibility of difficult mask ventilation or tracheal intubation.

17.4.2.2 Tracheal Intubation

1. Aims of Tracheal Intubation
    (a) Maintain airway patency.
    (b) Ensure effective gas exchange.
    (c) Reduce respiratory work.
    (d) Prevent regurgitant aspiration.
    (e) Mechanical ventilation required.
    (f) Administer inhalation anesthesia.
2. Preparation Before Intubation
    (a) Tracheal intubation tools: oxygen mask, oropharyngeal and nasopharyngeal air-

way, suction tube, suction tool, (video) laryngoscope, fiberoptical bronchoscope, tube holding forceps, stylets, bite blocks, adhesive tape, etc.
   (b) Anesthetic drugs: intravenous anesthetics, inhalation anesthetics, muscle relaxants.
   (c) Other equipment: anesthetic machines, simple ventilators, air sources, monitors, emergency drugs, etc.
3. Nasotracheal Tube

   In orthognathic surgery, where the operation site is deep and the position of the head changes frequently, transnasal intubation is often chosen to facilitate fixation of the tracheal tube away from the intraoral area. Before intubation, nasal vasoconstriction such as ephedrine and furacilin nasal drops can be used to prevent bleeding. A shaped tracheal tube, such as a Ring-Adair-Elwyn tube (RAE) or a wired tracheal tube, is used to maximize exposure of the surgical area for surgical operation. After induction of anesthesia, the tube which is lubricated by petrolatum is gently inserted into the anterior nostril and advanced perpendicular to the face. The catheter is delivered through the posterior nasal aperture to the oropharyngeal cavity and into the voice box in plain view. After intubation, both lungs are auscultated and observed to confirm that the end-expiratory carbon dioxide waveform is regular, that is, the tracheal tube is in the trachea and the cuff is inflated (pressure usually not exceeding 25 cmH_2O) [9].
4. Blind Nasoendotracheal Intubation

   It is often used in patients who have difficulty with mask ventilation or intubation during pre-anesthetic airway assessment. This method does not require special instruments and is relatively simple and practical. During intubation, the head is tilted back and the shoulders are elevated, and the head position can be adjusted according to the sound of the breath at the tube end (tilted back to lying down to forward flexion). Patients with skull base fractures, coagulation disorders, nasal or paranasal sinus malformations should avoid this intubation method.
5. Fiberoptic Laryngoscope-Guided Intubation

   It is endotracheal intubation guided by a fiberoptic laryngoscope and is indicated for patients with predicted difficult airway. It can be performed nasally or orally, yet it might be compromised when there is bleeding or a large amount of secretion in the intubation routes.
6. Retrograde Intubation

   This refers to the placement of a thin introducer tube (usually an extradural guiding tube) through the cricothyroid membrane puncture to tract the tube into the trachea. It is very effective in patients with severe maxillofacial deformities and temporomandibular joint ankylosis. Modified retrograde tracheal intubation is performed at the level of the cricoid cartilage, allowing the catheter to be tractioned into the trachea more easily and avoiding complications such as vocal cord injury and bleeding.
7. Laryngeal Mask Airway (LMA) Ventilation or LMA-Guided Intubation

   A laryngeal mask can effectively solve upper airway obstruction and maintain voluntary or positive pressure ventilation by forming a closed circle around the patient's laryngeal inlet, but the mask is not effective in preventing regurgitation of gastric contents and aspiration. LMA-guided intubation guarantees safer and more effective airway management. In addition, the laryngeal mask facilitates retrograde intubation and fiberoptic laryngoscope-guided tracheal intubation.
8. Blind Tracheal Intubation Instrument-Guided Intubation

   The Ninth People's Hospital affiliated to Shanghai Jiaotong University School of Medicine has developed a successful tracheal intubation guide device, which is the first of its kind in China and has obtained a utility model patent. The device is designed for patients with difficult tracheal intubation, in which the tube is prone to slip into the esophagus. The performer first places the esophagus tracheal tube into the esophagus, then aligns the oblique opening at the front end of the tube with the glottis, inserts the light wand into the airway through the lumen of the tube and the oblique opening, and finally completes intubation under the guidance of the light wand [10, 11].

9. Complications of Endotracheal Intubation

   The process of endotracheal intubation, placement of oropharyngeal or nasopharyngeal airways and tracheal tubes can cause damage to the capillaries and soft tissue mucosa in the teeth, mouth, and nasopharyngeal cavity, resulting in complications such as post-intubation nasal bleeding, hoarseness, sore throat, and dislocation of the arytenoid cartilage. Therefore, tracheal intubation should be performed gently and without violence.

17.4.2.3 Maintenance of Anesthesia

1. Combined Intravenous and Inhalation Anesthesia

   A balanced anesthetic technique is currently advocated, whereby different anesthetic drugs and methods are used to minimize the amount of anesthetic drugs required to carry out the procedure, in order to minimize their adverse effects on the patient. Intraoperative maintenance of anesthesia is often achieved by combined intravenous and inhalation anesthesia, such as isoflurane, desflurane, sevoflurane, or nitrous oxide inhalation anesthetic drugs combined with intravenous anesthetic analgesics and nondepolarizing muscle relaxants. The purpose of using muscle relaxants is not simply to relax muscle sufficiently, but to facilitate mechanical ventilation and to enhance intraoperative respiratory management. Inhaled anesthetics have a good central muscle relaxing effect and their combination with nondepolarizing muscle relaxants can have a synergistic effect, reducing the amount of the latter. Inhalation of nitrous oxide has a good analgesic effect and reduces the amount of intraoperative narcotic analgesic.

2. Total Intravenous Anesthesia (TIVA)

   This refers to the use of a combination of intravenous anesthetics to maintain the appropriate depth of anesthesia in the patient. The most common combination of sedative-analgesic-muscarinic agents used in clinical practice is isoproterenol-fentanyl, remifentanil/sufentanil-vecuronium bromide or atracurium. The advantage of TIVA is that it avoids the adverse effects and contamination of inhaled anesthetics and is particularly suitable for patients with pulmonary disease. The main disadvantage of TIVA is that the dose and the administering time cannot be adjusted precisely. Target controlled infusion (TCI) is a drug infusion system for the precise administration of TIVA in which a microcomputer processor can adjust the drug infusion rate in real time according to the patient's age, weight, and the set target drug concentration in the target effect site (plasma or effect compartment).

17.4.3 Perioperative Monitoring and Management

17.4.3.1 Respiratory Monitoring and Management

As the patient's head is occupied by the operator and sterile towel during surgery, and the head position is often changed during surgery, and the anesthetist can only operate from a distance, the tracheal tube should be closely monitored intraoperatively to avoid abnormalities such as over-deepening, folding, twisting, and dislodging of the breathing loop. After completion of tracheal intubation, the appropriate anesthetic drug should be selected for intraoperative maintenance according to individual circumstances. Gas flow, tidal volume, respiratory rate, and respiratory ratio should be accurately set and the upper and lower airway pressure alarm limits should be adjusted before mechanical ventilation is administered. Continuously monitor the patient's pulse oximetry, partial pressure of end-expiratory carbon dioxide, and the concentration of all types of inhaled gases, and closely observe the color of the patient's skin mucosa and the oozing blood from the wound. For prolonged major surgery, arterial blood gases should be reviewed regularly to avoid disturbances in the patient's internal environment due to hypoxia, carbon dioxide accumulation, and imbalance in acid-base balance.

17.4.3.2 Circulatory Function Monitoring

1. Electrocardiogram (ECG) Monitoring

   It is a routine monitoring program for clinical anesthesia, reflecting the presence of arrhythmias and myocardial ischemia in patients and providing a basis for treatment and management.
2. Ambulatory Blood Pressure Monitoring (ABPM)

   Blood pressure reflects the patient's cardiac contractility, peripheral vascular resistance, blood volume, and perfusion of the organs. Controlled hypotension is often required during orthognathic surgery and invasive blood pressure monitoring should be performed in order to obtain timely and accurate ambulatory blood pressure. The radial or dorsalis pedis artery is often used for invasive arterial pressure monitoring in patients undergoing orthognathic surgery.
3. Central Venous Pressure (CVP) Monitoring

   The normal value of central venous pressure is 5–12 cmH_2O (0.5–1.2 kPa), which reflects the heart's ability to pump out the venous return and indicates the adequacy of venous return [12]. The main puncture routes for the central veins include the internal jugular, femoral, and subclavian veins. For orthognathic surgery patients, the femoral vein is chosen because the head, face, and neck are sterile areas for surgery.
4. Urinary Output Monitoring

   It may reflect the perfusion of organs and tissues. If the duration of surgery is estimated to be shorter than 4 h, no preoperative urethral catheterization is required. However, when the operation is estimated to be longer and a lot of bleeding would be caused, a catheter should be placed to prevent urinary retention and bladder distention. Urinary output monitoring reflects the patient's circulating capacity and renal perfusion and the intraoperative urinary output should be less than 0.5 ~ 1 mL/kg/h [13].

17.4.3.3 Temperature Monitoring

Prolonged perioperative exposure, massive infusion of replacement fluids, and suppression of the patient's thermoregulatory capacity by anesthetic drugs can lead to changes in body temperature. Perioperative hypothermia could cause delayed awakening and increase the risk of postoperative complications. Therefore, body temperature should be one of the parameters routinely monitored intraoperatively, especially for those who have long surgery duration. Nasopharyngeal, rectal, or esophageal temperatures are usually chosen to continuously monitor the patient's temperature changes for early detection of complications such as malignant hyperthermia.

17.4.3.4 Neuromuscular Monitoring and Management

It can instruct the administration of clinical medicine, maintain appropriate muscle relaxant effect to facilitate surgery, particularly fine surgical operations. Muscle relaxant monitoring can provide evidence for deciding the timing of reversal of muscle relaxants and the dose of antagonists, preventing residual risk of muscle relaxants and identifying the cause of postoperative respiratory depression. A reliable method of perioperative evaluation of neuromuscular conduction is to stimulate the motor nerve with a peripheral nerve stimulator and determine the mechanical or electromyographic effects of the muscle contraction to determine the nature and extent of the neuromuscular block. Commonly monitored sites include the ulnar nerve, median nerve, peroneal nerve, and facial nerve.

17.4.3.5 Anesthesia Depth Monitoring

While administrating general anesthesia, it is essential to maintain the appropriate depth of anesthesia. If it is too deep, it may cause neurological sequelae to patients or even threaten their lives. If it is too light, it may inhibit noxious stimulation, causing pain or body movements, or even triggering intraoperative awareness. In the past, the depth of anesthesia was judged according to the patient's physical signs, such as respiration, heart rate, blood pressure, tears, and body movements. At present, commonly used methods to monitor the patient's consciousness are: bispectral index (BIS), entropy index, auditory evoked potential (AEP), etc.

17.4.4 Estimation of Intraoperative Blood Loss and Blood Conservation

The most common complication of orthognathic surgery in the perioperative period is intraoperative hemorrhage due to the deep and complex anatomy of the area, the various types of maxillary Le Fort osteotomy, and the mandibular ascending branch. As there are no venous valves in the maxillofacial vasculature, intraoperative hemorrhage is likely to occur and cannot be easily stopped. The arteries of the maxillofacial region can be injured, resulting in acute hemorrhage in a short period of time, and the blood volume should be replenished in time to ensure perfusion of the tissues and organs.

1. Estimation of Intraoperative Blood Loss

   Blood volume is 5%–8% of a normal person's body weight. When blood loss is greater than 20% of blood volume, it may cause decompensation and trigger hypovolemic shock. The anesthetist can estimate blood loss by observing the amount of blood lost from the trauma and the degree of blood soaked in the dressing, etc. to develop a volumetric treatment plan and to control the timing and amount of blood transfusion. The formula for calculating blood loss is as follows:

   Calculated estimated blood loss = (Predelivery HCT − postdelivery HCT)/predelivery HCT × weight(g) × 7% [14].
2. Ways to Reduce Intraoperative Blood Transfusion

   Using anesthetic techniques appropriately and manipulating the anesthetic depth; infiltration of wounds with local anesthetic containing vasoconstrictors; using coagulants appropriately; and rational use of plasma substitutes.

   The more commonly used artificial colloids in clinical practice include succinylated gelatin, dextran, and hydroxyethyl starch.
3. Acute Hemodilution

   This refers to the use of colloids or crystalloids solution to dilute the blood after induction of anesthesia and before surgery, to make the red blood cells loss remain at minimum level for the same amount of bleeding.
4. Using controlled hypotension techniques to reduce intraoperative bleeding and the need for blood transfusions.

17.4.5 Controlled Hypotension

Controlled hypotension is the technique of "using physiological or pharmacological methods to reduce systemic perfusion pressure to 80–90 mmHg systolic pressure or 50–65 mmHg mean arterial pressure to avoid ischemic and hypoxic damage to vital organs, and to allow blood pressure to return to normal level rapidly after termination of hypotension [15]." The main objectives of controlled hypotension include reducing intraoperative bleeding and keeping the surgical field clean, which enables the operator to observe vital tissue structures clearly and quickly.

1. Indications, contraindications, and complications of controlled hypotensive techniques
   (a) Indications

   (1) The bleeding is severe and hard to stop under normal pressure anesthesia, even interrupting the surgery; (2) massive blood transfusion is a contraindication; (3) the patient refuses blood transfusion for some reason.

   (b) Contraindications

   Insufficient cardiovascular blood supply, myocardial ischemia, renal disease, anemia, and hypovolemia are absolute contraindications and inexperience of the anesthetist is a relative contraindication.

   (c) Complications

   (1) Cerebral thrombosis and cerebral hypoxia; (2) inadequate coronary artery

supply, embolism, heart failure, cardiac arrest; (3) renal insufficiency; (4) persistent hypotension; (5) vascular embolism; (6) reactive hemorrhage; (7) respiratory dysfunction; (8) post-emergence mental disorder, delayed emergence, blurred vision, etc.

2. Considerations for Controlled Hypotension

   An indicator for safe controlled hypotension is a pressure that guarantees the perfusion of all organs. The level of hypotension should be adjusted flexibly according to specific situations. When the bleeding is significantly reduced in the surgical field, the blood pressure should not be lowered anymore. If the mean pressure needs to be lowered to 50 ~ 60 mmHg (6.7 kPa ~ 8 kPa) in the operation, the duration should not exceed 30 min.

3. Controlled Hypotension Techniques
   (a) Physiological techniques include physiological methods such as changing body position, heart rate and blood volume in the body circulation, and the hemodynamic effects of mechanical ventilation, in conjunction with antihypertensive drugs to bring blood pressure down to the required level.
   (b) Pharmacological techniques include combined administration of anesthetic drugs, sympathetic nerve blockers, or vascular smooth muscle relaxants. Antihypertensive drugs commonly used in orthognathic surgery are: inhalational anesthetics; intravenous antihypertensive drugs (including sodium nitroprusside, adenosine triphosphate (ATP), nitroglycerin, labetalol, esmolol, Urapidil Hydrochloride, nicardipine, etc) [16].

4. Monitoring of Controlled Hypotension

   Controlled hypotension is part of anesthetic management. Ambulatory blood pressure should be monitored continuously during controlled hypotension, while blood gas analysis should be monitored intermittently. Intensive ECG monitoring and monitoring of ST segment can help to detect inadequate myocardial perfusion due to abnormal hypotension. In addition, it is important to observe skin color and bleeding in the surgical field where there should be a minimal oozing of blood.

17.4.6 Post-Anesthesia Care Unit (PACU)

Before the patient is transferred to the PACU after surgery, the anesthetists should make sure that the patient has recovered spontaneous breathing or is adequately oxygenated with assisted ventilation and the hemodynamics is stable. During the transfer, the patient should be monitored by a portable monitor and provided with oxygenation.

Upon arrival in the PACU, the patient's airway, vital signs, and oxygenation should be quickly confirmed; blood pressure, pulse, and respiratory rate should be monitored intermittently every 5 min; pulse oxygen saturation should be continuously monitored and the recovery of neuromuscular function should be assessed. Removal of the tracheal tube can only be considered when the patient is awake, muscle strength restores, reflexes are active, hemodynamics are stable, and there is no significant hematoma or active bleeding in the intraoral wound. If the floor of the mouth and perimandibular soft tissues swell evidently, tracheal tube should be left in place until the tissue edema subsides. For patients who have difficulty with intubation or mask ventilation, extubation should be conducted carefully, to prevent airway crisis after extubation and reintubation.

17.4.7 Anesthetic Complications

1. Respiratory Complications

   Generally, 72 h after orthognathic surgery is a period embracing high incidence of complications, particularly on the day after surgery. Complications related to anesthesia are most likely to be respiratory system problems, which can progress rapidly and become life-threatening if not treated timely [17]. Therefore, patients' airway management after surgery is extremely important.

   Postoperative airway obstruction after orthognathic surgery is commonly caused by: (1) glossoptosis before recovery from anesthesia; (2) significant obstruction of the airway by bleeding from the wound, blood clots, secretions, or foreign bodies left in the mouth; (3) edema of the nasal cavity, maxillary sinus, larynx, and tracheal mucosa caused by tracheal intubation or maxillary operations; (4) hematoma of the perimandibular soft tissues or mouth floor, elevation of the tongue and glossoptosis caused by genioplasty, resulting in airway obstruction; (5) the displacement of the maxilla and mandible narrows the nasal and oral cavity and removes the tongue, leading to ventilatory disorder; (6) patients have difficulty opening their mouths due to entanglement of the jaw and neck with dressings, intermaxillary ligation, and temporomandibular joint dysfunction, which significantly increases the risk of postoperative airway obstruction [18]. Therefore, it is important to strictly control the indications for extubation in orthognathic surgery patients, to closely monitor the patient after extubation, and to reintubate or perform a tracheotomy immediately if any airway abnormality is detected.

2. Unstable Circulatory Function

   Patients' circulatory function may be unstable during surgery. Hypotension may lead to inadequate perfusion to vital organs; thus, once identified, its etiology should be actively sought and promptly treated. Patients with high blood pressure before surgery are more likely to have elevated arterial blood pressure in the perioperative period than normal patients. In patients with postoperative hypertension, the first thing is to eliminate the cause and give appropriate sedative and analgesic medication and, if necessary, appropriate vasodilators.

3. Delayed Emergence

   After the cessation of administering anesthetic drugs for general anesthesia (including inhalation, total intravenous, and combined anesthesia), the patient generally wakes up within 60–90 min, and recovers orientation, reaction to commands, and preoperative memory. In addition to the patient's own physiological and pathological state, the emergence time is also related to the types, doses, and effects of drugs administered during anesthesia induction and maintenance. If the patient's emergence is delayed, anesthetists should continue the life support while seeking the causes and remedying them [19].

4. Postoperative Agitation

   Some patients' emotions may change significantly during recovery from general anesthesia, mainly taking the form of uncontrollable agitation. In addition to preoperative and intraoperative medication, postoperative agitation may also relate to postoperative hypoxemia, hypercapnia, pain, urinary retention, and flatulence. Therefore, these potential factors should be excluded clinically.

5. Postoperative Vomiting

   Postoperative vomiting is the most common clinical complication of anesthesia. Postoperative vomiting can be caused by anesthetic drugs, pain, anxiety, and overfilling of the bladder, which can damage and contaminate the repaired tissues of the maxillofacial region, and cause regurgitation and aspiration, leading to airway obstruction. Therefore, after surgery, the patient can be suctioned with an indwelling gastric tube and treated with drugs such as haloperidol and 5-hydroxytryptamine receptor antagonists.

6. Hypothermia

   Perioperative hypothermia may be associated with low temperature in the operating room, massive blood loss, and fluid transfusion. It may cause delayed emergence from anesthesia, prolonged bleeding time, vasoconstriction, and shivering. Patients with hypothermia should be oxygenated and infused fluids that have been warmed.

7. Cerebrovascular Accident

   Normally, clinicians would take actions when delayed emergence, conscious disturbance, or special signs triggered by dysfunction in the relevant areas appeared. Patients with cerebrovascular disease history are prone to develop perioperative stroke. In the event of a cerebrovascular accident, it is important to maintain a patent airway and hemodynamic stability, consult a specialist, and manage the situation together.

8. Malignant Hyperthermia

   Malignant hyperthermia is a rare genetic skeletal muscle dysfunction disease that is commonly seen in children and young adults. It is caused by uncontrollable increases in calcium levels of intracellular myocytes due to sarcoplasmic reticulum dysfunction. It is often manifested clinically by elevated body temperature, tachypnea, tachycardia, arrhythmia, cyanosis, skeletal muscle rigidity, and hematuria. With the exception of nitrous oxide, all inhaled anesthetics and suxamethonium, a depolarizing muscle relaxant, are potential triggers of malignant hyperthermia. The only test currently available to diagnose malignant hyperthermia is an abnormal contracture response of muscle specimens to halothane and caffeine. For susceptible population, inhalational anesthetics (other than nitrous oxide) and suxamethonium must be contraindicated; nitrous oxide, narcotic analgesics, barbiturates, and nondepolarizing muscle relaxants can be used clinically [20].

References

1. Giannini L, Galbiati G, Cressoni P, Esposito L. Bad oral habits: a review of the literature. J Biol Regul Homeost Agents. 2021;35(1):403–6. https://doi.org/10.23812/20-577-L.
2. Grippaudo C, Paolantonio EG, Antonini G, Saulle R, La Torre G, Deli R. Association between oral habits, mouth breathing and malocclusion. Acta Otorhinolaryngol Ital. 2016;36(5):386–94. PMID: 27958599; PMCID: PMC5225794. https://doi.org/10.14639/0392-100X-770.
3. Thongrong C, Sriraj W, Rojanapithayakorn N, et al. Cleft lip cleft palate and craniofacial deformities care: an Anesthesiologist's perspective at the Tawanchai Center. J Med Assoc Thai. 2015;98(Suppl 7):S33–7.
4. Goloborodko E, Foldenauer AC, Ayoub N, et al. Perioperative safety and complications in treatment of oral and maxillofacial surgery patients under general anesthesia with obstructive sleeping disorders. J Craniomaxillofac Surg. 2018;46(9):1609–15.
5. Kheterpal S, Healy D, Aziz MF, Shanks AM, et al. Multicenter perioperative outcomes group (MPOG) perioperative clinical research committee. Incidence, predictors, and outcome of difficult mask ventilation combined with difficult laryngoscopy: a report from the multicenter perioperative outcomes group. Anesthesiology. 2013;119(6):1360–9.
6. Langeron O, Masso E, Huraux C, Guggiari M, Bianchi A, Coriat P, Riou B. Prediction of difficult mask ventilation. Anesthesiology. 2000;92(5):1229–36. https://doi.org/10.1097/00000542-200005000-00009.
7. Harjai M, Alam S, Bhaskar P. Clinical relevance of Mallampati grading in predicting difficult intubation in the era of various new clinical predictors. Cureus. 2021;13(7):e16396. https://doi.org/10.7759/cureus.16396.
8. Hu R, Liu JX, Jiang H. Dexmedetomidine versus remifentanil sedation during awake fiberoptic nasotracheal intubation: a double-blinded randomized controlled trial. J Anesth. 2013;27(2):211–7.
9. Ahmed RA, Boyer TJ. Endotracheal tube. In: StatPearls [Internet]. Treasure Island, FL: StatPearls; 2022. https://www.ncbi.nlm.nih.gov/books/NBK539747/. Accessed 2 May 2022.
10. Wuhua M, Xiaoming D, Mingzhang Z, Ming T, Zhen H, Juan L, Jie Y, Xue G, Hongguang B. Guidelines for difficult airway management. Beijing: Chinese Society of Anesthesiology, Chinese Medical Association; 2017.
11. Sun Y, Liu JX, Zhu YS, Xu H, Huang Y, Jiang H. Nasotracheal intubation using the blind intubation device in anaesthetised adults with Mallampati class 3: a comparison with the Macintosh laryngoscope. Eur J Anaesthesiol. 2011;28(11):774–80.
12. Shah P, Louis MA. Physiology, central venous pressure. In: StatPearls [Internet]. Treasure Island, FL: StatPearls; 2022. https://www.ncbi.nlm.nih.gov/books/NBK519493/. Accessed 14 Sep 2021.
13. Klein SJ, Lehner GF, Forni LG, Joannidis M. Oliguria in critically ill patients: a narrative review. J Nephrol. 2018;31(6):855–62. https://doi.org/10.1007/s40620-018-0539-6.
14. Conner SN, Tuuli MG, Colvin R, Shanks AL, Macones GA, Cahill AG. Accuracy of estimated blood loss in predicting need for transfusion after delivery. Am J Perinatol. 2015;32(13):1225–30. https://doi.org/10.1055/s-0035-1552940.
15. Weiliu Q. Theory and practice of oral and maxillofacial surgery. Beijing: People's Medical Publishing House; 1998.
16. Shen G, Bing F. Orthognathic surgery. Hangzhou: Zhejiang Science and Technology Publishing House; 2012.
17. Steel BJ, Cope MR. Unusual and rare complications of orthognathic surgery: a literature review. J Oral Maxillofac Surg. 2012;70(7):1678–91.
18. Apfelbaum JL, Hagberg CA, Caplan RA, et al. Practice guidelines for management of the difficult airway: an updated report by the American Society of Anesthesiologists Task Force on Management of the Difficult Airway. Anesthesiology. 2013;118(2):251–70.
19. Cook TM, Woodall N, Harper J, et al. Major complications of airway management in the UK: results of the fourth National Audit Project of the Royal College of anaesthetists and the difficult airway society. Part 2: intensive care and emergency departments. Br J Anaesth. 2011;106(5):632–42.
20. Fang S, Xu H, Zhu Y, Jiang H. Continuous veno-venous hemofiltration for massive rhabdomyolysis after malignant hyperthermia: report of 2 cases. Anesth Prog. 2013;60(1):21–4.

18 Anesthesia for Nasal and Antral Surgery

Jingjie Li

18.1 Introduction

Surgical procedures involving the nasal cavity and the antral cavity are both commonly performed. Septoplasty and rhinoplasty are conducted as outpatient procedures, often at a freestanding hospital. The septoplasty procedure may be performed to relieve nasal obstruction or accompany rhinoplasty surgery to alter the appearance of the nose. Rhinoplasty, on the other hand, is performed cosmetically or for reconstructive purposes. Functional endoscopic sinus surgery (FESS) is the most used phrase for antral surgery, or sinus surgery. In the early years of nasal endoscopy, it was mostly used for diagnostic purposes. A minimal amount of trauma was involved in providing appropriate airway drainage and aeration. The increasing development of surgical procedures over the last few decades has led to an expanding range of options.

J. Li (✉)
Department of Anesthesiology, Shanghai Ninth People's Hospital Affiliated to Shanghai Jiao Tong University School of Medicine, Shanghai, China
e-mail: chenx1853@sh9hospital.org.cn

18.2 Anatomy

18.2.1 Nose

18.2.1.1 Skeletal Structure

The skeleton structure of the external nose consists of both bony and cartilaginous components. The bony component locates superiorly and is comprised of contributions from the nasal bones, maxillary bone, and frontal bone while the cartilaginous component locates inferiorly and is comprised of the two lateral cartilages, two alar cartilages and one septal cartilage. There are also smaller alar cartilages present.

While the skin over the bony part of the nose is thin, that overlying the cartilaginous part is thicker and carries many sebaceous glands. Skin overlying the cartilaginous components extends into the vestibule of the nose via the nares, where there are hairs that function to filter air as it enters the respiratory system.

18.2.1.2 Muscles

There are numerous small muscles inserting into the external nose and contributing to facial expression, which are all innervated by branches of the cerebral nerve VII, also known as the facial nerve.

The procerus muscle originates in the fascia overlying the nasal bone and lateral nasal cartilage and inserts into the inferior forehead. Its

H. Jiang, M. Xia (eds.), *Anesthesia for Oral and Maxillofacial Surgery*,
https://doi.org/10.1007/978-981-19-7287-4_18

contraction can depress the medial eyebrows and can wrinkle the skin of the superior dorsum.

The transverse portion of the nasalis muscle assists the procerus muscle in this action. In addition, the alar part of nasalis arises from the maxilla and inserts into the major alar cartilage. This allows the muscle to dilate the nares.

18.2.1.3 Vessels and Lymphatics

The external nasal vein converges into the internal and external jugular veins mainly through the internal canthal vein and the facial vein. Since the internal canthal vein connects to the intracranial cavernous sinus from the superior and inferior ophthalmic veins and the facial vein has no valves, blood can flow up and down. The blood supply to the tip of the nose is limited by the anatomical features of the nose. It has been found that the blood supply to the nasal tip vessels can be divided into four types: (1) receiving blood supply from the lateral artery; (2) receiving blood supply from the dorsal nasal artery; (3) receiving blood supply from the contralateral vessels; and (4) receiving blood supply from the contralateral nasal artery. The main sources of blood supply to the nasal tip are the lateral nasal artery and the dorsal nasal artery, with a portion coming from the lateral nasal branch. The lateral nasal artery and the dorsal nasal artery are distributed at the tip of the nose in the fascial layer or thin fatty layer. This artery supports the nasal tip form through the top nasal cartilage, closer to the cartilage.

The lymphatic drainage of the nose is through superficial lymphatic vessels that accompany the facial veins. These vessels, like all lymphatic vessels in the head and neck, eventually drain into the deep lymph nodes of the neck.

18.2.1.4 Nasal Cavity Divisions

The nasal cavity is the highest part of the respiratory tract. It extends from the vestibule of the nose to the nasopharynx and has three divisions: vestibule, respiratory region, olfactory region. The vestibule is the area surrounding the anterior external opening to the nasal cavity; the respiratory region is lined by a ciliated pseudostratified epithelium, interspersed with mucus-secreting goblet cells; and the olfactory region is located at the apex of the nasal cavity, lined by olfactory cells with olfactory receptors.

18.2.1.5 Nasal Conchae

Curved shelves projecting out of the lateral walls of the nasal cavity are called conchae (or turbinates). There are three conchae—inferior, middle, and superior.

Conchae project into the nasal cavity, creating four pathways for the airflow. These pathways are called meatuses: the inferior meatus is between the inferior concha and the floor of the nasal cavity; the middle meatus is between the inferior and middle concha; the superior meatus is between the middle and superior concha, and the spheno-ethmoidal recess lies superiorly and posteriorly to the superior concha.

The conchae functions to increase the surface area of the nasal cavity, which increases the amount of inhaled air that can come into contact with the cavity walls. They also make the flow of the air slow and turbulent. The air spends longer in the nasal cavity, so that it can be humidified.

18.2.1.6 Vasculature

The nose has a very rich vascular supply, which allows it to effectively change the humidity and temperature of inhaled air. The nose receives blood from both the internal and external carotid arteries. The internal carotid arteries include the anterior ethmoidal artery and the posterior ethmoidal artery, while the external carotid arteries include the sphenopalatine artery, the greater palatine artery, the superior labial artery, and the lateral nasal arteries.

The ethmoidal arteries are a branch of the ophthalmic artery. They descend into the nasal cavity through the cribriform plate.

In addition to the rich blood supply, these arteries form anastomoses mutually, especially in the anterior portion of the nose.

The veins of the nose tend to follow the arteries. They drain into the pterygoid plexus, facial vein, or cavernous sinus.

In some people, some nasal veins are connected to the sagittal sinuses (double venous sinuses). This also means that the infection can spread from the nose to the cranial cavity, which is a potential route of infection.

18.2.1.7 Innervation

The olfactory nerve is formed by the nerve fibers of the olfactory cells in the mucosa of the nasal cavity and reaches the olfactory bulb through the sieve plate. The olfactory nerve is surrounded by a tubular sheath, which is connected to the dura mater.

The sensory nerves mainly come from the first branch of the trigeminal nerve (ophthalmic nerve) and the branches of the second branch (maxillary nerve).

The ophthalmic nerve divides into the anterior septal nerve via the nasociliary nerve, which is distributed in the anterior part of the nasal septum and lateral wall of the nasal cavity.

The maxillary nerve forms the pterygopalatine ganglion in the pterygopalatine fossa and divides into the posterior superior nerve, which is distributed in the nasal cavity and sinuses above the middle turbinate, and the posterior inferior nerve, which is distributed in the nasal cavity below the middle nasal passage.

The maxillary nerve also divides into the posterior branch of the superior alveolar nerve, which is distributed in the maxillary sinus and alveolus, and the inferior orbital nerve, which is distributed in the nasal vestibule, nasal floor, and anterior part of the inferior nasal passage.

The vegetative nerves include sympathetic and parasympathetic nerves.

Sympathetic nerve fibers cause vasoconstriction of the nasal mucosa and decrease secretion by the deep rock nerve from the sympathetic plexus of the internal carotid artery, the pterygopalatine nerve, and the pterygopalatine ganglion distributed in the blood vessels and secretory glands in the nasal cavity.

Parasympathetic nerve fibers cause vasodilation of nasal mucosa and increase secretion, which are distributed to the nasal cavity by the large superficial rock nerve and pterygopalatine nerve from the facial nerve to the pterygopalatine ganglion, and then the postganglionic fibers.

18.2.2 Sinus

The human skull has four pairs of sinuses. They are air-filled cavities adjacent to the nasal region and collectively may be referred to as the paranasal sinuses. The four sinuses are: the frontal sinus, the sphenoidal sinus, the ethmoidal sinus, and the maxillary sinus (also referred to as the antrum of Highmore or maxillary antrum).

The following picture illustrates the anatomical position of the sinuses. The maxillary sinus is a large pyramidal chamber within the maxillary bone and is lined with respiratory epithelium. Its function is uncertain, but it has been suggested that it moistens inhaled air, lightens the skull, and possibly provides vocal resonance. The terms maxillary sinus and antrum of Highmore are used synonymously, while maxillary sinus is the preferred terminology.

The anatomical locations of the above four sinuses are shown in Fig. 18.1.

The maxillary sinus is also known as the antrum of Highmore, but is more commonly referred to as the maxillary sinus. The maxillary sinus is located within the maxilla and is covered with a layer of respiratory epithelium. Its function is unclear; it is thought to moisten inhaled air, reduce the weight of the skull, and possibly provide vocal cord resonance.

The maxillary sinus has a pyramidal shape, with its base on the palate, three sides (lateral nasal wall, posterior antral wall, and anterior maxillary wall), and its apex laterally in the zygomatic process. The roof of the sinus forms part of the floor of the orbit and is therefore related to the infraorbital vessels and nerves. The base of the sinus can project between the roots of the maxillary premolar and molar teeth. The sinus is separated from the nasal cavity by a thin wall of bone/cartilage medially, and it drains through ciliary action into the nose high on the lateral wall through an ostium in the middle meatus. The height of this ostium means that sinus drainage is poor in the presence of inflammation or after the surgical intervention. Traditionally, increasing the size of this ostium was a routine part of ENT (ears, nose, and throat) surgery to improve drainage from the maxillary sinus. However, this

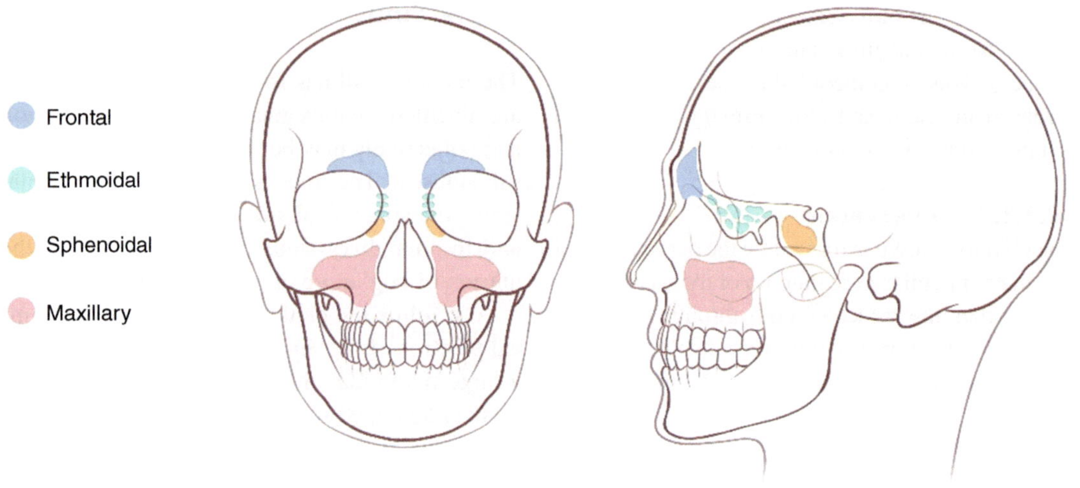

Fig. 18.1 The anatomical position of the sinuses

causes damage to the ciliary motion, thus compromising natural sinus drainage. The development of minimal access surgery (functional endoscopic nasal surgery) largely avoids the need for invasive surgery [1].

The maxillary sinus is the largest of the four sinuses, with an average volume of 13 ml and five walls. Its anterior wall is called canine fossa, and it is central thin and concave fossa; above the fossa and 12 mm below the infraorbital rim is the infraorbital foramen, through which the infraorbital nerve and blood vessels pass. Its posterior outer wall is adjacent to the pterygopalatine fossa and the inferior fossa of the hazel; the maxillary artery can be ligated through this foramen. Its medial wall is the lower part of the lateral wall of the nasal cavity. In the posterior part of the middle nasal passage, there is a fissure named "maxillary hiatus," the lower boundary of which is the attachment of inferior turbinate, the posterior boundary is the vertical plate of palatine bone, the anterior boundary is the lacrimal process of inferior turbinate and lower end of lacrimal bone, and the upper boundary is the parietal wall of maxillary sinus connected with sieve sinus. This bony sinus opening is separated into four quadrants by a cross-shaped connection of the hooked process and the septal process of the inferior turbinate, of which only the anterior superior quadrant is the true natural sinus opening of the maxillary sinus. The natural maxillary sinus opening varies in size, averaging 2.8 mm, and is not easily visible on routine anterior rhinoscopy. Its superior wall is the floor wall of the orbit, so maxillary sinus disease and intraorbital disease can interact with each other. Its basal wall is the alveolar process. The basal wall is often lower than the nasal floor and is closely related to the second bicuspid and the first and second molars, so root infection can sometimes cause odontogenic maxillary sinusitis.

When there is infection, blockage of the lacrimal duct and occlusion of the maxillary antral space may cause epiphora (excessive tear formation), decreased ocular movement, and/or exophthalmos. The proximity of the infraorbital nerve and superior alveolar nerves results in pain, which can be quite severe. However, if there is direct nerve injury due to trauma or neoplasia there may be anesthesia, altered sensation, and/or pain. Pain in the region of the maxillary sinus may be due to a number of causes including sinusitis, tumor, myofascial pain, trigeminal neuralgia, atypical facial pain, or periodic migrainous neuralgia [1].

Increasing pneumatization with age concomitant with any alveolar ridge resorption due to loss of teeth may result in little bone between the dental alveolus and the base of the maxillary antrum.

The ethmoid sinus, also known as the ethmoid labyrinth, is the anatomical structure with the most complex anatomical relationships, the most variation in itself, and the closest connection to adjacent organs of the four groups of sinuses. The septal sinus airspaces vary from 4–17 to 18–30 depending on their degree of development. The septal sinuses are divided by the middle turbinate substrate into an anterior group of septal sinuses, which open into the middle nasal tract, and a posterior group of septal sinuses, which open into the upper nasal tract.

The sphenoid sinus resides within the pterygoid bone, and the size and morphology of the two sinus cavities differ due to differences in the location of the septum and the development of the pterygoid sinus itself. It is located in the posterior, inner and lower part of the posterior septal sinus. There is no uniform classification standard.

Hammer [2] classifies the pterygoid sinus into three types, i.e., mesenteric (3%), presaddle (11%), and saddle (86%). The posterior border of the sinus cavity is in line with the vertical line of the saddle node (anterior to the saddle), and there is still thick bone between the posterior border of the sinus cavity and the vertical line of the saddle node (anterior to the saddle); the anterior saddle sinus has better gasification and development than the A-type, but not as good as the saddle type. The entire base of the pterygoid saddle is separated from the pterygoid sinus by a thin bone plate. The walls of the pterygoid sinus, especially the lateral, superior, and posterior walls, have complex adjoining relationships and are the most dangerous areas for conventional sinus surgery and endoscopic sinus surgery.

18.3 Nasal Surgery and Anesthesia

18.3.1 Types of Nasal Surgery

Turbinoplasty and septoplasty are the two most common nasal procedures.

Turbinoplasty is indicated for hyperplasia of the inferior turbinate and is chosen when other treatments are ineffective. Excessive removal of the inferior turbinate is contraindicated in order to prevent the nasal cavity from becoming too wide and forming atrophic rhinitis, causing crusting and odor in the nasal cavity and increasing the patient's pain. If ventilation is still poor after healing, reoperation may be considered. Occasionally it is necessary to perform sinus surgery and rhinoplasty together with colleagues from rhinology or facial plastic surgery.

Septoplasty is mainly used for deviated septum, which can cause nasal congestion, headache, and affect the sinus openings when septoplasty is required. The septoplasty is usually performed under general anesthesia. The cartilage is then incised slightly backward 1 cm from the original incision, separated with a stripper to the contralateral lesion, and the cartilage and bony parts of the lesion are trimmed with scissors until there is no deviation, and the cartilage membrane of the bilateral septum is repositioned. Check for perforation and hematoma, etc. The expansion sponge is filled with bilateral nasal cavities and saline is injected into the expansion sponge and the procedure is finished after expansion.

There are also rhinoplasties for cosmetic purposes. Rhinoplasty can reduce or increase the size of the nose, reduce the nostrils, change the angle between the nose and the upper lip, etc. Sometimes it can also correct some breathing problems.

18.3.2 Anesthesia for Different Types of Nasal Surgery

18.3.2.1 Turbinate Reduction Surgery

Turbinate reduction surgery is a surgical procedure for enlarged turbinates. Enlarged turbinates are usually the result of edema caused by inflammation of the internal nasal tissues, and patients usually experience clinical symptoms such as poor breathing and decreased oxygen levels in the body. If the symptoms are mild, the patient can be treated with medications that improve congestion. If the condition is severe, patients may be treated with ionic ablation to reduce the internal volume of the nose and improve ventilation, while generally causing less damage to the nose.

Enlarged turbinates can cause chronic nasal congestion that interferes with normal nasal breathing, thus forcing patients to breathe through their mouths and having an impact on their daily activities. Also, headaches and sleep disorders such as snoring and obstructive sleep apnea may occur because the nasal airway, the normal pathway for breathing during sleep, is affected. Turbinate reduction surgery is usually performed in conjunction with septal surgery.

Routine practice of turbinate reduction surgery is the injection of local anesthetics. The pain is tolerable in such applications, although it is noted that the septal contact of instruments such as the nasal speculum and aspirator entering the nasal passage during the procedure discomforts patients and reduces their tolerance. The idea of a further local anesthetic injection to the nasal septum is also abandoned due to the possibility of reduced patient cooperation. A pledget containing a mixture of lidocaine and prilocaine would be more effective, and so adopted such an approach.

1. Premedication

   Premedication for turbinate reduction surgery could be to prevent nausea, reduce stomach acid, or help the patient to relax if the patient seems to be anxious.
2. Local Anesthesia

   In turbinate reduction surgery, local anesthetics are usually applied to the inside of the nostrils. The most commonly used local anesthetic is Lidocaine, which is usually injected. Recently, the eutectic mixture local anesthetics (EMLA) cream is also introduced to perform surface anesthesia.

   Clinical practice now routinely employs EMLA cream. It contains 25 mg lidocaine and 25 mg prilocaine in 1 g. Skin and mucosa can be anesthetized effectively and safely with this solution. After applying EMLA cream to the skin, the cream starts to work within 2 h. Through mucosal surfaces, it absorbs faster, but loses its effect sooner. When applied to mucous membranes, it produces a strong analgesic effect within 15 min. Most common side effects of the cream are edema, redness, and temporary paleness, which are rare but mild. Methemoglobinemia can occur in newborns if the cream is used. A clinical test has been conducted on its application to the nasal mucosa, and no serious side effects have been reported. It was found that neither the cream nor the injection had any significant side effects [3–5].

   The intraoral and intranasal application of EMLA cream has been studied in several clinical papers. During the functional turbinate operations with a neodymium-doped yttrium aluminum garnet (Nd:YAG) laser, Di Carlo reported analgesic effects of the cream on nasal mucosa within 15 min before the procedure [6]. It was shown in a study by Joki-Erkkilä et al. [7] that EMLA had a faster effect during maxillary sinus puncture when compared with cotton-tip applicators moistened with lidocaine-adrenalin solution. Many patients reported success with the cream after just 5 min, according to the authors. The EMLA cream was less painful than local anesthetic injections for nasal fracture reductions.

   In a study with radiofrequency turbinate tissue reduction using cream anesthetics and lidocaine, Martellucci et al. reported that choking and pain (visual analogue scale) VAS scores were not significantly different. Furthermore, it may enhance both the surgeon's and patient's comfort, thereby increasing procedural success. As liquid anesthetics undergo injection, they might enter the patient's throat, and we consider that the identified difficulty swallowing and choking sensation could result from oropharyngeal and hypopharyngeal hypoesthesia occurring after the swallowing of such liquids [3, 8].

   In our experience, the effect of the cream does not interfere with the procedure overall, although drug residues within the nasal passage after the pledget is removed may pollute the optics and obstruct endoscopic vision. That said, such disadvantage can be easily eliminated through the aspiration of drug residues. Additionally, plasma concentrations of anesthetics were not measured in either of the groups, and no verification could be made of the systemic absorption amount of these drugs, which may be considered as a limitation.

3. Sedation

   Sedation is often used in combination with local anesthesia. It reduces the patient's awareness of the surgery and discomfort. Sedation is usually given through an intravenous cannula.

4. General Anesthesia

   General anesthetics often cause postoperative nausea and vomiting. In overweight or obese patients, risks associated with general anesthesia increase. A general anesthetic can be combined with local anesthetic into the surgical wound for pain relief after surgery.

18.3.2.2 Septoplasty and Rhinoplasty

Septoplasty and rhinoplasty are both commonly performed surgical procedures, mostly as outpatient surgeries. Septoplasty can be performed as a relief to symptoms of nasal obstruction; it can also be performed as a component of rhinoplasty, and is often combined with turbinate reduction surgery. To facilitate use of continuous positive airway pressure (CPAP), patients with obstructive sleep apnea (OSA) may undergo septoplasty. On the other hand, rhinoplasty is usually performed for cosmetic or reconstructive purposes to alter the appearance of the nose [9]. In other words, the indication for surgery may be purely cosmetic, post-trauma, reconstructive after tumor resection, or to improve nasal breathing.

1. Local Anesthesia with Sedation

   Nasal procedures can usually be performed under local anesthesia with sedation, which avoids airway instrumentation, positive pressure ventilation, and inhaled anesthetics, at the same time requires less intravenous medication administration.

   When an endotracheal tube is inserted in the wrong place, there is higher possibility of coughing, bucking, or straining, all of which bring the risk of bleeding from the surgical site. Fewer nausea and vomiting are observed with less intravenous administration of opioids and no inhaled anesthetic administration; however, local anesthesia with sedation has disadvantages including patient awareness, the possibility of patient movement, pain with inadequate block, oversedation resulting in hypoventilation, and even potential for loss of the airway [10]. This approach probably needs emergency airway management in the setting of unexpected or brisk intraoperative bleeding leading to aspiration or frank obstruction, as the airway is not secure and the patient has an altered sense of awareness, which is another risk.

   For vasoconstriction of the nasal mucosa, cocaine, phenylephrine, or oxymetazoline may be applied. Also, soaking gauze in local anesthetic and injecting submucosal local anesthetic with epinephrine may be performed to shrink the nasal mucosa and decrease intraoperative bleeding. Most commonly, the medication contains 1% lidocaine (10 mg/mL) and 1:1,00,000 or 1:2,00,000 epinephrine. Once the patient has been lightened, a short-acting anesthetic can be administered, such as propofol [11]. Rhinoplasty requires a steady flow of local anesthetic in order to avoid distortion and interfere with the assessment of cosmetic results; therefore, the amount of local anesthetic should be controlled. Sedatives can be used in conjunction with other medications; however, patients can become disoriented and uncooperative when given sedatives, so care must be taken not to oversedate them. A nasal cannula or face mask in proximity to an open oxygen delivery system with a high oxygen concentration while electrocautery is present poses a risk of surgical fire when the face is being operated on under sedation. Patients undergoing sedation should receive supplemental oxygen at the same time as several precautions to prevent a fire should be taken. An overall rule of thumb is that surgical drapes should be designed to minimize the accumulation of oxygen, flammable skin preparation solutions should be allowed to dry before drapes are applied, and gauze and sponges should be moistened prior to use in proximity to electrocautery. It may be necessary to use a sealed oxygen delivery system, such as an endotracheal tube or supraglottic airway, if the procedure requires moderate or deep sedation or if the patient displays oxygen dependence. For fire prevention, oxygen should be stopped or reduced to the minimum required before electrocautery is used. The person managing the airway should then wait a few minutes for oxygen to disperse before using electrocautery. Furthermore, medical air can be insufflated and suction can be used to scavenge the operative field of oxygen.

Perioperative time has been shown to be shorter for patients undergoing surgery under local anesthesia with sedation when compared with those under general anesthesia. There may also be less emesis, epistaxis, and nausea as well as earlier discharge times.

Local analgesia and sedation in septoplasties is a good and safe technique for ambulatory surgery, but it requires cooperation between the surgeon and the anesthesiologist.

Septoplasty under local anesthesia could be a good and safe technique for outpatient surgical care as well, but the surgeon should have a central role in the overall patient management, including the local analgesia and pain management.

Anatomy, availability of the caudal septum, as well as possibility for adequate local analgesia are the mainstay for further treatment.

The advantages of sedation under local anesthesia in an outpatient environment in adequately selected patients are a smooth postoperative course, shorter medical procedure, and shorter recovery time.

Furthermore, this procedure gives a possibility to avoid potential side effects of general anesthesia and sedation.

2. General Anesthesia

When the procedure is longer, more extensive, or when large-volume blood loss is anticipated, general anesthesia may be preferred. General anesthesia provides total patient analgesia and immobility, less patient cooperation requirement, and control of the airway by intubation or laryngeal supraglottic airway; it also reduces the risk of aspiration of secretions, blood, or irrigation fluids. However, there also exist some disadvantages, including the potential for coughing on the endotracheal tube upon emergence, more nausea and vomiting, higher doses of intravenous medications, a longer recovery, and postoperative disorientation. General anesthesia may be performed with either supraglottic airway devices or endotracheal tubes. During induction of anesthesia and mask ventilation an oral airway may be needed to alleviate the effects of the nasal obstruction if significant septal deviation is present.

Maintenance of anesthesia can be performed with volatile inhaled anesthetics, total intravenous anesthesia (TIVA), or a balanced anesthesia technique. A continuous intravenous opioid-based technique with alfentanil or remifentanil reduces the total amount of volatile anesthesia given and significantly blunts the tracheal response to the endotracheal tube. This also improves hemodynamic stability and rapid smooth emergence. Remifentanil, especially if given as a bolus, may cause a significant opioid-induced bradycardia, which may lead to decreased cardiac output and hypotension [12]. A propofol infusion decreases blood pressure and the incidence of postoperative nausea and vomiting; in addition, it is rapidly metabolized, resulting in a quicker emergence. Inhalational anesthesia can be used and also provides the advantage of decreasing blood pressure, thus lessening blood loss. During emergence, there might appear bucking or coughing on the endotracheal tube, increasing venous pressure and increasing bleeding and swelling. This should be avoided if possible.

Patients may be disorientated after general anesthesia and may attempt to rub their nose. As this can disrupt the surgical sutures the patient should be watched very carefully until they are back to their baseline mental status.

It is accepted that volatile anesthetics (compared to intravenous anesthetics) are well-established risk factors for postanesthetic agitation. In addition to the anesthesia technique, some risk factors cause emergence agitation development. Otorhinolaryngologic and ophthalmologic surgery, male sex, age, severe postoperative pain, smoking, the presence of additional diseases, and urinary catheterization are the main risk factors for emergence agitation development after extubation [13]. According to Liu's analysis [14] of 674 nasal surgery patients, the emergence agitation frequency was 23.15%, and male gender, age, inhalation anesthesia, preoperative anxiety, postoperative pain, the tracheal tube, and the presence of a urinary catheter all correlated with emergence agitation. In 80 patients undergoing nasal surgery, Jo et al. [15] compared the effects of external anesthesia combined with that of inhalation anesthesia. According to RASS, the emergence agitation frequency immediately after extubation was 20% in the inhalation group, and 2.5% in the TIVA group. In this study, there were no differences between the groups in terms of age, gender, and smoking. None of the patients underwent urinary catheterization or premedication. All patients underwent the same number of tracheal tubes and underwent the same postoperative analgesia protocols. According to our study, the emergence agitation frequency after general anesthesia was higher than the literature (35.6%). The emergence agitation frequency has not been studied in rhinoplasty patients before; therefore, we believe that emergence agitation after rhinoplasty may be more common than other nasal surgeries.

Low-flow anesthesia has many advantages in terms of decreasing atmospheric pollution, cost effects, and efficient maintenance of airway temperatures and humidification. In 1994, Baker [16] used the following classification for low-flow anesthesia: minimal flow <500 mL fresh gas flow (FGF) per minute, low-flow >0.5–1 L/min, medium flow 2–4 L/min FGF, and very high-flow >4 L/min of FGF. Stevanovic et al. [17] evaluated 60 patients who underwent laparoscopic cholecystectomy under low-flow sevoflurane anesthesia and TIVA. The frequency of postoperative agitation and nausea and vomiting were not different between groups, but extubation times and early emergence times were longer in the TIVA group.

18.4 Antral Surgery and Anesthesia

18.4.1 Surgical Considerations for Antral Surgery

Early attempts to combat sinus pathology were founded on the appreciation that healthy sinus functional states required normal ventilation and drainage of sinus secretions without obstruction due to mucosal swelling, inflammation, or other mechanical impediments. The most common type of antral surgery, functional endoscopic sinus surgery (FESS), strives to enable direct examination in situ with subsequent correction of encountered chronic changes and barriers which limit sinus drainage and ventilation. Operative goals are reduction of abnormal tissue mass, creation of effective drainage via larger sinus passages, or complete obliteration of smaller sinuses. FESS is a relatively safe surgical procedure, although the limited evidence available suggests that FESS has not been demonstrated to be superior to medical treatment in chronic rhinosinusitis.

18.4.2 Anesthetic Management

18.4.2.1 Preoperative Considerations

The issue with sinusitis and upper respiratory infection (URI) is of particular importance to the surgeries discussed here. Infection should be controlled with the appropriate antibiotics before these elective antral surgeries. Clinical opinions differ on how to best treat uncomplicated URIs; however, the majority of clinicians recommend proceeding with surgery, provided that there is no fever, severe wheezing, infected secretions, or any other sign or symptom of active infection (as in bacterial sinusitis or pneumonia) [18].

18.4.2.2 Intraoperative Management

1. Anesthetic Technique

   While many intranasal procedures can be performed without a general anesthetic with adequate patient selection, general anesthesia is increasingly being integrated into the daily surgical pattern due to the availability of anesthesiologists, the minimally adverse effects of the newer anesthetic agents, the increasing number of pediatric and elderly patients, widespread training of surgeons in fast-track general anesthesia techniques, and the increased importance placed on patient satisfaction.

2. Anesthetic Goals

   (a) Patient Immobility

   FESS requires nasal puncture, but if the patient has intraoperative somatic movements—either voluntary or involuntary—the risk of deviation increases dramatically, and nasal puncture, if deviated, can affect the surrounding cranial structures dangerously. Therefore, in order to successfully perform FESS superficially in the nasal cavity, the patient needs to be rendered immobile intraoperatively, and rendering the patient immobile is one of the early goals of FESS anesthesia. An early goal of anesthesia is to immobilize the patient in order to allow FESS to be performed superficially in the nasal cavity. Local vasoconstrictors and anesthetics combined with sedatives or general anesthetics are better able to achieve this goal.

   (b) Dryness of the Surgical Field

   After avoiding risks, the quest is for better surgical results. The operative field of FESS is very close to the airway, so in case of bleeding or secretions, the lenses of the device may be contaminated, thus affecting the visualization and accuracy of the operation and prolonging the operative time [19]. Also, a study related to the reduction of surgical estimated blood loss (EBL) and the use of various anesthetic techniques to increase surgical visualization showed that the amount of blood loss during FESS, but perhaps not much in terms of volume, can cause difficulties in practice, leading to delays in treatment and compromising surgical outcomes.

   (c) Rapid and Smooth Postoperative Discharge

   The awakening after general anesthesia may be accompanied by various problems, commonly such as coughing, postoperative nausea and vomiting, and bleeding. Today, FESS can be performed under outpatient conditions and commonly uses the supraglottic airway (SGA) technique and fast-tracking of total intravenous anesthesia (TIVA) with the application of propofol and short-acting anesthetics. The aforementioned approach is also able to optimize the operative field, which in turn requires the combined efforts of two teams: the anesthesiologist who maintains a low heart rate and applies a combined local/injectable vasoconstrictor with local anesthetics, positioned to optimize the drainage of the surgical area, and the surgeon who performs the operation with great skill [20].

3. Total Intravenous Anesthesia

   TIVA with spontaneous respiration and propofol/remifentanil may be the most effective method to avoid emergence problems, decrease nausea, vomiting, and EBL, and ensure rapid induction and emergence [21]. Numerous studies have shown that it facilitates hemodynamic conditions, reduces EBL, and optimizes surgical conditions, visibility, and efficiency. While topical and injected local vasoconstrictor are useful to minimize blood loss from the soft tissue, penetration into the ossified structures can be limited, and hemodynamic methods are more effective in reducing bleeding from resected bone. The amounts of EBL during FESS typically range from 1–200 ml of blood and are therefore relatively unimportant to patient welfare [11]. Blood in the surgical field, however, is a concern to surgeons, as it limits their visibility and extends the length of surgery. Monitoring of EEG (i.e., the bispectral index (BIS)) provides continuous TIVA drug delivery and anesthetic depth control, especially when the intravenous infusion site is not readily accessible, as when arms are tucked away from the anesthesia provider for better access to the surgeon. Even over expertly managed endotracheal intubation techniques using TIVA, inhalational anesthetics, endotracheal topical anesthesia, and deep extubation, many of the advantages (due to anesthesia alone) may be small or negligible. LTA kits can facilitate smooth extubation in short, less than 20–30 min procedures by introducing an anesthetic at induction. When still effective, topical anesthetics mitigate reflex responses during positioning, intraoperatively, and at extubation. Anesthesia provider, hospital and surgeon assessment will ultimately determine the anesthetic technique to be used, specifically in light of patient-specific considerations.

4. Supraglottic Airway Devices

   SGA devices reduce coughing during and after the procedure, especially compared to the use of endotracheal tubes (ETT). In addition, routine extubation can be performed under anesthesia with the SGA. It is also important to note that there are some contraindications for SGA, namely patients infected with cancer, those with severe obesity, and those with insufficient lower esophageal sphincters.

   To reduce the adverse effects of tracheal tubes, the SGA is often substituted for them. Although its use in properly selected patients has been documented as having no increased adverse event rates, it does not mechanically prevent fluid penetration from the lower respiratory tree. Significant gastroesophageal reflux, obesity, and hiatal hernia are among the most commonly cited exclusions for SGA.

   The SGA will normally seal the airway adequately intraoperatively while enabling controlled extubation with minimal anesthesia to avoid coughing, hypertension, or significant pulmonary bleeding from the field. As with SGAs, they are also intended for use in spontaneously breathing patients, where lower intrathoracic pressures are thought to reduce venous stasis. As long as the SGA seals the airway adequately intraoperatively, controlled extubation with minimal anesthesia is possible, so coughing, hypertension, or significant pulmonary bleeding are avoided. SGAs are also intended to reduce venous stasis in patients with spontaneous breathing, where lower intrathoracic pressures may reduce venous stasis. The larger diameter of SGAs allows for lower mean intrathoracic pressure and a greater tidal volume during air exchange, compared with ETTs. When the surgery progresses from anesthetized tissues to normally sensitive tissues after light levels of anesthesia, spontaneous respiration techniques are limited by intraoperative movement of the patient.

5. Anesthetic Emergency Techniques

   In addition to emergence, extubation is one of the challenging objectives of ESS. In order to optimize emergence, the surgeon and patient should discuss emergence plans preoperatively. In order to pack the nasal cavity postoperatively, oral breathing will be required. After being anesthetized with local anesthetics, even the most complicated neurosurgical procedures are painless. It is important to stress both facts as reassuringly as possible in preoperative communication. When SGAs are used, airways can be removed while the patient is awake without stressful coughing, hypertension, or venous congestion. Before leaving the operating room, the bleeding should be controlled carefully, and all packing and blood removed. When intubating the trachea, it is important to pay attention to the details so that emergence is maximized. An adequate spontaneous respiratory rate (at the surgical planes of anesthesia) is also necessary to avoid tracheal stimulation from oral secretions or surgical bleeding during extubation. In patients who are fasted and at minimal risk of aspiration of gastric contents, as well as those who possess a reasonable likelihood of spontaneous breathing without requiring significant supportive measures, deep extubations should be performed. When there is a surgical concern with pressure on the nose, positioning patients in a lateral and head-dependent position is useful for draining secretions from the mouth. In the event that spontaneous breathing is not maintained by the patient after the oral airway is inserted, consideration should be given to installing a possible oral airway to ensure ventilation. Furthermore, this will prevent airway obstruction caused by clenching on the ETT, as well as ETT removal. Frequently, and especially for the shortest procedures requiring intubation, the utilization of laryngotracheal anesthesia (LTA) kits during intubation to distribute 4% lidocaine into the trachea can effectively obtund cough reflexes for periods of 20–30 min and allow complete emergence without significant stimulation from the ETT, facilitating awake extubation and maintenance of a spontaneous airway patency. Topical intratracheal lidocaine can also help facilitate a smooth emergence after prolonged surgical procedures.

After surgery, there are several methods that provide effective intratracheal topical anesthesia. To allow lidocaine to diffuse into the adjacent mucosa, 4–10% lidocaine is instilled into the ETT cuff at intubation. Effectiveness is usually obtained after up to 60 min. The significant drawback of this technique is that only the tissue in contact with the cuff will be anesthetized. Furthermore, an adequate deflation of the cuff at extubation requires special attention during injection and especially withdrawal of the solution. An endotracheal tube can inject lidocaine in situ via topical administration of lidocaine. When active topical agents are administered in this manner, the patient may cough unless there is effective anesthesia and immobilization by neuromuscular blocking agents at the time of injection. With specially designed laryngotracheal instillation of topical anesthesia (LITATM) tubes (Sheridan Catheter Corp, Argyle, NY), one can administer the solution over and above the ETT cuff since they spray the solution circumferentially at both sites via an integral port. A different type of endotracheal tube (TaperGuard Evac™-Mallinckrodt™, Tyco Healthcare™, Pleasanton, CA, USA) with low suction but can still deliver above the cuff only can reduce silent aspiration by long-term intubated patients. ETTs and cuffs, however, do not require manipulation for injectate delivery. If a significant depth of anesthesia is not given, the injection of the solution itself may still trigger cough reflexes, causing movements and intrathoracic pressure changes. Furthermore, these specialty ETTs are costlier by three or four times than standard ETTs.

18.4.2.3 Sphenoidotomy

An endoscopic sphenoidotomy corrects conditions affecting the sphenoid sinus and can be performed with or without an ethmoidectomy. Sphenoid sinuses are accessed either by widening the natural ostium or by making another opening through the posterior ethmoid sinuses. It is most obvious on axial and sagittal reformatted CT images when there is widened communication between the sphenoid and ethmoid sinuses. The process of marsupialization consists of exteriorizing the affected sinus to treat chronically infected sphenoid sinuses [21].

Moreover, sphenoid drilling out is also a procedure that is used to treat chronic sinusitis and is considered a middle-ground alternative to sphenoidotomy and marsupialization. It is imperative to improve sphenoid sinus aeration, regardless of which technique is used.

18.4.2.4 Balloon Sinuplasty

It involves dilation of the paranasal ostia while minimizing mucosal damage during a minimally invasive endoscopic procedure. By blowing the inflated balloon, the bone surrounding sinus outflow is delicately displaced, microfractured, and molded. Conventional endoscopic surgery may be performed as a stand-alone procedure or in conjunction with balloon surgery. The contrast-filled balloon, which appears radiopaque under fluoroscopic guidance, can be seen in position and expanded under fluoroscopic guidance [22].

18.4.2.5 Sinonasal Debridement

It is possible to treat invasive fungal sinusitis with endoscopic sinus surgery and nasal irrigation with antifungal agents. As part of an endoscopic surgical intervention, necrotic sinonasal mucosa and bone may be removed along with fungal debris. After debridement for invasive fungal sinusitis, CT is challenging to interpret as there may be sinonasal opacification, which can make it difficult to distinguish between bleeding, irrigation fluid, and packing material [23]. A MR imaging image may be more useful in identifying fungal infections that sometimes coexist with neoplasms because of the possibility of neoplasms within the sinonasal cavity. A MR scan can also be used to assess the extent of disease in the orbits and intracranial compartments early on.

18.4.2.6 Transsphenoidal Pituitary Surgery

The transcranial approach is a common surgical method used to remove lesions found in the ventricles of the brain. The transsphenoidal sinus technique was developed in the early twentieth century, prior to which transcranial techniques were mostly used for ventricular lesions, but they were relatively more invasive and less safe. Once developed, the transsphenoidal technique was rapidly promoted. Although the transsphenoidal technique was sometimes controversial in the century that followed, the advent of modern microsurgery and endoscopic techniques has contributed to its acceptance today as a high priority technique for resection of lesions in the pterygoid sinus region.

In general, the transsphenoidal sinus technique consists of two main types: (1) the sublabial approach, which involves incising the gingiva below the upper lip and then crossing the nasal septum; and (2) the transnasal approach, which involves using microsurgical or endoscopic instruments inserted through the nostril and through the nasal wall. To manipulate CSF levels in the lumbar region, a CSF drain can be inserted in either of these methods. Through the drainage tube, saline or air may be injected into the spinal colon in order to lower the lesion into the surgical region. A lumbar drainage tube opening may assist with the reduction of postoperative CSF leakage. As a result of removing the tumor, the spine is reconstructed in order to restore its integrity. An autologous fat graft from the abdomen is usually used to fill the spine if there is CSF leakage detected by a Valsalva maneuver. In our institution, intranasal techniques are generally preferred, with sublabial approaches reserved for patients with small nostrils or for whom the transnasal approach is difficult.

The anesthetic management of patients undergoing transsphenoidal resection of pituitary tumors requires not only consideration for surgical aspects of the procedure, but also a firm understanding of the unique implications that the underlying neuroendocrine pathology may have in terms of their secondary effect on various body systems. Headache, nausea/vomiting, or visual disturbances can be observed in most patients presenting for transsphenoidal pituitary tumor resection; these are symptoms of mass effect produced by a nonfunctioning endocrine tumor. Alternatively, some patients will have some pituitary abnormality of hypo- or hypersecretion warranting a thorough evaluation by an endocrinologist prior to surgery.

Nasotracheal intubation should be avoided due to the nature of the surgical approach. For patients who are difficult to ventilate and intubate, for example, patients with acromegaly or Cushing's disease, alternative intubating techniques such as awake fiberoptic intubation may be indicated. The endotracheal tube should be secured to the left side of the mouth once the patient is intubated. Avoid tape over the upper lip to maximize operating conditions for the surgeon. The surgeon often places a throat pack to minimize drainage into the oropharynx.

Those with coexisting heart disease or hypertension that is poorly controlled may benefit from placement of a second peripheral intravenous line and invasive monitoring of blood pressure, typically via radial artery catheterization. When patients have adequate peripheral access, central venous lines are not necessary unless cardiovascular comorbidities are present.

Using phenylephrine or epinephrine and local anesthetic after intubation assists the surgeon in decreasing bleeding and optimizing surgical conditions. These agents are absorbed systemically with minimal side effects; however, they may be injected intravenously inadvertently, resulting in cardiac arrhythmias or severe hypertension. During this stage of the procedure, you should be vigilant about monitoring your EKG and blood pressure. Hypertension may be worsened using nonselective b-blockers, which cause unopposed alpha activity of epinephrine. The use of direct-acting vasodilators and/or phentolamine may be considered in these situations.

When a patient is positioned supine with the upper torso elevated, venous return helps the body to eliminate waste products. Despite the elevated angle of head in this semisitting position, the risk of venous air embolism (VAE) is not high enough to warrant placing an intracardiac air detection device such as a transesophageal echo or precordial Doppler. As per our institution's practice, Mayfield pins allow for a midline approach by the right-handed surgeon by slightly extending the patient's neck. After anesthesia is administered, a circuit is secured on the left side of the patient, anticipating that fat grafts will be harvested in the right abdominal area. It is imperative that peripheral intravenous lines, monitoring wires, and the anesthesia breathing circuit are arranged carefully prior to draping so that the patient's head can be accessed freely.

Maintaining hemodynamic stability, maximizing surgical conditions, and maintaining cerebral perfusion and oxygenation are among the goals of anesthetic management for transsphenoidal pituitary resection. Due to the close proximity of the brain tissue and neurovasculature to the surgical field, the transsphenoidal approach poses specific challenges to these goals, including increased stimulation compared to the transcranial approach. When necessary, short-acting opioids may be administered intravenously in titrations of short-acting to maintain adequate surgical conditions with inhaled volatile agents. While inhaled agents may be beneficial in some patients, they can also increase CSF pressure. Compared to inhaled gas-based techniques, total intravenous anesthesia with propofol and opioid infusions provides acceptable surgical conditions while preventing an increase in CSF pressure. We commonly administer an opioid infusion (remifentanil) along with an inhaled gas with a low solubility (sevoflurane). Remifentanil is used during surgery to prevent rapid hemodynamic instability and to allow rapid emergence. Alternative narcotic infusions that can provide clinically apparent smooth emergence from anesthesia include fentanyl infusion 2 mg/kg/h or sufentanil infusion 0.4 mg/kg/h [24].

The surgeon may use a packing to plug the nasal cavity at the end of the procedure, which is effective in stopping bleeding and preventing fluid from leaking into the oropharynx. If the patient meets the criteria for extubation, extubation should be performed immediately. Prior to extubation, the mouth should be carefully suctioned. To prevent packing displacement due to coughing, a low-dose infusion of remifentanil or an intravenous lidocaine bolus (0.5 mg/kg) may be administered immediately prior to extubation. If the patient has OSA, a transoral airway may be required [25]. Immediately after extubation, oxygen is administered through a face mask. However, it is important to note that positive pressure ventilation through the face mask should be avoided due to the presence of nasal packing. Preoperative use of 5HT-3 receptor antagonists or butyrophenones may prevent nausea/vomiting, and implementation is based on patient risk factors.

References

1. Renton T, Durham J, Hill C. Oral surgery II: Part 2. The maxillary sinus (antrum) and oral surgery. Br Dent J. 2017;223:483–93.
2. Hammer G, Radberg C. The sphenoidal sinus. An anatomical and roentgenologic study with reference to transsphenoid hypophysectomy. Acta Radiol. 1961;56:401–22.
3. Ata N. Advantages of Emla cream over lidocaine injection for radiofrequency reduction of the inferior turbinate. Am J Otolaryngol. 2021;42(3):102850. Epub 2020 Dec 17. https://doi.org/10.1016/j.amjoto.2020.102850.
4. Ata N, Bülbül T, Demirkan A. Comparison of Emla cream and lidocaine injection for local anaesthetic before radiofrequency reduction of the inferior turbinates. Br J Oral Maxillofac Surg. 2017;55(9):917–20. Epub 2017 Sep 28. https://doi.org/10.1016/j.bjoms.2017.06.010.
5. Erol O, Buyuklu F. Comparison of the efficacy of two different local anesthetics in inferior turbinate reduction. Am J Otolaryngol. 2020;41(6):102712. Epub 2020 Sep 2. https://doi.org/10.1016/j.amjoto.2020.102712.
6. Di Carlo R, Lombardo P, Modugno V, Pastore A. Eutectic Mixture of Local Anaesthetics (EMLA):

valutazione dell'efficacia analgesica nella turbinoplastica al laser Neodymio: ittrio-alluminio-granato (Nd: Yag) [Eutectic mixture of local anesthetics (EMLA): evaluation of the analgesic effectiveness during ND: YAG laser turbinoplasty]. Acta Otorhinolaryngol Ital. 2001;21(5):287–9. Italian
7. Joki-Erkkilä VP, Penttilä M, Kääriäinen J, Rautiainen M. Local anesthesia with EMLA cream for maxillary sinus puncture. Ann Otol Rhinol Laryngol. 2002;111(1):80–2. https://doi.org/10.1177/000348940211100113.
8. Martellucci S, Pagliuca G, de Vincentiis M, Greco A, Fusconi M, De Virgilio A, Rosato C, Gallo A. EMLA(®) cream as local anesthetic for radiofrequency turbinate tissue reduction. Eur Arch Otorhinolaryngol. 2014;271(10):2717–22. Epub 2014 Feb 21. https://doi.org/10.1007/s00405-014-2940-7.
9. Park CY, Hong JH, Lee JH, Lee KE, Cho HS, Lim SJ, Kwak JW, Kim KS, Kim HJ. Clinical effect of surgical correction for nasal pathology on the treatment of obstructive sleep apnea syndrome. PLoS One. 2014;9(6):e98765. https://doi.org/10.1371/journal.pone.0098765.
10. Tobias JD, Leder M. Procedural sedation: a review of sedative agents, monitoring, and management of complications. Saudi J Anaesth. 2011;5(4):395–410. https://doi.org/10.4103/1658-354X.87270.
11. Abdelmalak B, Doyle, J. (Eds.). Anesthesia for otolaryngologic surgery. Cambridge: Cambridge University Press; 2012. https://doi.org/10.1017/CBO9781139088312.
12. Vasian HN, Mărgărit S, Ionescu D, Keresztes A, Arpăşteuan B, Condruz N, Coadă C, Acalovschi I. Total Intravenous Anesthesia-Target Controlled Infusion for colorectal surgery. Remifentanil TCI vs sufentanil TCI. Roman J Anaesth Intensive Care. 2014;21(2):87–94.
13. Lee SJ, Sung TY. Emergence agitation: current knowledge and unresolved questions. Korean J Anesthesiol. 2020;73(6):471–85. https://doi.org/10.4097/kja.20097.
14. Liu GY, Chen ZQ, Zhang ZW. Comparative study of emergence agitation between isoflurane and propofol anesthesia in adults after closed reduction of distal radius fracture. Genet Mol Res. 2014;13(4):9285–91. https://doi.org/10.4238/2014.January.24.9.
15. Jo JY, Jung KW, Kim HJ, Park SU, Park H, Ku S, Choi SS. Effect of total intravenous anesthesia vs volatile induction with maintenance anesthesia on emergence agitation after nasal surgery: a randomized clinical trial. JAMA Otolaryngol Head Neck Surg. 2019;145(2):117–23. PMID: 30489620; PMCID: PMC6440219. https://doi.org/10.1001/jamaoto.2018.3097.
16. Baker AB. Back to basics—a simplified non-mathematical approach to low flow techniques in anaesthesia. Anaesth Intensive Care. 1994;22(4):394–5. https://doi.org/10.1177/0310057X9402200413.
17. Stevanovic PD, Petrova G, Miljkovic B, Scepanovic R, Perunovic R, Stojanovic D, Dobrasinovic J. Low fresh gas flow balanced anesthesia versus target controlled intravenous infusion anesthesia in laparoscopic cholecystectomy: a cost-minimization analysis. Clin Ther. 2008;30(9):1714–25. https://doi.org/10.1016/j.clinthera.2008.09.009.
18. Ah-See KW, Evans AS. Sinusitis and its management. BMJ (Clin Res Ed). 2007;334(7589):358–61. https://doi.org/10.1136/bmj.39092.679722.BE.
19. Gan EC, Alsaleh S, Manji J, Habib AR, Amanian A, Javer AR. Hemostatic effect of hot saline irrigation during functional endoscopic sinus surgery: a randomized controlled trial. Int Forum Allergy Rhinol. 2014;4(11):877–84. Epub 2014 Aug 18. https://doi.org/10.1002/alr.21376.
20. Auanet.org. Optimizing Outcomes in Urological Surgery: Pre-Operative Care for the Patient Undergoing Urologic Surgery or Procedure - American Urological Association. [online]. 2022. <https://www.auanet.org/guidelines/guidelines/optimizing-outcomes-in-urological-surgery-pre-operative-care-for-the-patient-undergoing-urologic-surgery-or-procedure>. Accessed 25 May 2022.
21. Radiology Key. Posttreatment imaging of the paranasal sinuses following endoscopic sinus surgery. [online]. 2022. https://radiologykey.com/posttreatment-imaging-of-the-paranasal-sinuses-following-endoscopic-sinus-surgery-2/. Accessed 25 May 2022.
22. Lofgren DH, Shermetaro C. Balloon sinuplasty. In: StatPearls [Internet]. Treasure Island, FL: StatPearls; 2022. https://www.ncbi.nlm.nih.gov/books/NBK546671/. Accessed 15 Dec 2021.
23. Joshi V. Imaging of paranasal sinuses, an issue of neuroimaging clinics 25–4. Philadelphia: Elsevier Health Sciences; 2015.
24. Zhang C, Huang D, Zeng W, Ma J, Li P, Jian Q, Huang J, Xie H. Effect of additional equipotent fentanyl or sufentanil administration on recovery profiles during propofol-remifentanil–based anaesthesia in patients undergoing gynaecologic laparoscopic surgery: a randomized clinical trial. BMC Anesthesiol. 2022;22:127.
25. Modica DM, Marchese D, Lorusso F, Speciale R, Saraniti C, Gallina S. Functional nasal surgery and use of CPAP in OSAS patients: our experience. Indian J Otolaryngol Head Neck Surg. 2018;70(4):559–65. Epub 2018 May 31. PMID: 30464916; PMCID: PMC6224838. https://doi.org/10.1007/s12070-018-1396-2.

19 Perianesthesia Monitoring

Ming Xia

19.1 Introduction

Monitoring is a core topic that is not limited to oral and maxillofacial surgeries—it can be said that where there is surgery, there is necessity of monitoring. Monitoring goes through the whole perioperative period. In this book, we focus on the "anesthesia" field, and therefore this chapter introduces mainly the perianesthesia monitoring, that is, monitoring in the operating room and the PACU.

19.2 Blood Pressure Monitor

Blood pressure monitoring is necessary both in the operating room and in the PACU.

Large fluctuations in blood pressure (either too high or too low) during surgery are one of the major causes of intraoperative emergencies. The causes of intraoperative hypertension are diverse and include primary hypertension, pheochromocytoma, hyperthyroidism, primary aldosteronism, coexisting disorders such as increased intracranial pressure, surgical exploration, anesthesia operations such as tracheal intubation, causing carbon dioxide accumulation, and drugs such as ketamine. Hypertension increases myocardial wall tension and decreases coronary blood flow, which results in increased demand and consumption of oxygen. In addition, acute episodes of hypotension, which are precursors to cardiac arrest, may occur after drug administration and should be given high priority. During acute hypotension, myocardial wall tone decreases, thereby reducing oxygen demand; however, coronary perfusion is reduced to a greater extent and the probability of an episode of cardiac disease rises. In addition to cardiac perfusion, brain and kidney concerns may be affected by large fluctuations in blood pressure and therefore also need to be maintained by monitoring blood pressure.

In the PACU, blood pressure is also one of the items that must be monitored, and it is an important criterion to determine whether the patient can be subsequently transferred back to the general ward/discharge from the PACU.

Continuous monitoring of blood pressure to prevent hemodynamic emergencies is most desirable; however, the most widely used method of continuous measurement, namely indwelling arterial catheters, is invasive. In the outpatient setting, the most common methods of blood pressure recording are noninvasive and intermittent, with various automated methods of measurement replacing manual methods.

M. Xia (✉)
Department of Anesthesiology, Shanghai Ninth People's Hospital Affiliated to Shanghai Jiao Tong University School of Medicine, Shanghai, China
e-mail: xiaming1980@xzhmu.edu.cn

H. Jiang, M. Xia (eds.), *Anesthesia for Oral and Maxillofacial Surgery*,
https://doi.org/10.1007/978-981-19-7287-4_19

19.2.1 Basis of Blood Pressure Monitoring

In traditional sphygmomanometry, the observer hears Korotkoff's sounds when the cuff-occluded blood pressure is released. Systolic blood pressure is the pressure recorded at the first sound. On further deflation of the cuff, the sounds cease. This is the diastolic pressure. Measurement accuracy depends on a number of factors. Getting an accurate reading of blood pressure depends on the relationship between arm circumference and cuff size. Miscuffing, specifically using small cuffs on large arms, is the most common blood pressure measurement error (84% of errors) in outpatient clinics. At least 40% of the arm circumference should be covered by the cuff, and the cuff length should equal 80% of the arm circumference [1]. Oversized cuffs cause falsely low readings, whereas undersized cuffs cause falsely high readings; however, because the error caused by an oversized cuff is smaller than the error caused by an undersized cuff, it is preferable to use a larger cuff.

It is also crucial to consider the site of the placement. Systolic pressure increases as monitor placement becomes more distal, while diastolic pressure decreases. Whenever possible, patients with peripheral vascular disease should have their pressure measured as close to their heart as possible because peripheral sites may give erroneously low pressure readings.

Measurements of blood pressure are greatly affected by the position of the arm. In order to accurately measure blood pressure, the cuff must be at the same level as the patient's heart. 7.5 mmHg must be added or subtracted from the reading for every 10 cm above or below the level of the heart [2]. The reading will be falsely elevated if the upper arm is positioned below the right atrium (such as when it is hanging down while the patient is sitting). A false low reading will also result if the arm is above the level of the heart. If the patient is positioned so that their back is unsupported or their legs are dangling, the reading will also be high due to isometric effects, as when they actively hold their arm up instead of passively supporting it.

19.2.2 Noninvasive Blood Pressure Monitoring

Blood pressure is measured most commonly using an automated noninvasive blood pressure monitor by measuring oscillations in cuff pressure using a pressure transducer. During arterial pulsation, pressure pulsations in the cuff are still present as the pump inflates it to a predetermined pressure. In order to determine the systolic blood pressure, the oscillations of the cuff are transmitted through the transducer to the transducer, which gauges the pressure at this point. In the occluded artery, blood is allowed to flow again by releasing the cuff pressure until there are no pulsations (oscillations) detected. This is the point at which diastolic pressure is determined by transmitting pressure oscillations through the cuff. Systolic, diastolic, and mean pressures are determined by measuring the magnitudes of these oscillations and comparing them with algorithms.

Blood pressure monitors that are automated offer convenience, safety, and sphygmomanometer placement precision that is not as crucial as it is with traditional sphygmomanometers. When peripheral vasoconstriction occurs, automated monitors can obtain accurate measurements without requiring venous drainage, which is required with traditional mercury-gravity manometers. Additionally, they are not sensitive to electrosurgical interference and can work in very noisy environments. In addition to complications and limitations associated with the use of automatic arterial blood pressure monitors, these devices may also fail to detect blood pressure in patients with dysrhythmias. Monitors that automatically measure blood pressure may also make it easier for anesthesiologists to lose vigilance.

It is also possible to monitor continuous blood pressure without invasive methods, but they are only commonly used in research. Penáz described a monitor in the 1970s that incorporated an inflatable finger cuff connected to an infrared photoplethysmograph for estimating blood flow through the finger artery under the cuff. You can feel a rise in blood volume in your digital artery during systole and a decrease in blood volume during diastole every time your heart beats. The pressure in the cuff is kept equal to the pressure in the artery and thus can be considered as no load on the vessel wall. The mean arterial set point needs to be maintained by fine-tuning the cuff volume by the amount of adjustment determined by the change in arterial wall pressure detected by the computer. This is the basis of the step-by-step blood pressure measurement [3].

Arterial dilatometry is another noninvasive method of continuous blood pressure monitoring that is characterized. Another method of noninvasive continuous blood pressure monitoring is achieved by externally placed sensors. The sensor is placed externally and senses the pulse rate, the maximum pulse amplitude, and the widest pulse pressure. These values are measured and then calibrated with previously recorded oscillometric brachial artery pressure measurements as a way to perform continuous calibration and measurement of blood pressure. The accuracy of such noninvasive detectors has been confirmed by research; however, further studies are needed to compare the data with standards to validate the use of these monitors in the clinical setting.

19.2.2.1 Tonometry Blood Pressure

Arterial blood pressure tonometry (TBP) is a new noninvasive technique for continuous arterial blood pressure monitoring. The principle is to obtain blood pressure values by applying appropriate pressure to a specially designed pressure transducer placed in the radial artery and detecting the maximum and minimum signals of arterial pulse. It is first developed by O'Rourke et al. in search of a noninvasive mechanism by which blood pressure waveforms (as opposed to numerical estimates) could be measured [4]. As shown by its name, tonometers "measure tone" by placing a sensor directly over an artery, as is shown by its name. Tonometers quantify and display this tactile information.

Tensys Medical (Irvine, CA) affixed a tonometer to a locking clamp that stabilizes the tonometer over the radial artery in the wrist–the T-line® in an effort to develop a more user-friendly and automated tonometer [5]. Once affixed over the radial artery, it can periodically locate the ideal measuring point and adjust the tonometric pressure transducer. This makes automated cuff-based blood pressure measurement possible, because this device can function with minimal intervention related to the operator and is analogous to the development of the oscillometer.

19.2.2.2 Pulse Wave Velocity

Pulse wave velocity (PWV) refers to the velocity of pressure wave transmission along the wall of the large arteries generated by each beat of the heart. It is a simple, effective, and economical noninvasive index to assess arterial stiffness, which can reflect the damage to blood vessels by various risk factors in a comprehensive manner and is an independent predictor of cardiovascular events. Pulse wave velocity can respond to the elastic state of the large and medium arterial systems, and is noninvasive, simple, effective, and reproducible, while reflecting real-time changes in arterial function.

The aortic vessels function as elastic reservoirs to maintain continuous blood flow in the arteries and buffer fluctuations in arterial blood pressure, and pulse waves are transmitted along the walls of the arteries. Pulse wave conduction velocity uses the principle that the conduction velocity of fluctuations (i.e., pulse waves) generated by blood output from the heart through the blood vessels is accelerated when atherosclerosis occurs, and the conduction velocity of fluctuations between two heartbeats is measured to determine the degree of vascular elasticity. It has also been demonstrated that systolic blood pressure, diastolic blood pressure, and mean arterial pressure all have a positive correlation with PWV [6].

19.3 Electrocardiogram

The contraction of the heart muscle is associated with electrical changes, which is also known as depolarization and repolarization. Depolarization refers to the movement of a cell's membrane potential to a more positive value while repolarization refers to the change in membrane potential, returning to a negative value. With electrodes at skin surface that is joined to the electrocardiograph (ECG) by wires, these changes can be detected. The ECG compares the electrical activity in each of the electrodes and forms a picture of the heart from different directions, and the picture is displayed in the pattern of ECG tracing that is characteristic from each view. This tracing can then be used to analyze the heart's electrical activity in detail.

An ECG is a 12-lead electrocardiogram, usually taken lying down, as discussed below. Some smartwatches can also record an ECG, such as Holter monitors, which can measure heart activity electrically. It is possible to record ECG signals with other devices in other contexts.

An ECG has 12 leads, each of which is connected to ten electrodes on the surface of the chest and on the limbs of the patient. Over a period of time (usually 10 s), twelve angles ("leads") are used to measure the overall magnitude of the heart's electrical potential. Through this method, each moment of the cardiac cycle can be captured as to the magnitude and direction of the heart's electrical depolarization.

ECGs are composed of three phases: P waves, representing depolarizations of the atria; QRS complexes, representing depolarizations of the ventricles; and T waves, representing repolarizations of the ventricles.

In addition to monitoring heart rate, the ECG can detect dysrhythmias, conduction defects, or other changes in myocardial electrical activity, such as ischemia or electrolyte imbalance. It is common to use standard leads I, II, and III during anesthesia in order to detect dysrhythmias. If there is ischemia in the inferior wall of the body, lead II can detect it. Furthermore, it provides an accurate diagnosis of dysrhythmias by revealing the maximal amplitude of P waves. Adding lead V allows the detection of ischemic damage to the anterior and lateral walls of the left ventricle, the most common and deleterious areas of ischemia. The appearance of dysrhythmias can therefore be anticipated by using a five-lead system in monitoring general anesthesia patients. When a normal rhythm is key, we can use the ECG to detect myocardial changes and intervene, but the ECG only provides information about electrical activity, not the heart's mechanical ability to pump. ECG monitors are best used in combination with pulse oximeters in order to monitor circulatory function.

In addition, ECG monitors are essential for diagnosing myocardial ischemia. Dysrhythmias during sedation are commonly caused by hypoxia and endogenous catecholamine release. Myocardial ischemia caused by hypoxia is indicated by reduced or elevated ST segment. An ECG tracing should contain an isoelectric ST segment, or a segment at the same level as the T wave and the next P wave. Infarction or acute myocardial injury may have caused the ST segment to be elevated. Detecting elevation in a lead indicates the part of the heart that has been injured. The entire heart is affected by pericarditis, which can also cause ST elevation. An ischemia-induced downward ST segment depression is usually more prevalent than an infarction-induced downward ST segment depression. It is also possible to have an ST segment depression due to downsloping ischemia, which may also be caused by digoxin treatment. Myocardial problems associated with horizontal and downsloping ST segment depressions are more ominous than those associated with upsloping ST segment depressions. Ischemia is also associated with changes in T wave; however, digoxin therapy and ventricular hypertrophy can also cause T wave inversions. Three of the four leads, III, VR, and V1, show normal T wave inversions. Various electrolyte abnormalities can also be detected in an ECG trace. T waves flatten in hypokalemia, while QRS complexes widen in hyperkalemia [7]. It is also common for nonspecific ST-T changes to occur regularly in the ST portion and the T wave; these changes are usually of no major significance. Although changes in the ST segment and T wave are not specific for ischemia, when these abnormalities are detected during anesthesia, they should be immediately investigated.

19.4 Respiratory System Monitoring

During anesthesia, insufficient ventilation contributes significantly to morbidity and mortality. In addition, ventilatory changes resulting from administered sedative medications tend to precede cardiovascular system depression. For the above reasons, respiratory system monitoring is an extremely important aspect of anesthesia management and involves visual methods and the use of monitoring devices. Auscultation of breath sounds during conscious and deep sedation can be performed with a precordial or suprasternal stethoscope. If the patient is undergoing endotracheal intubation, or nitrous oxide/oxygen anesthesia, movement of the reservoir bag and visualization of thoracic activity should be continually monitored, as should the color of the mucous membranes. However, these observational methods alone are not sufficient for assessing respiratory adequacy. The use of pulse oximetry and capnography is recommended, which has greatly increased the safety of anesthesia care.

19.4.1 Basic Tools for Monitoring

Various complications and emergencies of the respiratory system can be better prevented, or better treatment provided, if detected early. To achieve this, various monitoring tools need to be integrated, the most basic of which are pulse oximetry and carbon dioxide monitoring.

19.4.1.1 Pulse Oximetry

When COVID-19 first broke out in early 2020, many people became concerned about pulse oximetry. This is because oxygen saturation (SpO_2) is the percentage of oxygen-bound hemoglobin (HbO_2) capacity in the blood to the total bound hemoglobin (Hb, hemoglobin) capacity, i.e., the concentration of oxygen in the blood is an important indicator to determine the severity of COVID-19. For prediction of postoperative pulmonary complications (PPCs), which are common complications in surgeries, it is found that almost one-third of the patients with $SpO_2 \leq 90\%$ developed at least one postoperative in-hospital pulmonary complication; therefore preoperative SpO_2 has been included in the ARISCAT PPCs prediction score [8].

In biological tissue optics, the spectral region in the 600–1300 nm band is often referred to as the "spectral window of the organism," and light in this band is of particular interest for many known and unknown spectral therapies and spectral diagnostics. In the infrared region, water becomes the dominant light-absorbing substance in biological tissues, so the wavelength used by the system must avoid the absorption peak of water to obtain better information about the light absorption of the target substance. Thus, in the near-infrared spectral range of 600–950 nm, the main components of human terminal tissues that can absorb light include water in the blood, O_2Hb (oxyhemoglobin), RHb (reduced hemoglobin), and peripheral skin melanin and other tissues. At the 940 nm wavelength, however, this phenomenon is reversed, which means HbO_2 absorbs more infrared light than does Hb, and Hb allows more red light to pass through than does HbO_2 [9]. Also, because MetHb (methemoglobin) absorbs light at both 660 nm and 940 nm, the R/IR ratio is once again erroneous, causing the calibrated saturation to read approximately 80%–85% depending on the percentage of MetHb present [10].

The role of hemoglobin is to carry oxygen to all parts of the body. We refer to the oxygen level of hemoglobin at any given moment as the oxygen saturation level. It is this oxygen saturation level that is measured by a finger oximeter. Hemoglobin has an oxygen-carrying state and an unloaded state. We call oxygen-carrying hemoglobin oxyhemoglobin and unloaded hemoglobin reduced hemoglobin.

Oxyhemoglobin and reduced hemoglobin have different absorption characteristics in the visible and near-infrared spectral range. Reduced hemoglobin absorbs more red frequency light and less infrared frequency light, while oxyhemoglobin absorbs less red frequency light and more infrared frequency light.

Therefore, the data of the emission spectrum can be analyzed to get the effective information of the concentration of the components to be measured in the tissue. When we get O_2Hb and RHb concentrations, we can know the oxygen saturation. Oxygen saturation (SpO_2) is the volume of oxygenated hemoglobin (HbO_2) bound by oxygen in the blood as a percentage of the volume of all available bound hemoglobin (Hb), i.e., the concentration of oxygen in the blood. SpO_2 is physiologically related to PaO_2; therefore, according to the oxyhemoglobin dissociation curve, in patients with PaO_2 higher than 60 mmHg, SpO_2 has low sensitivity for detection of hypoxemia [11]. For nonsmokers HbCO levels will be less than 2%; for smokers HbCO levels can be 20% higher than normal; and for patients who have been exposed to carbon monoxide, these levels can be 40% higher than normal [12].

During each cardiac cycle, contraction of the heart causes a rise in blood pressure within the aortic root vessels, which in turn causes the vessel walls to expand outward, and conversely, diastole of the heart causes a fall in blood pressure within the aortic root vessels, which in turn causes the vessel walls to contract. As the cardiac cycle repeats, the changing blood pressure in the aortic root vessel is transmitted to the downstream vessels connected to it and even to the entire arterial system, resulting in the continuous expansion and contraction of the entire arterial vascular wall. In other words, the periodic beating of the heart generates pulse waves in the aorta, which propagate forward in waves along the vessel wall to the entire arterial system. Each time the heart expands and contracts, a pressure change occurs in the arterial system, which generates a periodic pulse wave. This is the process we normally refer to as pulse wave generation. The waveform characteristics of the pulse wave reflect some physiological information such as heart, blood pressure, blood flow, etc., and can provide important information for the noninvasive detection of specific body parameters. In medicine, pulse waves are usually divided into two types: pressure pulse waves and volume pulse waves. Pressure pulse waves primarily characterize blood pressure transmission, while volumetric pulse waves characterize periodic changes in blood flow. Compared to the pressure pulse wave, the volumetric pulse wave will contain more important cardiovascular information such as human blood vessels and blood flow, and the noninvasive detection of the volumetric pulse wave can be realized by the photoelectric volumetric pulse wave tracing method. A specific wave of light is used to irradiate the body measurement site, and the light beam is reflected or transmitted to the photoelectric sensor, and the received light beam will carry the effective characteristics of the volumetric pulse wave information. As the blood volume changes periodically with the expansion and contraction of the heart, when the heart is diastolic, the blood volume is the smallest, and the absorption of light by the blood is if the sensor detects the maximum light intensity; when the heart is contracted, the volume is the largest, and the sensor detects the minimum light intensity.

19.4.1.2 Capnography

A definition of the components of the analysis and measurement of carbon dioxide in the respired air is required for carrying out this process. Capnometry is measurement of CO_2 concentrations during the respiratory cycle, and capnography is the graphic record of the measured CO_2 concentrations. The capnometer analyzes the gases and displays the readings, and capnography is usually displayed graphically on a monitor screen.

Capnogram is normally rectangular in shape and divided into four phases. Phase I represents the cessation of inspiration and the beginning of expiration, the exhaled gas is the invalid lumen gas from the duct, and the carbon dioxide partial pressure is zero; Phase II represents the mixing process of invalid lumen gas and alveolar gas, and the carbon dioxide level rises rapidly; Phase III the expiratory plateau, which is a horizontal line, represents the alveolar gas mixture containing carbon dioxide gas being continuously exhaled, and the highest point at the end of it is the carbon dioxide partial pressure value at the end of expiration displayed by the instrument; Phase IV for the inspiratory descending branch. It is often used to understand the airway and ventilation, blood perfusion, and other conditions. The capnogram is often one of many other displayed parameters on a large multipurpose monitor in the operating room; however, there are portable battery-powered end-tidal CO_2 ($ETCO_2$) monitors that are used for monitoring during transport.

Monitoring of $ETCO_2$ concentration or its partial pressure ($PETCO_2$) reflects pulmonary ventilation and also pulmonary blood flow. In the absence of significant cardiopulmonary disease and a normal V/Q ratio, $PETCO_2$ reflects arterial blood carbon dioxide ($PaCO_2$). When using ventilators and anesthesia, ventilation is adjusted based on $PETCO_2$ measurements to keep $PETCO_2$ close to preoperative levels. Its waveform also determines whether the tracheal tube is in the airway. And for those who are on mechanical ventilation, if there is a malfunction such as air leak, catheter twist, or tracheal obstruction, $PETCO_2$ digital and morphological changes and alarms can appear immediately to help doctors detect and deal with it in time.

What is also worth mentioning is that for anesthetists, $ETCO_2$ can be used as a sign for the guidance of intubation, on which our institute, Shanghai Ninth People's Hospital, Department of Anesthesiology has already got a patent of invention.

19.4.1.3 Precordial/Pretracheal Stethoscope

The precordial/pretracheal stethoscope allows for practical and inexpensive monitoring of the circulatory and respiratory systems during anesthesia. It consists of a weighted stethoscope head connected by a transducer to a custom-molded monaural earpiece. When placed in the precordial region, the head of the stethoscope should be placed on the chest wall between the sternotomy and the left nipple to monitor cardiac and breath sounds, and when placed in the cervical region above the trachea, it monitors breath sounds. Arguably, the use of a stethoscope in an anterior tracheal position is ideal for monitoring respiration during ambulatory anesthesia for oral surgery because the commonly used sedative drugs depress respiration and cause much lower chances of changes in cardiovascular function that can be diagnosed by auscultation. However, the use of the stethoscope has declined dramatically in the last decade due to its limitations: although respiratory sounds can be heard, it is not possible to determine the adequacy of tidal volume through the stethoscope. For this reason, it needs to be used in combination with other oxygen saturation monitors such as pulse oximetry.

19.4.1.4 Other Tools

Current evidence supports the potential role of protective low tidal volume ventilation in healthy lungs during general anesthesia in decreasing the incidence of PPCs. The role of PEEP level is still controversial. However, ongoing large prospective observational and randomized controlled studies will provide further information.

19.4.2 Respiratory Mechanics

Measurement of airway pressure and compliance may be helpful during the intraoperative period to determine the right tidal volume, plateau pressure, and PEEP. There are some circumstances, such as postoperative intra-abdominal surgery, obesity, and patients with increased intra-abdominal pressure (IAP), where respiratory compliance is affected not only by the lungs, but also by the chest wall. Thus, the airway pressure might not accurately reflect the real stress and strain on the lungs. During preoperative esophageal catheter placement, high-risk patients can be measured for transpulmonary pressure (Ptp), work of breathing, and intrinsic PEEP [13]. A balloon placed in the esophagus can measure the esophageal pressure, which can be used to determine the pressure required for alveolar recruitment, tidal volume, and safe plateau pressure, in addition to determining the level of PEEP during the perioperative period. Hence, the measurement of esophageal pressure can aid in better titration and optimization of the pressure required for alveolar recruitment, tidal volume, etc. Furthermore, monitoring of esophageal pressure can be done in the postoperative period to minimize patient-ventilator asynchrony, especially in patients suffering from COPD.

19.4.2.1 Hemodynamics and Respiration

In the twentieth century, recent developments in mini-invasive hemodynamic measurement techniques have enabled continuous monitoring of cardiac output and other parameters at the bedside, and timely information about the role of hemodynamics in respiratory failure. Several of these methods are based on pulse pattern analysis, which can be done during or after major surgery with a peripheral arterial line. It has been proposed recently that a completely noninvasive alternative exists, but its effectiveness is being debated. Transpulmonary thermodilution is a minimally invasive technique for estimating extravascular lung water (EVLW) and EVLW index (EVLWi). In addition to measuring cardiac output, transthoracic echocardiography can also assess stroke volume variation, which is increasingly useful in assessing fluid responsiveness in patients.

Most studies conclude that hemodynamic goal-directed therapy can improve outcome in high-risk surgical patients, especially in terms of reduction of postoperative complications, while mortality reduction is significant only in very high-risk surgical patients.

19.5 Temperature Monitoring

For intubated, anesthetized patients and those who are not intubated, the American Association of Oral and Maxillofacial Surgeons (AAOMS) anesthesia guidelines advise recording patients' temperatures. A way of continuously monitoring the body temperature of anesthesia patients should be readily available. If changes in body temperature are expected or suspected, a continuous monitoring method should be used. The normal methods of regulating a patient's body temperature are impaired under general anesthesia. It is, however, critical to measure continuous temperature in patients under sedated anesthesia whenever there is a suspicion that it may differ from normal preoperatively since hypothermia and hyperthermia may lead to negative outcomes; both are discussed in more detail later in this section.

The decrease in body temperature is expected in pediatric patients, whose surface area to mass ratio is greater, in patients undergoing large amounts of intravenous fluid, and in patients undergoing major surgery involving the body cavity. As a result of hyperthermia, adverse outcomes can occur, such as prolonged recovery, wound infection, and increased cardiac morbidity. A patient's ability to tolerate stress decreases as their body temperature increases, while their respiratory and cardiovascular systems work harder. Hyperthermia can indicate serious physiological disturbances such as drug reactions, transfusion reactions, hyperthyroidism, and malignant hyperthermia. Anesthetics containing volatile anesthetics or depolarizing muscle relaxants should be monitored constantly when they may cause malignant hyperthermia; however, even if these agents are not used, a method should be readily accessible for monitoring body temperature.

Various technologies are used to display accurate temperature measurements in temperature monitors. An element that measures temperature, a thermistor, exhibits a large change in resistance in proportion to a small change in temperature. Low cost, accuracy, sensitivity to small temperature changes, disposable probes, and sensitivity to small temperature changes are among its advantages. A thermocouple also uses an electrical current to determine temperature, like a thermistor. Two dissimilar metals are welded together to form the cable. There are some similarities between thermocouples and thermistors; however, thermocouples do not detect small temperature changes as well as thermistors. Temperature-dependent electrical resistance is found in both the thermistor and thermocouple. A platinum wire thermometer is accurate, continuous, and inexpensive, just like a thermistor or thermocouple. This type of thermometer employs a probe enclosed inside a casing to protect it from contact with body fluids.

An organic compound melts and recrystallizes at specific temperatures in a liquid crystal thermometer. The strips are placed on the skin using adhesive backs. They are a convenient, inexpensive, disposable, noninvasive, and portable method of monitoring temperature. Their readings can, however, be influenced by factors in the environment, such as humidity or presence of a heating lamp. Although infrared thermometers are only convenient for intermittent measurements, they are accurate and noninvasive. An infrared camera records the amount of infrared radiation emitted by objects, including ear canals. It is a technique-sensitive thermometer, and its accuracy depends on how well it is aimed and penetrated into the ear canal.

A nasopharynx, an esophagus, a tympanic membrane, an oral cavity, a rectum, a bladder, and a trachea are all commonly measured as part of a routine general anesthetic. Oral surgery is more unique in nature than other surgeries in that, on the one hand, the surgeon shares the airway with the anesthesiologist and, on the other hand, because various instruments are placed in the oral cavity or nasopharynx, this may cause the thermometer probe to shift when temperature monitoring is performed. In addition, irrigation may interfere with monitoring, resulting in inaccurate readings. Patients may be less tolerant under sedation; therefore, during general anesthesia, measurements may be taken using areas such as the skin and axilla, or an LCD thermometer may be placed on the forehead to measure skin temperature.

There are certain limitations of temperature monitors, mainly inaccurate readings. Inaccurate readings can be caused by various reasons, including incorrect probe connection, improper probe placement, and machine malfunction. To prevent excessive readings, the internal probe connections must be kept dry. Also, body temperature monitors have some potential hazards—if they catch fire due to high temperatures, they can cause damage to the monitoring site. The body temperature probe acts as a ground for electrosurgical equipment and can catch fire. In addition, body temperature probes can lead to perforation of the rectum, tympanic membrane, and esophagus.

19.6 Neuromuscular Transmission Monitoring

As well as facilitating endotracheal intubation, reducing patient movement, and promoting a more favorable surgical environment, muscle relaxants are frequently used during anesthesia. Each of the above uses may require different levels of neuromuscular blockade (NMB). Since patients respond to muscle relaxants differently, monitoring NMB is a critical aspect of maintaining the desired level of relaxation. Nerve stimulation with electrical current and measurement of muscle response are two ways to assess the level of NMB. Usually the adductor pollicis muscle adducts the thumb and stimulates the ulnar nerve at the wrist with 20–60 mA current. Using electrical stimulation to stimulate the facial muscles reflects the response of the airway musculature and can give a good indication that NMB is adequate for intubation. An ideal way to determine intubation readiness is to stimulate the facial nerve, but the adductor pollicis usually responds adequately.

Nerve stimulators are used during anesthesia induction to determine whether the vocal cords are relaxed enough to permit the passage of the endotracheal tube. It is necessary to maintain a moderate depth of anesthesia during maintenance of anesthesia in order to prevent patient movement, but not to reach such a depth that postoperative respiratory support is necessary. Nerve stimulators allow anesthetists to determine if NMB is reversible at the end of the procedure and to what extent it can be reversed. At this point, the ideal approach is to monitor peripheral muscles, such as the thumb adductor, because this muscle is one of the last to recover and its recovery status gives a good indication of the recovery status of the respiratory muscles.

The pattern of stimulation and response is usually performed as a single twitch, train-of-four (TOF), or tetanus, and can be used to determine the readiness for intubation by comparing the post-stimulation measurements with control values. Depolarizing and nondepolarizing muscle relaxants inhibit the response in the same way. Therefore, the anesthesiologist cannot distinguish between depolarizing and nondepolarizing blocks using a single twitch stimulus.

A TOF stimulation pattern consists of 4 identical twitches delivered over a period of about 2 s as a means of distinguishing depolarizing and nondepolarizing blocks. The height of all four twitches will be equally lowered with a depolarizing muscle relaxant. The twitches will slowly fade as the antidepolarizing muscle relaxant establishes deep blockade, causing the fourth twitch to disappear, followed by the third, and so on. A major advantage of TOF stimulation is its lack of control response and its ability to monitor NMB effectively compared to single twitches.

Repeated single twitches are part of tetanic stimulation; usually between 30 and 100 signals per second are delivered. In the absence of NMB, sustained contractions are observed. Depolarizing drugs sustain tetanic contractions but depress them uniformly; nondepolarizing drugs depress and do not sustain tetanic contractions. By stimulating NMB with tetanic stimulation, deeper levels of NMB can be monitored when a single twitch or TOF does not produce a response. In addition to being painful, it can only be used when the patient is anesthetized.

19.7 Depth of Sedation Monitoring

Maintaining the patient's safety while providing the best experience requires evaluating the depth of sedation. Apart from maintaining an appropriate level of amnesia, analgesia, and anxiolysis, it is also important to prevent respiratory depression, laryngospasm, and circulation problems, such as hypotension.

For evaluating the level of sedation in a patient, subjective measures (scores) are available; however, monitoring the patient's level of responsiveness requires repeatedly waking them or disturbing them. This scale is indicated whenever sedative medication is administered. The Ramsay Sedation Scale is one of the most common subjective scales used for sedation assessment. It grades sedation based on the patient's response. Patients undergoing NMB cannot be assessed with Ramsay Sedation Scales since they require a response. Also available are a variety of clinical assessments, including the Observer's Assessment of Alertness/Sedation Scale, the Riker Sedation-Agitation Scale, and the Motor Activity Assessment Scale. Patients on sedative medications are assessed on these scales based on their alertness. They can be limited by the fact that they rely on individual interpretations of measurement criteria and definitions.

References

1. Muntner P, Shimbo D, Carey R, Charleston J, Gaillard T, Misra S, Myers M, Ogedegbe G, Schwartz J, Townsend R, Urbina E, Viera A, White W, Wright J. Measurement of blood pressure in humans: a scientific statement from the American Heart Association. Hypertension. 2019;73(5):e35.
2. Beevers G, Lip GY, O'Brien E. ABC of hypertension. Blood pressure measurement. Part I-sphygmomanometry: factors common to all techniques. BMJ (Clin Res Ed). 2001;322(7292):981–5. https://doi.org/10.1136/bmj.322.7292.981.
3. Truijen J, van Lieshout JJ, Wesselink WA, Westerhof BE. Noninvasive continuous hemodynamic monitoring. J Clin Monit Comput. 2012;26(4):267–78. https://doi.org/10.1007/s10877-012-9375-8.
4. O'Rourke MF, Adji A. An updated clinical primer on large artery mechanics: implications of pulse waveform analysis and arterial tonometry. Curr Opin Cardiol. 2005;20(4):275–81. https://doi.org/10.1097/01.hco.0000166595.44711.6f.
5. 2022. [online]. https://medaval.ie/device/tensys-t-line-tl-200/. Accessed 26 May 2022.
6. Koo HS, Lee HS, Hong YM. Methylenetetrahydrofolate reductase TT genotype as a predictor of cardiovascular risk in hypertensive adolescents. Pediatr Cardiol. 2008;29(1):136–41. Epub 2007 Oct 5. https://doi.org/10.1007/s00246-007-9103-1.
7. Weiss J, Qu Z, Shivkumar K. Electrophysiology of hypokalemia and hyperkalemia. Circ Arrhythm Electrophysiol. 2017;10(3):e004667.
8. Canet J, Gallart L, Gomar C, Paluzie G, Vallès J, Castillo J, Sabaté S, Mazo V, Briones Z, Sanchis J. Prediction of postoperative pulmonary complications in a population-based surgical cohort. Anesthesiology. 2010;113(6):1338–50.
9. Medicine.uiowa.edu. Pulse oximetry basic principles and interpretation | Iowa Head and Neck Protocols. 2022. https://medicine.uiowa.edu/iowaprotocols/pulse-oximetry-basic-principles-and-interpretation. Accessed 27 May 2022.
10. Chan ED, Chan MM, Chan MM. Pulse oximetry: understanding its basic principles facilitates appreciation of its limitations. Respir Med. 2013;107(6):789–99. Epub 2013 Mar 13. https://doi.org/10.1016/j.rmed.2013.02.004.
11. Collins J, Rudenski A, Gibson J, Howard L, O'Driscoll R. Relating oxygen partial pressure, saturation and content: the haemoglobin–oxygen dissociation curve. Breathe. 2015;11(3):194–201.
12. Van Gastel M, Stuijk S, De Haan G. Camera-based pulse-oximetry—validated risks and opportunities from theoretical analysis. Biomed Opt Express. 2017;9(1):102–19. PMID: 29359090; PMCID: PMC5772567. https://doi.org/10.1364/BOE.9.000102.
13. Sun X, Zhou J. Esophageal pressure and transpulmonary pressure monitoring. Zhonghua Wei Zhong Bing Ji Jiu Yi Xue. 2018;30(3):280–3; Chinese. https://doi.org/10.3760/cma.j.issn.2095-4352.2018.03.018.

20 Postoperative Pain Management in Oral and Maxillofacial Surgery

Ming Xia

20.1 Introduction

Oral and maxillofacial surgery involves the nasopharyngeal cavity, tongue root, mouth floor, and regiones colli anterior, which are prone to cause postoperative edema, lymphatic reflux disorders, swelling of reconstructed flaps, compression of the airway, etc. Over half of patients reported moderate or severe pain after oral and maxillofacial surgery [1]. The pain felt by patients during perioperative period may increase the risk of complications happening after surgery, and thus impeding the recovery of patients. Hence, postoperative pain management is critical in the process of surgical treatment and postoperative recovery. Also, it is clinicians' ethical responsibility to minimize patients' pain. Fortunately, multimodal analgesia has been introduced and developed currently and organizations have launched expert consensus and guidelines. It is expected that OMFS patients could receive better pain management. In this chapter, we will present postoperative analgesic strategies and their optimization.

M. Xia (✉)
Department of Anesthesiology, Shanghai Ninth People's Hospital Affiliated to Shanghai Jiao Tong University School of Medicine, Shanghai, China
e-mail: xiaming1980@xzhmu.edu.cn

20.2 Strategies for Postoperative Pain Management

20.2.1 Standardized Analgesia

Postoperative analgesia of oral and maxillofacial surgery can be incorporated into the postoperative pain management framework of the whole hospital. The establishment of a hospital-wide or anesthesiology-based acute pain service (APS) group, including surgeons and nurses, can effectively improve the quality of perioperative analgesia in oral and maxillofacial surgery. The work scope and purpose of APS group include: (1) treating perioperative pain, evaluating and recording analgesic effect, and dealing with adverse reactions and problems in analgesic treatment; (2) carry out education on the necessity of postoperative analgesia and related knowledge; (3) improve the comfort and satisfaction of surgical patients; (4) reduce postoperative pain-related complications.

20.2.2 Preventive Analgesia

Modern pain management concept advocates preventive analgesia, that is, giving effective anesthesia or nerve block before operation, and giving enough analgesics [such as selective cyclooxygenase-2(COX-2) inhibitors] before the

H. Jiang, M. Xia (eds.), *Anesthesia for Oral and Maxillofacial Surgery*,
https://doi.org/10.1007/978-981-19-7287-4_20

onset of pain, so as to reduce traumatic stress, prevent central sensitization, lower pain threshold, reduce the dosage of postoperative analgesics, and prolong the analgesic time.

20.2.3 Multimodal Analgesia

Multimodal analgesia refers to the combined application of analgesic drugs with different analgesic methods and different action mechanisms, taking effect on different parts, phases, and targets of pain by different administration routes, so as to achieve the purpose of additive or synergistic analgesic effects and reduce adverse drug reactions. Multimodal analgesia is an ideal perioperative analgesia management scheme at present.

The recommended combination regimen in clinical practice includes the combination of opioids with selective COX-2 inhibitors, nonsteroidal anti-inflammatory drugs (NSAID) and/or acetaminophen, etc. It is proposed to combine various analgesic drugs on the basis of ultrasound-guided nerve block or intraspinal analgesia for general perioperative multimodal analgesia is advised. For patients who use self-controlled analgesia devices, it is still recommended for them to concurrently take NSAID orally or intravenously to relieve postoperative residual pain.

20.2.4 Individualized Analgesics

Patients suffer from different pain degrees in the same kind of surgery, not to mention in different ones. Furthermore, there are individual differences in the response of patients to pain and analgesic drugs. Individualized analgesics are necessary to precise pain management. It refers to the selection of analgesic methods such as oral or intravenous administration, epidural analgesia, and patient-controlled analgesia (PCA) according to the patient's pain degree, type, duration, etc. Individualized analgesia should comprehensively consider various factors and formulate the optimal pain management plan. In addition, it should also analyze patient factors, so that clinicians can achieve the best analgesic effect with the smallest drug dose. If permitted, the gene polymorphism can be detected, the degree of pain can be managed hierarchically, and the use of opioids can be guided.

20.3 Pharmacological Aspect of Pain Management

20.3.1 Simple Analgesics

There are three drugs in this category: paracetamol, NSAIDs, and COX-2 inhibitors.

Cochrane recently reevaluated the effect of single-dose oral analgesics on moderate and severe pain. Figure 20.1 shows that a majority of data were collected from patients who had their third molars extracted. In general, with increasing doses and types of analgesics, the number needed to treat (NNT) decreased. Analgesic supplementation was required by patients who consumed NSAIDs along with paracetamol when compared with any drug taken alone [3]. All patients who are postoperative are recommended to consider this combination [4].

COX-1 inhibition induced by chronic NSAIDs has been shown to adversely affect the digestive, renal, and cardiovascular systems, as well as platelet aggregation. In nearly half of the patients who take NSAIDs regularly, gastric erosions were present, and ulcers were seen on endoscopy in nearly 30% of these patients. It is estimated that upper gastrointestinal events occur in approximately 3%*4.5% of patients, with serious events occurring in about 1.5%. There are several factors that lead to increased risk of upper gastrointestinal events, including previous ulceration, chronic anticoagulation, coexisting corticosteroids, and increased NSAID dosage. In addition to proton pump inhibitors like omeprazole, COX-2 inhibitors such as celecoxib can also reduce these adverse effects.

Additionally, NSAIDs can negatively impact the renal system as well. Because NSAIDs inhibit vasodilatory renal prostaglandin synthesis, which is normally increased in cases of hypotension or

Single dose analgesic		NNT (95% CI)
Ibuprofen 400 mg + Paracetamol 1000 mg	BEST	1.5 (1.4 to 1.7)
Ibuprofen 200 mg + Paracetamol 500 mg		1.6 (1.5 to 1.8)
Paracetamol 1000 mg + Oxycodlone 10 mg		1.8 (1.6 to 2.2)
Diclofenac potassium 100 mg		1.9 (1.7 to 2.3)
Diclofenac potassium 50 mg		2.1 (1.9 to 2.5)
Ibuprofen 400 mg		2.1 (1.9 to 2.3)
Paracetamol 1000 mg + Codeine 60 mg		2.2 (1.8 to 2.9)
Ibuprofen 400 mg + Oxycodlone 5 mg		2.3 (2.0 to 2.8)
Naproxen 500 mg		2.7 (2.3 to 3.3)
Paracetamol 1000 mg		3.6 (3.2 to 4.1)
Tramadol 100 mg		4.6 (3.6 to 6.4)
Tramadol 50 mg		9.1 (6.1 to 19)
Codeine 60 mg	WORST	12 (8.4 to 18)

Fig. 20.1 Number needed to treat (NNT) to achieve at least 50% reduction in maximal postoperative pain (moderate or severe) over 4–6 h [2]. NNT of 2–5 is considered useful. (Reproduced with permission from S.W. Evans, R.A. McCahon. Management of postoperative pain in maxillofacial surgery. Br J Oral Maxillofac Surg, 2019, 57(1):4–11)

hypovolemia to preserve renal perfusion, their use can result in progressive acute kidney injury, and may worsen the progression of chronic renal failure. Patients at risk include those with pre-existing renal impairment, hypovolemia, heart failure, cirrhosis, multiple myeloma, and those who are taking ACE inhibitors, angiotensin II receptor antagonists, or diuretics [5].

20.3.2 Opioid Analgesics

Opioids once have been popular in treating moderate to severe postoperative pain whereas their acute side effects including nausea, constipation, itching, drowsiness, respiratory depression, and death from overdose have been realized to a greater extent. Therefore, they are viewed as a course of treatment that will be reduced as appropriate and many countries enact regulations on the use of opioid [6]. Clinicians and patients should fully understand opioid abuse before taking them regularly.

20.3.2.1 Weak Opioids

Codeine phosphate and tramadol are two of the most common opioids prescribed in UK practice, both of which have a low relative potency compared with morphine. Neither is particularly effective in the absence of other opioids (Fig. 20.1). Because codeine is metabolized differently by different people, it can have severe adverse effects, including respiratory depression, in people metabolizing it slowly. Codeine should not be administered to patients known to have hyperactive CYP2D6 metabolizing enzymes or to children under 12 years of age [7]. Due to its stimulatory effects on serotonergic receptors, tramadol is contraindicated in patients with poorly controlled epilepsy.

20.3.2.2 Strong Opioids

Analgesia after surgery is generally achieved with morphine, oxycodone, and fentanyl. In comparison with morphine, oxycodone's relative potency is 1.5–2 times greater. High doses of fentanyl can lead to respiratory depression, as it is ten times stronger than morphine.

As intravenous analgesics or oral preparations (oxycodone, morphine), strong opioids are typically administered intravenously. The slow onset of action and lack of rapid titratability make transdermal delivery unsuitable for acute pain relief. When parenteral delivery is necessary, patient-controlled opioids should only be administered intravenously rather than orally [8].

20.3.2.3 Chronic Use of Opioids

Addiction and drug tolerance are caused by chronic opioid use [9]. In addition, they have a higher risk of developing chronic pain following surgery, and they require more postoperative analgesia [10, 11]. They need their usual dose of analgesia to treat their chronic pain and additional doses to manage their acute pain. In these cases, postoperative analgesia should be handled with a multidisciplinary approach, and should begin preoperatively.

The efficacy of the analgesic regimen should be evaluated preoperatively and be optimized timely. Whether transdermal opioid patches should continue to be used in the perioperative period is controversial because during surgery, various modalities are used to keep patients warm to maintain their body temperature, and the rate of drug delivery may increase in such cases, but may decrease if the patch is applied to poorly infiltrated skin. In addition, high doses of buprenorphine can antagonize full opioid receptor agonists and morphine and lead to analgesic failure and withdrawal. The current view is that transdermal administration of buprenorphine (less than 70 g/h) is unlikely to interfere with all-opioid agonists used to treat acute postoperative pain. That is, perioperative transdermal administration of fentanyl and buprenorphine should be continued, with the addition of oral opioids or as patient-controlled analgesia postoperatively [11]. If the patch is discontinued preoperatively, it needs to be replaced with an oral immediate-release opioid in a graded fashion for 72 h.

20.3.2.4 Opioid-Induced Hyperalgesia

It can result either in hyperalgesia or allodynia, which are painful responses to non-painful stimuli. Pain will be exacerbated by higher dosages, unlike opioid tolerance.

Specifically, remifentanil is associated postoperatively with opioid-induced hyperalgesia that can be observed [12]. In particular, its use during surgery can result in more intense pain in the first 24 h after surgery, and a moderate increase in the need for morphine. Thus, local anesthetics and nonsteroidal anti-inflammatory drugs can be used to reduce the dosage by using opioid-sparing techniques.

20.3.3 Local Anesthetic

A variety of trigeminal nerve branches can be numbed with local anesthetics by using regional anesthesia in maxillofacial surgery. These are recommended as part of a multimodal approach to postoperative analgesia, and are strongly recommended for techniques that are specific to the surgical site [8]. Continuous delivery through a catheter is preferable to a single-bolus dose if the duration of postoperative pain is likely to be longer than the duration of action of the drug used—for example, when harvesting rib grafts [13]. An overview of when and how postoperative analgesia is provided or supplemented in maxillofacial surgery is presented in Table 20.1.

To reduce the need for perioperative opioids, lidocaine has been infused intravenously during surgery. During bimaxillary osteotomies, lidocaine was given intraoperatively and reduced pain scores for eight hours [14]. Systemic lidocaine infusion during bimaxillary surgery reduces postoperative pain, analgesic consumption, and facial swelling [15].

There are cardiovascular and neurological complications associated with local anesthetic toxicity, such as circumoral tingling, tonic-clonic convulsions, and cardiac arrhythmias. As long as

Table 20.1 Regional anesthetic techniques used in maxillofacial practice for postoperative analgesia (Reproduced with permission from S.W. Evans, R.A. McCahon. Management of postoperative pain in maxillofacial surgery. Br J Oral Maxillofac Surg, 2019, 57(1):4–11)

Target or local anesthetic (LA) technique, or both	Study	Outcome, findings, and comment
Inferior alveolar nerve block + buccal infiltration	Split mouth, randomized Bilateral third molar extraction under GA	2% lidocaine (1:80,000 adrenaline) improves pain VAS compared with control Pain VAS significantly lower for 0.5% bupivacaine at 3–8 h postoperatively compared with 2% lidocaine (1:80,000 adrenaline); no difference thereafter. Patients preferred bupivacaine over lidocaine
	2% lidocaine (1:80,000 adrenaline) cf. control (*n* = 52) 2% lidocaine (1:80,000 adrenaline) cf. 0.5% bupivacaine (*n* = 68)	
Dental LA:	Cochrane review of use of dental LA in patients <17 years (*n* = 1152)	Unable to establish effect because of clinical and methodological heterogeneity of studies
• Intraligamental injection • Topical • Infiltration		
Anterior iliac crest donor site	Triple blind RCT of 0.5% bupivacaine:	Subperiosteal delivery of bupivacaine through catheter has considerable benefits with respect to dynamic analgesia, at-rest analgesia, and time to first mobilization
	Single shot femoral nerve block Single shot subcutaneous injection Repeated bolus through subperiosteal catheter	
	RCT of 0.2% ropivacaine (*n* = 17) cf. 0.25% bupivacaine (*n* = 17) infusions through periosteal catheter	0.2% ropivacaine provides comparable analgesia to 0.25% bupivacaine
	Retrospective cohort study:	Compared with infiltration alone, BAS + infiltration offered considerable benefits in terms of acute pain, need for opioids, time to first mobilization, and duration of stay
	– Bupivacaine infiltration (*n* = 89)	No studies have compared catheter-based techniques with BAS
	– Bupivacaine infiltration + bupivacaine-soaked absorbable sponge (BAS), (*n* = 118)	
Mandibular nerve block (MNB)	Blinded RCT of preinduction MNB (*n* = 21) cf. control (*n* = 21) in patients having partial glossectomy or transmandibular lateral pharyngectomy	MNB reduced mean consumption of opioids by 56% and 45% at 12 h and 24 h, respectively, postoperatively. The incidence of severe pain was significantly lower in the MNB group on the first postoperative day (3 cf. 10)
	Pilot study of preoperative MNB in patients with unilateral mandibular angle fracture (*n* = 6)	Trismus relieved, and a 12-fold reduction in VAS pain scores after MNB block
Maxillary nerve block	Double-blind RCT of bilateral suprazygomatic maxillary nerve block with 0.2% ropivacaine cf. placebo for cleft palate repair in children (*n* = 60)	The cumulative dose of intravenous morphine at 48 h postoperatively was 50% less in the maxillary nerve block group

(continued)

Table 20.1 (continued)

Target or local anesthetic (LA) technique, or both	Study	Outcome, findings, and comment
Infraorbital nerve block	Cochrane review of infraorbital nerve block in cleft lip repair ($n = 353$)	Low to very low-quality evidence that infraorbital nerve block reduces postoperative pain more than placebo or intravenous analgesia
	Retrospective study of infraorbital nerve block + subciliary infiltration to provide anesthesia for isolated orbital floor fracture ($n = 135$)	Able to assess globe movement during operation. Conversion to general anesthesia in four patients. Mean VAS for pain and discomfort
Scalp nerve block:	Meta-analysis of seven RCTs ($n = 320$) of scalp nerve block for pain after craniotomy	Studies are of limited methodological quality. However, postoperative pain is consistently reduced by scalp nerve block. This is associated with a concomitant reduction in opioid use in the first 24 h postoperatively
• Supratrochlear nerve • Supraorbital nerve • Auriculotemporal nerve • Great auricular nerve • Greater, lesser, and third occipital nerves		
Other blocks:		
• Palatine nerves—analgesia for cleft palate repair • Mental nerve—analgesia for surgery on lower lip, skin of chin • Superficial cervical plexus—anesthesia of external pinna, post-auricular, and temporoparietal areas of scalp, anterior neck and supraclavicular region		

Note: *cf* compared with, *LA* local anesthetic, *GA* general anesthetic, *RCT* randomized controlled trial, *VAS* visual analogue scale

doses are within recommendations [16] and susceptible patients are identified (the elderly, children, women in pregnancy, and those with a reduced level of alpha-1 antitrypsin), the risk can be reduced significantly.

20.3.4 Ketamine

NMDA receptors mediate central sensitization caused by nociceptive stimuli which are antagonized by ketamine. Thus, it reduces postoperative nausea and vomiting, rescue analgesia, patient-controlled opioid consumption, and the intensity of pain; and its effects last beyond its pharmacological duration [17–19]. 0.5 mg/kg is the lowest dose that has been shown to minimize psychokinetic effects. In addition to being increasingly used in anesthetic practice (particularly for painful operations), ketamine can reduce the need for opioids in opioid-tolerant patients and also have a beneficial effect in managing opioid-induced hyperalgesia [20, 21]. In dental practice, ketamine 0.5 mg/kg considerably reduces postoperative pain after the extraction of third molars whether it is given topically, submucosally, or intravenously [22–24].

20.3.5 Gabapentinoids

Patients at risk of severe acute postoperative pain are purported to benefit from gabapentin's and pregabalin's antineuropathic analgesic effects. Despite these findings, two meta-analyses of gabapentin and pregabalin use during surgery showed only marginal improvements in postoperative analgesia and increased risks of side effects [25, 26]. With pre-emptive pregabalin, there was a reduction in postoperative pain scores and opioid requirements following bimaxillary surgery ($n = 60$ patients) [27]. However, there is little evidence supporting the routine use of gabapentinoids following surgery.

20.3.6 Corticosteroids

Preoperative administration of corticosteroids, including dexamethasone and methylprednisolone, was suggested in oral surgery such as orthognathic and third molar surgery to decrease edema and pain, with no higher risk of infection and with a minimum risk of other side effects [28–30].

20.3.7 $\alpha 2$ Adrenoceptor Agonists

In addition to dexmedetomidine, clonidine is another common $\alpha 2$ agonist. A direct effect of their activity on $\alpha 2$ adrenoceptors in the central and peripheral nervous systems is the inhibition of pain transmission and sympathetic activity. The effects produced by these drugs include anxiolysis, analgesia, sympatholysis, sedation, and hypnosis on a pharmacological level. Combined use of these drugs, either orally or intravenously, orally or intravenously, reduced postoperative morphine consumption by 25% and 30%, respectively, according to a meta-analysis in 2012. Furthermore, both drugs significantly reduced visual analogue scores for acute pain, but this benefit dissipated within 48 h. The heterogeneity of the included studies prevented the meta-analysis from establishing optimal dosing regimens.

Clonidine was associated with clinically significant hypotension and bradycardia in the POISE-2 trial ($n = 10{,}010$). A planned subanalysis by the authors demonstrated that clonidine 0.2 mg given orally did not improve pain scores and did not increase morphine consumption; higher doses may provide analgesic benefits, but may also cause hypotension and bradycardia. The use of clonidine perioperatively was not justified based on the meta-analysis of the previous studies. Nevertheless, studies in 2013 found that dexmedetomidine in the operating room reduced postoperative pain and opioid consumption, though use of dexmedetomidine might be associated with a high risk of bradycardia.

20.4 Psychological and Physical Aspect of Pain Management

20.4.1 Relaxation

Relaxation techniques may be useful in managing postoperative pain, but more research is needed.

20.4.2 Hilotherapy

At 48–72 h postoperatively, heliotherapy, which applies cold compression through a facemask at a regulated temperature of 15 °C, significantly reduces pain and swelling. The efficacy of the therapy and its optimal duration need to be established in clinical trials.

20.4.3 Acupuncture

There are studies that examined oral and maxillofacial surgery patients who were treated with acupuncture postoperatively. Acupuncture has been shown to enhance endogenous opioids, such as daunorphan, endorphins, and enkephalins, and to release corticosteroids that relieve pain and accelerate the healing process [31].

20.5 Perioperative Pain Management Techniques

20.5.1 Patient-Controlled Analgesia, PCA

PCA is an analgesic device in which the healthcare provider pre-sets the mode of analgesic drug delivery according to patients' pain degree and other factors, and then leaves it to patients to control it by themselves. Among them, patient-controlled epidural analgesia (PCEA) and patient-controlled intravenous analgesia (PCIA) are the most widely used devices.

20.5.1.1 PCEA

PCEA uses a PCA device to deliver drugs into the epidural cavity and is primarily indicated for analgesia for pain in the chest and back region and below. In the PCEA protocol of local anesthetics compounded with opioids, the commonly used local anesthetics are 0.1% to 0.15% ropivacaine or 0.1%–0.12% bupivacaine, and the commonly used opioids and their usage are shown in Table 20.2. Specifically, 0.1% bupivacaine +2 μg/mL fentanyl or 0.3 μg/mL sufentanil is used as an example, and 0.9% saline is used to dilute to 250 mL. Analgesic pump parameters were set to an infusion rate of 2–5 mL/h, a single dose of 2–5 mL administered, and a lock time of 10–20 min.

20.5.1.2 PCIA

PCIA uses a PCA device to administer analgesics via the intravenous route, with more drugs available. However, due to systemic medication of PCIA, it has more adverse effects and its analgesia effect is slightly weaker than PCEA. Analgesic regimens for commonly used opioids in PCIA are shown in Table 20.3. For non-opioid-tolerant patients, setting a background dose for administration is not recommended, and instead multimodal analgesia is preferred.

Table 20.2 Commonly used opioids in PCEA

Opioids	Loading dose	Concentration (μg/mL)
Morphine	1–2 mg	20–40
Fentanyl	50–100 μg	2
Hydromorphone	0.2–0.5 mg	8–16
Sufentanil	10–20 μg	0.3–0.5

Table 20.3 Commonly used opioids in PCIA

Opioids	PCA bolus dose	Setting time (min)
Morphine	0.5–2.5 mg	5–10
Fentanyl	10–20 μg	4–10
Hydromorphone	0.05–0.25 mg	5–10
Oxycodone	0.2–0.4 mg	8–10
Sufentanil	2–5 μg	6–10

20.5.2 Ultrasound-Guided Nerve Block Technique

Nerve block analgesia reduces the central afferent of injurious stimuli with few adverse effects, and with the popularity of ultrasound technology, it has been widely used for general surgical perioperative analgesia [32]. Puncture site infection, severe deformity, and allergy to local anesthetics are contraindications to ultrasound-guided nerve blocks. Cervical plexus blocks provide excellent postoperative analgesia for head and neck surgery.

20.6 Summary

Patients and healthcare systems are affected significantly by acute postoperative pain. There is a growing body of evidence that supports multimodal analgesia, the use of two or more analgesics with different modes of action delivered through the same or different mechanisms. Postoperative complications, distress, duration of stay, and chronic postsurgical pain can be reduced substantially if patients are identified early, coordinated multidisciplinary interventions are implemented, and multimodal analgesia is administered.

Standardized and individualized perioperative pain management can help reduce patients' pain and accelerate their early feeding and activity, while lowering the incidence of postoperative complications. In clinical practice, effective perioperative pain management in oral and maxillofacial surgery requires the participation and collaboration of a multidisciplinary team of anesthesiologists, surgeons, and nurses to develop an individualized postoperative pain management plan based on different surgical procedures and the patients' own conditions, so that surgical patients can receive safe, effective, comfortable, and satisfactory analgesic treatment.

References

1. Coulthard P, Haywood D, Tai MA, et al. Treatment of postoperative pain in oral and maxillofacial surgery. Br J Oral Maxillofac Surg. 2000;38:588–92.
2. Moore RA, Derry S, Aldington D, et al. Single dose oral analgesics for acute postoperative pain in adults—an overview of Cochrane reviews. Cochrane Database Syst Rev. 2015;2015(9):CD008659. https://doi.org/10.1002/14651858.CD008659.pub3.
3. Ong CK, Seymour RA, Lirk P, et al. Combining paracetamol (acetaminophen) with nonsteroidal anti-inflammatory drugs: a qualitative systematic review of analgesic efficacy for acute postoperative pain. Anesth Analg. 2010;110:1170–9.
4. Gupta A, Bah M. NSAIDs in the treatment of postoperative pain. Curr Pain Headache Rep. 2016;20:62.
5. Non-steroidal anti-inflammatory drugs (NSAIDS): reminder on renal failure and impairment. Medications and Healthcare Products Regulatory Agency; 2009. https://www.gov.uk/drug-safety-update/non-steroidal-anti-inflammatory-drugs-nsaidsreminder-on-renal-failure-and-impairmen.
6. Hermanowski J, Levy N, Mills P, et al. Deprescribing: implications for the anaesthetist. Anaesthesia. 2017;72:565–9.
7. Drugs—codeine phosphate. In: British National Formulary. National Institute for Health and Care Excellence. n.d. https://bnf.nice.org.uk/drug/codeine-phosphate.html.
8. Chou R, Gordon DB, de Leon-Casasola OA, et al. Management of postoperative pain: a clinical practice guideline from the American Pain Society, the American Society of Regional Anesthesia and Pain Medicine, and the American Society of Anesthesiologists' Committee on Regional Anesthesia, Executive Committee, and Administrative Council. J Pain. 2016;17:131–57.
9. Coluzzi F, Bifulco F, Cuomo A, et al. The challenge of perioperative pain management in opioid-tolerant patients. Ther Clin Risk Manag. 2017;13:1163–73.
10. Pluijms WA, Steegers MA, Verhagen AF, et al. Chronic post-thoracotomy pain: a retrospective study. Acta Anaesthesiol Scand. 2006;50:804–8.
11. Simpson GK, Jackson M. Perioperative management of opioid-tolerant patients. BJA Educ. 2017;17:124–8.
12. Fletcher D, Martinez V. Opioid-induced hyperalgesia in patients after surgery: a systematic review and a meta-analysis. Br J Anaesth. 2014;112:991–1004.
13. Anantanarayanan P, Raja DK, Kumar JN, et al. Catheter-based donor site analgesia after rib grafting: a prospective, randomized, double-blinded clinical trial comparing ropivacaine and bupivacaine. J Oral Maxillofac Surg. 2013;71:29–34.
14. Kranke P, Jokinen J, Pace NL, et al. Continuous intravenous perioperative lidocaine infusion for postoperative pain and recovery. Cochrane Database Syst Rev. 2015;(7):CD009642.
15. Lee U, Choi YJ, Choi GJ, et al. Intravenous lidocaine for effective pain relief after bimaxillary surgery. Clin Oral Investig. 2017;21:2645–52.
16. Christie LE, Picard J, Weinberg GL. Local anaesthetic systemic toxicity. BJA Educ. 2015;15:136–42.
17. Wu CL, Raja SN. Treatment of acute postoperative pain. Lancet. 2011;377:2215–25.
18. Bell RF, Dahl JB, Moore RA, et al. Perioperative ketamine for acute postoperative pain. Cochrane Database Syst Rev. 2006;1:CD004603.
19. Gorlin AW, Rosenfeld DM, Ramakrishna H. Intravenous sub-anesthetic ketamine for perioperative analgesia. J Anaesthesiol Clin Pharmacol. 2016;32:160–7.
20. Farrington M, Hanson A, Laffoon T, et al. Low-dose ketamine infusions for postoperative pain in opioid-tolerant orthopaedic spine patients. J Perianesth Nurs. 2015;30:338–45.
21. Barreveld AM, Correll DJ, Liu X, et al. Ketamine decreases postoperative pain scores in patients taking opioids for chronic pain: results of a prospective, randomized, double-blind study. Pain Med. 2013;14:925–34.
22. Landari E, Hustveit O, Trumpy IG, et al. Ketamine as single dose analgesics on acute postoperative pain in both genders following surgical removals of third molars. J Oral Maxillofac Surg. 2013;71:e38.
23. Gönül O, Satilmis T, Ciftci A, et al. Comparison of the effects of topical ketamine and tramadol on postoperative pain after mandibular molar extraction. J Oral Maxillofac Surg. 2015;73:2103–7.
24. Hadhimane A, Shankariah M, Neswi KV. Pre-emptive analgesia with ketamine for relief of postoperative pain after surgical removal of impacted mandibular third molars. J Maxillofac Oral Surg. 2016;15:156–63.

25. Fabritius ML, Geisler A, Petersen PL, et al. Gabapentin for post-operative pain management—a systematic review with meta-analyses and trial sequential analyses. Acta Anaesthesiol Scand. 2016;60:1188–208.
26. Fabritius ML, Strøm C, Koyuncu S, et al. Benefit and harm of pregabalin in acute pain treatment: a systematic review with meta-analyses and trial sequential analyses. Br J Anaesth. 2017;119:775–91.
27. Ahiskalioglu A, Ince I, Aksoy M, et al. Effects of a single-dose of preemptive pregabalin on postoperative pain and opioid consumption after double-jaw surgery: a randomized controlled trial. J Oral Maxillofac Surg. 2016;74(53):e1–7.
28. Lima CA, Favarini VT, Torres AM, et al. Oral dexamethasone decreases postoperative pain, swelling, and trismus more than diclofenac following third molar removal: a randomized controlled clinical trial. Oral Maxillofac Surg. 2017;21:321–6.
29. Dan AE, Thygesen TH, Pinholt EM. Corticosteroid administration in oral and orthognathic surgery: a systematic review of the literature and meta-analysis. J Oral Maxillofac Surg. 2010;68:2207–20.
30. Ngeow WC, Lim D. Do corticosteroids still have a role in the management of third molar surgery? Adv Ther. 2016;33:1105–39.
31. Patil S, Sen S, Bral M, Reddy S, Bradley KK, Cornett EM, Fox CJ, Kaye AD. The role of acupuncture in pain management. Curr Pain Headache Rep. 2016;20(4):22. https://doi.org/10.1007/s11916-016-0552-1.
32. Rawal N. Current issues in postoperative pain management. Eur J Anaesthesiol. 2016;33(3):160–71.

21 Oral and Maxillofacial Surgical Intensive Care Unit

Ming Xia

21.1 Introduction

Surgical intensive care unit (SICU) is defined as a hospital unit designated for care of critically ill surgical patients. The SICU is a dedicated center for the treatment of critically ill surgical patients, located in the surgical ward, where surgical skills and equipment are pooled to provide treatment for critically ill surgical patients, such as severe hemorrhagic shock, serious surgical infections, post-surgical treatment, and organ transplants. The establishment of the SICU provides a strong guarantee for the treatment of critically ill surgical patients. As a relatively new concept, SICU differs from ICU in various aspects, which could be summarized as:

SICU: mainly for surgical patients, serious patients for relatively short period of stay, generally after the surgery, 1–2 days immediately can be transferred out of the ICU, but the condition of these patients changes a lot, especially after cardiac surgery of such patients, to the cardiac surgery SICU, from the monitoring should be very important, including postoperative bleeding. Because postoperative patients are most afraid of bleeding, low blood pressure, to strengthen monitoring, the first time to take appropriate treatment measures, to be able to minimize, reduce the time of post-surgical patients in the ICU.

ICU: usually a comprehensive ICU for both medical and surgical patients, but there may be more medical patient, and these patients may require long-term stay in ICU for resuscitation treatment.

This chapter focuses on the postoperative care in SICU, especially procedures that are required because of the characteristics of oral and maxillofacial surgeries.

21.2 Postoperative Care

21.2.1 Monitoring in the SICU

The main content of SICU work is to apply advanced monitoring and life support techniques to continuously and dynamically monitor the physiological functions of patients qualitatively and/or quantitatively, to assess their pathophysiological status, severity of illness and urgency of treatment, to provide standardized, high-quality life support, and to improve the success rate of life-saving treatment. Purposes of monitoring in the SICU are:

M. Xia (✉)
Department of Anesthesiology, Shanghai Ninth People's Hospital Affiliated to Shanghai Jiao Tong University School of Medicine, Shanghai, China
e-mail: xiaming1980@xzhmu.edu.cn

H. Jiang, M. Xia (eds.), *Anesthesia for Oral and Maxillofacial Surgery*,
https://doi.org/10.1007/978-981-19-7287-4_21

1. Early detection of high-risk factors that seriously threaten patients' lives and timely interventions to avoid further deterioration of the disease state are especially important for high-risk patients.
2. Continuous evaluation of organ function status to discover early evidence of organ function damage and to provide a basis for prevention and treatment of organ function damage.
3. To assess the severity of the primary disease. Through continuous and dynamic monitoring and examination combined with medical history, more accurate assessment of disease severity and its changes can predict the development trend and prognosis of critically ill patients.
4. To guide the diagnosis and differential diagnosis of diseases based on monitoring data and biochemical information.
5. Adopt goal-directed therapeutic approach to readily adjust the treatment plan (e.g., treatment and intervention strategies, drug dose and rate, etc.) based on continuously monitored physiological parameters and their response to treatment, with a view to achieving target physiological status. For example, goal-directed therapy in patients with severe systemic infections and infectious shock is a way to achieve a significant reduction in morbidity and mortality in patients with severe infections by using certain target physiological parameter values to guide the continuous revision of the treatment approach [1]. Goal-directed therapy based on close monitoring of critically ill patients is one of the important features of SICU treatment.

21.2.2 Special Postoperative Treatment Required for Oral and Maxillofacial Surgical Patient

After the removal of intraoral lesion, patients need to keep their mouth clean and use mouthwash for oral care: if necessary, intraoral fasting should be replaced by nasal fluid: local braking should be applied to the head for free flap repair to prevent torsion or compression of the vascular tip: the color change of the flap should be observed regularly to correctly determine the vascular crisis, and once the vascular crisis occurs, surgical exploration should be performed in a timely manner. After the formation of dead space after lesion removal, attention should be paid to the correct establishment of drainage to prevent the formation of effusion and infection of the surgical wound, and the amount and color change of the drainage fluid should be observed, and salivary fistula and celiac leakage, even the occurrence or formation of celiac chest, should be paid attention to during the neck surgery. When the flap survives, it needs to be treated with proper pressure dressing according to the situation to eliminate the dead cavity and deal with salivary fistula or celiac leakage. Fasting and parenteral nutrition are required in cases of celiac disease.

21.2.3 Hypoproteinemia

Hypoproteinemia after oral and maxillofacial surgery is commonly caused by the following factors: (1) insufficient protein intake or malabsorption; (2) reduced protein synthesis; as surgery puts the body in a state of stress, the liver synthesizes more acute temporal proteins, while plasma proteins and other synthesis are reduced, causing hypoproteinemia in the mouth of the patient; (3) large amounts of protein loss: oral and maxillofacial surgery has large traumatic surfaces and more tissue exudate, which can lead to large amounts of plasma protein loss; (4) accelerated protein catabolism: After surgery, the body is in a state of stress, energy is obtained by large amounts of protein catabolism, urinary nitrogen excretion increases, branched chain amino acids in the blood are elevated, and there is a negative nitrogen balance.

Hypoproteinemia can cause a decrease in plasma colloid osmotic pressure, causing a large amount of fluid to be retained in the interstitial space of tissues, reducing the effective circulating blood volume, leading to an increase in blood viscosity, further promoting microcirculatory disorders, seeking insufficient perfusion of important organs, and causing multi-organ insufficiency. In addition, a decrease in serum albumin can lead to a decrease in various enzymes required for antibody synthesis and a decrease in enzyme activity, resulting in a decrease in the immunity of the organism, an increase in the chance of infection, difficulty or delay in wound healing, and even aggravation of the disease.

After surgery, the plasma albumin level should be routinely monitored. Severe hypoproteinemia requires intravenous plasma or human albumin 10 g/d, high-protein food, preferably high-quality vegetable protein, and high-energy food are recommended, so that the daily intake of protein cluster 60–80 g can be guaranteed [2].

21.2.4 Nutritional Considerations

Oral and maxillofacial surgery patients are often restricted from eating normally because the surgical site is mostly related to the oral cavity, and as we all know, the first step of human digestion process is carried out in the oral cavity. Therefore, once the disease occurs in the oral cavity, the digestive function of the oral cavity will not be carried out normally. However, the secretion of digestive juices and intestinal absorption function of such patients are no different from those of normal people, which requires that the diet for patients with oral diseases must be configured according to these characteristics. For example, the food should be made fine and soft, so that it can be swallowed directly without chewing, but the required amount of nutrition should be ensured, which is related to the success of the surgery and the recovery of the wound and physique after the surgery.

1. High-calorie, high-protein meal. The surgery can lead to heat consumption regardless of the size; therefore, the supply of energy must be increased for patients. Protein is the raw material for renewal and repair of wounded tissues. Due to the increase of protein exuded from wound surface and surgical catabolism after surgery, if protein intake is not paid attention to, it will lead to the decrease of blood volume, plasma protein, wound healing ability, and immune function. Therefore, a high-calorie, high-protein meal must be supplied after surgery.
2. Sufficient carbohydrates. Carbohydrates are the main source of energy, accounting for 60–70% of the total caloric energy: if the intake of carbohydrates is not paid attention to after surgery, dietary protein can be consumed as caloric energy, which is unfavorable to the patient's recovery [3]. In addition, carbohydrates are easy to digest and absorb, which is especially suitable for those with poor digestive function after surgery.
3. Vitamins and minerals are indispensable. Vitamins are closely related to the healing of trauma and surgical wounds. In patients with good nutritional status, the postoperative water-soluble vitamins are 2–3 times larger than normal, while the supply of fat-soluble vitamins need not be too much [4]. B vitamins are closely related to carbohydrate metabolism and have great influence on wound healing. Minerals are indispensable for maintaining normal physiological function and metabolism. Surgery results in protein loss and increased excretion of some elements; thus special attention should be paid to patients' vitamin and mineral supplementation after surgery and during recovery.

21.3 Handoff

Intensive care units are more likely than other units to experience adverse events as a result of medical errors, especially due to insufficient handoffs with healthcare providers from the operating room to the intensive care unit. Aside from invasive hemodynamic monitoring and high-risk medications, SICU patients are also subjected to frequent surgical procedures. The failure of communication was found to be responsible for nearly 15% of adverse events after surgery. Standards-based checklist-driven handoff processes can improve the quality of information exchange during handoff, as well as minimize extraneous diagnostic testing and procedures [5]. In addition, handoffs among healthcare providers can provide opportunities for clinical review and teaching. In order to ensure patient safety, precise communication between the teams is crucial.

In order to promote patient safety and improve the quality of handoff, structured reporting tools are required to facilitate information transfer and sequenced tasks. In order to ensure a seamless and safe transition in care, a comprehensive handoff allows for a review of perioperative events and development of a shared understanding of what to expect after the operation. Formalized verbal communication can be facilitated by written handoff documents. With these communication scripts, teams are able to avoid omissions and know exactly what information they should provide and at what time. Having the right teamwork can help to shift the focus of healthcare to safety, as stated by TeamSTEPPS (Team Strategies & Tools to Enhance Performance & Patient Safety) [6]. By documenting critical points of the verbal handoff, a written report provides subsequent caregivers with a full understanding of the patient's procedure and plan.

Postoperative patient handoffs have been shown to improve patient safety in a systematic review conducted by Segall et al. [7]. They also noted that identifying ways to improve the handoff process and studying its effects were necessary in order to determine whether poor-quality handoffs are associated with adverse events. A study conducted by another group [8] evaluated the results through direct observation and focus groups rather than anonymous surveys. They concluded that they:

> … were unable to examine the effects of the [handover] redesign process on patient outcomes. However, improved team behaviors, reduced workload, and improved staff satisfaction … have all been linked to improved quality of care and patient outcomes in other care settings.

A SICU's handoff process also requires a close understanding of human factors science and engineering. It is unlikely that training on postoperative handoff alone will result in changes in behavior and improve patient safety. Changing people's behavior is not the same as fixing problems according to human factors science. Instead, it is about changing the design of the system in order to assist people in their work. Creating a new postoperative handoff structure through the intervention changed the system. Roles were assigned, tools were created, and visual cues were provided that redesigned the framework in which postoperative handoff occurred.

The current consensus is that patient safety cannot be achieved without leadership support, communication, and teamwork, and that this requires multidisciplinary collaboration. Therefore, wherever such interventions need to be attempted, a multidisciplinary approach to design and implementation should be taken to best achieve success.

21.4 Ethical Issues

The development of the modern SICU brings with it not only the opportunity to survive for the critically ill patient, but also a complex set of interpersonal relationships that look very different from the traditional surgeon-patient relationship. The most prominent players in decision-making regarding SICU patients include the patients themselves, the surgeons, and the intensivists. New interpersonal relationships create new ethical issues, and at the heart of the most challenging ethical situation in the SICU is the question of when to transition from curative to palliative care models for postoperative patients nearing the end of life. In this decision, the judgment of both the surgeon and the intensivist is based on the relationship that exists between them and the patient, and in the next section, the elements related to this decision are elaborated.

21.4.1 Ethical Issues Between the Patient and the Surgeon

Surgeons' work ethic and personality traits have been extensively studied. There is a high level of time commitment required in surgical residencies, as they are among the longest in duration and hours. The surgeon also has direct contact with his or her patients, so he or she has a strong sense of personal responsibility for the surgical outcomes.

Under what circumstances do the surgeon and patient meet significantly shapes their relationship. Emergency surgery is clearly distinguished from elective surgery. Outpatient consultations are required by surgeons in preparation for elective cases. There is a high likelihood of patients being ambulatory, cognitively intact, and able to participate actively in discussions about surgery. The surgeon becomes familiar with the patient as a whole person through the process. The surgeon listens to how the patient describes themselves—where they are from, what they do, and who they trust to accompany them; they also hear their clinical and personal history, which will inform the surgeon's interactions with them.

In addition, a patient's autonomous decisions play a role in balancing health risk and health benefit. The risk of short-term respiratory compromise and death may outweigh the benefit of long-term cancer-free survival, for example, if a patient with chronic lung disease refuses all mechanical ventilation during the postoperative period. The report shows that some surgeons refuse to perform surgery altogether when a patient requests that life-sustaining postoperative treatments be limited. Patients with terminal illnesses may be allowed more rights to limit life-sustaining therapies by individual surgeons than those with better prospects. The patient's autonomy may be compromised by these judgments, as the patient has no option to modify his or her treatment goals in response to postoperative results.

The surgeon-patient relationship must also consider surgical error. A surgeon's perception of error has a profoundly negative psychological effect that has been known for some time. Work ethic plays a critical role in assuming full responsibility for complications and patient ownership. At morbidity and mortality conferences, Bosk described an atmosphere in which the attending surgeon is expected to apologize for his failure to achieve a better clinical outcome. The act of wearing a hair shirt is referred to as "wearing the hair shirt" by Bosk. According to the 1995 Institute of Medicine report, To Err is Human [9], medical errors have devastating effects on healthcare in the United States, which have contributed to the success of patient safety movements and resident work hour restrictions. According to a nationwide survey, surgeon burnout and suicidal ideation are linked to emotional distress caused by perceived medical errors.

A surgeon's relationship with a critically ill patient is established in a rather different context when they meet in the emergency department. This encounter presents two particularly challenging aspects. The first thing to note is that time is often limited due to the urgent need for assessment and intervention in surgical emergencies. Second, surgeons and patients are usually meeting for the first time in an emotional situation with no prior understanding of each other. When a previously healthy patient is found to have a disease that can be cured by surgery, emergency surgery is usually favored. However, when a surgical emergency occurs in an elderly patient or a patient with severe, preexisting chronic illnesses, surgical decision-making is more complex.

In emergency situations, preoperative protocols may change, and personal responsibility for the outcome of the procedure may be diminished because the surgeon does not have a good understanding of the patient's underlying disease process and overall level of recovery at the time of intake—for example, the thought may arise that "because of lack of knowledge, there's nothing that can be done about it." Often, it is natural for surgeons to want to communicate with members of the surgical team and the patient's family about possible postoperative complications and the need for extended life support after surgery, but this may be less likely to be done fully in the acute care setting. Given the emotions of the patient and family, some surgeons may avoid detailing all possible outcomes, preferring instead to emphasize the need for immediate surgery to come and keep the patient alive to avoid creating a tense atmosphere. However, others may exaggerate the risks and shift the blame for negative outcomes to the decision maker, excusing the surgeon. If the prognosis for surgery is not favorable or if the postoperative response is poor, patients should also be able to accept the option of undergoing surgery first while retaining the goal of diversionary care. Interestingly, there is evidence that physicians performing high-risk surgery are indeed more comfortable withdrawing life-sustaining therapies after emergency surgery than after elective surgery.

21.4.2 Ethical Issues Between the Patient and the Intensivist

There are two physicians who manage SICU patients, the surgeon and the intensivist, and the two are partners in medical decision-making. Decades ago, the number of intensivists with basic anesthesiology or surgical training was small, and that the number has not risen very significantly to date. However, regardless of education, the role they play in patient management as intensivists is unique.

A critical care physician often manages multiple critically ill patients at the same time, and therefore may refuse to transfer a patient to the SICU if he or she determines that the patient does not meet certain criteria for clinical severity, a judgment that takes into account available resources. Beds, care, medications, and supplies are important resources, but they are limited in number and must be reserved for those who would benefit most, thus requiring appropriate triage to minimize the mortality of patients entering the SICU. Arguably, critical care physicians will more often weigh the duty to promote what is beneficial, normal, and respectful, and also more often take into account the fourth bioethical principle, justice.

Unlike surgeons, intensivists fight more against pain than against death. In their view, if there is difficulty in extending life, then extending life for a patient is not a heroic act, but rather a disrespect for life, as well as a huge expense to the patient and his or her family. This view values the quality of life over the quantity of life. However, judgments about quality of life are inherently subjective, and what the intensivist thinks is not representative of the patient, and sometimes even detrimental to the patient's rights—because the patient's right to decide what constitutes "quality of life" is taken away from him or her.

In addition, shifts are common in the SICU, and this shift system creates a unique feature of the ICU-patient relationship in that the ICU physician has less time to actually see the patient. In contrast, a surgeon performing elective surgery meets with the patient during the preoperative interview and also sees his or her illness firsthand in the operating room and follows up postoperatively. In addition, the varying management styles of intensivists, coupled with the fact that there is rarely a standard household handoff between intensivists, make it possible for the medical service plan to change significantly from week to week. This has led some to propose continuity of care as an indicator of quality of end-of-life care in the intensive care unit. Some evidence does suggest that fragmentation of care, i.e., the proportion of care provided by physicians other than the primary resident, can significantly increase length of stay. However, like surgeons, intensivists face ethical pressures: they need to provide the best possible care while preventing fatigue from uninterrupted work.

21.4.3 Ethical Issues Between the Surgeon and the Intensivist

The organizational structure of the SICU determines the dynamic relationship between the surgeon and the intensivist. If the SICU has a more open organizational structure, the surgeon remains in charge of the patient's postoperative care and the intensivist is responsible for making recommendations, whereas in a closed or intensivist-dominated organizational structure, the intensivist takes over the primary care of the patient and the responsibility for making recommendations is divided between the surgeons. In addition, there is a hybrid organizational structure that allows two primary care physicians to collaborate in the patient's care. The closed organizational structure has been found to reduce mortality and improve resource utilization based on previous experience; however, it can also lead to divergent physician opinions—in closed SICUs, 60% of surgeons report conflicts, while in open SICUs, only 41% report conflicts [10]. Intensivist-led care is now increasingly being used as a measure of quality, and thus surgeons and intensivists will need to work together more often in the future.

Suppose an elderly patient with multiple medical conditions undergoes a high-risk elective procedure and develops complications that require intensive care management. Two weeks have passed with no improvement in ventilator settings and a tracheotomy must be considered. Start manual feeding or initiate total parenteral nutrition via a central line. Small doses of vasoconstrictor, intermittent dialysis, or other intensive therapy may also be required. This is a classic case that can cause a difference of opinion between surgeons and intensivists [11]—whether the goal of medical care is to cure the patient's disease or to ensure the patient's comfort. In this case, the surgeon adheres to the preoperative protocol and does his best to get the patient through the dangerous postoperative period and to restore the quality of life to the extent possible. However, in the opinion of the intensivist, the patient's limited baseline functional status is unlikely to be restored, while other patients may benefit more from intensive care resources, so they are not inclined to allocate resources such as care, medications, and transfusions to a patient with a poor expected outcome, a practice that could be considered wasteful or even futile in their view.

Perhaps it should also be noted that today, the number of intensivists is still steadily increasing, and this trend may finally bridge the divide between surgeons and intensivists. Medical care in the SICU, led by intensivists, can reduce post-trauma mortality. Based on their education and training, intensivists may have a better understanding of surgical pathology, details of intraoperative procedures, and expected outcomes. Also, as physicians with specialized training in critical care management, they may have a better understanding of the limited resources of the SICU and the pain caused by repeated invasive procedures of unknown benefit. Arguably, and perhaps as some have suggested, surgical intensivists may be uniquely qualified to select management plans for critically ill surgical patients. However, further research is still needed to understand surgical intensivists' negotiation of end-of-life issues and the relatively new relationship between primary surgeons and surgical intensivists [10].

References

1. Hotchkiss RS, Moldawer LL, Opal SM, Reinhart K, Turnbull IR, Vincent JL. Sepsis and septic shock. Nat Rev Dis Primers. 2016;2:16045. https://doi.org/10.1038/nrdp.2016.45.
2. Liumbruno GM, Bennardello F, Lattanzio A, Piccoli P, Rossettias G, Italian Society of Transfusion Medicine and Immunohaematology (SIMTI). Recommendations for the use of albumin and immunoglobulins. Blood Transfusion = Trasfusione del sangue. 2009;7(3):216–34. https://doi.org/10.2450/2009.0094-09.
3. Lim HS, Kim YJ, Lee J, Yoon SJ, Lee B. Establishment of adequate nutrient intake criteria to achieve target weight loss in patients undergoing bariatric surgery. Nutrients. 2020;12(6):1774. https://doi.org/10.3390/nu12061774.
4. Molnar JA, Underdown MJ, Clark WA. Nutrition and chronic wounds. Adv Wound Care. 2014;3(11):663–81. https://doi.org/10.1089/wound.2014.0530.
5. Talley D, Dunlap E, Silverman D, Katzer S, Huffines M, Dove C, Anders M, Galvagno S, Tisherman S. Improving postoperative handoff in a surgical intensive care unit. Crit Care Nurse. 2019;39(5):e13–21.
6. Wolk CB, Stewart RE, Cronholm P, Eiraldi R, Salas E, Mandell DS. Adapting TeamSTEPPS for school mental health teams: a pilot study. Pilot Feasibility Stud. 2019;17:5–148. PMID: 31890260; PMCID: PMC6918659. https://doi.org/10.1186/s40814-019-0529-z.
7. Segall N et al. Operating room-to-ICU patient handovers: a multidisciplinary human-centered design approach. Jt Comm J Qual Patient Saf. 2016;42(9):400–14. https://doi.org/10.1016/S1553-7250(16)42081-7.
8. Rosen MA, DiazGranados D, Dietz AS, Benishek LE, Thompson D, Pronovost PJ, Weaver SJ. Teamwork in healthcare: key discoveries enabling safer, high-quality care. Am Psychol. 2018;73(4):433–50. https://doi.org/10.1037/amp0000298.
9. Stelfox HT, Palmisani S, Scurlock C, Orav EJ, Bates DW. The "To Err is Human" report and the patient safety literature. Qual Saf Health Care. 2006;15(3):174–8. https://doi.org/10.1136/qshc.2006.017947.
10. Sur MD, Angelos P. Ethical issues in surgical critical care: the complexity of interpersonal relationships in the surgical intensive care unit. J Intensive Care Med. 2016;31(7):442–50. Epub 2015 May 19. https://doi.org/10.1177/0885066615585953.
11. Tandukar S, Palevsky PM. Continuous renal replacement therapy: who, when, why, and how. Chest. 2019;155(3):626–38. https://doi.org/10.1016/j.chest.2018.09.004.

22 Nursing Considerations for Oral and Maxillofacial Surgical Patient

Yuelai Yang

22.1 Introduction

Painless surgery is now possible thanks to anesthesia. Anesthesia as a specialty was first practiced by nurse anesthetists in the 1800s when they administered anesthesia to wounded soldiers on the battlefields of the American Civil War [1]. During every surgical procedure, the surgical team will consider all aspects of the patient's well-being. A nurse anesthetist will be available to closely monitor the patient's vital signs when the surgeon is removing a mass, for example. During the surgical procedure, the anesthetist and surgeon will communicate with one another to ensure that the patient is responding well. A nurse anesthetist, however, does much more than the example written above. Nurse anesthetists are involved in the whole perioperative period, and this chapter explains in detail a nurse anesthetist's role in oral and maxillofacial surgeries.

Y. Yang (✉)
Department of Intensive Care Unit, Shanghai Ninth People's Hospital Affiliated to Shanghai Jiao Tong University School of Medicine, Shanghai, China

22.2 Pre-anesthesia Visit and Care for Oral Surgery

22.2.1 Pre-anesthesia Visit

Pre-anesthesia visit of nurse anesthetists mainly includes pre-anesthesia assessment and pre-anesthesia education. Every patient is nervous and fearful of surgical anesthesia, so the key to successful treatment is to fully mobilize the patient's subjective initiative and make them cooperate with anesthesia and surgery actively. The nurse anesthetist needs to make a pre-anesthesia visit 1 day before surgery to make another comprehensive assessment of the patient's condition, and the pre-anesthesia visit is also a good time to communicate with the patient.

22.2.1.1 Purpose of Pre-anesthesia Visit

1. Through the pre-anesthesia visit, the nurse anesthetist can conduct a comprehensive pre-anesthesia assessment of the patient, and provide personalized pre-anesthesia education to the patient according to the risk factors in the assessment results.
2. Through effective communication, the patients are guided to cooperate with anesthesia and informed of relevant precautions during the perianesthesia period, thus their pre-anesthesia anxiety and fear can be relieved.

H. Jiang, M. Xia (eds.), *Anesthesia for Oral and Maxillofacial Surgery*,
https://doi.org/10.1007/978-981-19-7287-4_22

3. Based on the assessment and mastery of the basic conditions of the patient, improve the pre-anesthesia preparation and formulate the corresponding perianesthesia care plan in order to implement proper care, take effective care measures, and actively prevent the occurrence of related complications.

22.2.1.2 Contents of the Pre-anesthesia Visit

1. Review medical history. Read the medical record, contact with the doctor in charge and the nurse in charge, and understand all the medical information and general conditions of the patient, including the diagnosis of the disease, the name of the proposed operation, the site of the operation, the duration of the operation, the mode of anesthesia, vital signs, etc., and ask the patient's personal history, past history, allergy history, current medical history, and the history of surgical anesthesia in a targeted manner.
2. Airway assessment. The most important part of a pre-anesthesia visit for oral surgery patients is to identify injuries to the upper airway or anatomical abnormalities of the upper airway. Adequate pre-anesthesia airway assessment is an important tool for timely detection of difficult airway, reducing the occurrence of unanticipated difficult airway, and is also a prerequisite for proper management of difficult airway and adequate preparation, especially for oral surgery patients, we need to do adequate and effective pre-anesthesia airway assessment.
3. Overall assessment. Establish a good nurse–patient relationship and strengthen the communication and interaction between the patient and the anesthesia nurse. Observe and examine the general physical condition of the patient, such as observing whether there is stunting, nutritional disorders, anemia, dehydration, swelling, fever, and impaired consciousness, measuring height and weight, understanding the recent weight change, asking female patients whether they are in menstruation, checking the functional status of important organs of the patient, and checking the laboratory test results. Overall assessment of the patient is performed to fully grasp the patient's situation and better prepare for surgical anesthesia. Assess the patient's psychological state and degree of cooperation, evaluate the patient's and family members' concerns and specific requirements about anesthesia and surgery, and provide timely and appropriate explanations.
4. Health education. Provide personalized pre-anesthesia education to patients and encourage patients to participate in the development of preoperative anesthesia care plans; encourage patients to improve their self-life skills and participate in postoperative care, such as abdominal breathing, coughing, and lying down, to enhance patients' confidence in surgical anesthesia and recovery, thereby accelerating postoperative recovery; clarify the exact duration of water and food fasting for patients; provide patients with humane care, and, for example, change the clothes and pants equipped by the hospital, do not wear jewelry or other accessories, remove the movable denture, and do not bring valuable items such as watches to the operating room.

After the visit, the risk of surgical anesthesia is combined with various patient information, including past medical history, physical and laboratory test results, and a comprehensive assessment is made to finally assess the patient's anesthetic tolerance and general condition. The best nursing care plan and crisis contingency plan measures are formulated for the possible foreseeable problems during the perianesthesia period, so as to lay a good foundation for guaranteeing the quality and safety of perianesthesia care [2].

22.2.2 Pre-anesthesia Psychological Care

Psychological care and pre-anesthesia preparation should be combined together, and the nurse anesthetist should take corresponding psychological care measures according to the individual. It is necessary to understand and assess the patient's anxiety and worry factors, and give the correct psychological care for the patient's anxiety and worry. Patients should be introduced to the necessity of anesthesia and surgery in easy-to-understand language, and the necessity of pre-anesthesia preparation should be explained to patients, and the anesthesia plan and the points that require patients' cooperation should be explained to patients in an individualized manner.

Oral surgery patients, especially those with congenital oral and maxillofacial deformities, often have obvious psychological barriers due to deformities in head and facial appearance or physiological dysfunction; for patients who have undergone surgical treatment several times, the painful experience and memories of surgical anesthesia can cause extreme fear and rejection of surgery again; elderly patients can become overly concerned about the development of their condition and health status, resulting in anxiety, depression, and other emotional changes. Therefore, for the many psychological problems that may occur in oral surgery patients, anesthesia nurses should pay great attention to them, do a good job of patient and detailed explanation, establish a good nurse-patient relationship with patients and their families, and obtain their cooperation.

For the psychological care of children, first of all, the psychological state of the child's family needs to be regulated. Nurse anesthetists need to understand the anxiety of the family and the fear of the child, put themselves in each other's shoes, and do a good job in the dual psychological care of the family and the child, which also requires that the nurse anesthetists involved in the preoperative visit must have high comprehensive quality. The nurse anesthetists can provide cartoon posters as well as picture books or animated videos for surgical anesthesia education to the family and the child, so that they can understand the family's concerns in time and make a good introduction. According to the dependence of the child on the family, especially the mother, the child's family is allowed to accompany the child in the waiting area to enhance the child's sense of security.

22.3 Preparation for Care Before Anesthesia for Oral Surgery

Safety of surgical patients is the most important issue in perioperative medicine and a key factor affecting surgical treatment. Starting from the perspective of anesthesia nursing, accurate and comprehensive preoperative assessment and risk prediction are the key measures to adequately prepare for surgery, develop effective anesthesia care plans to cope with various risks, and thus reduce the complication and morbidity and mortality rates during the perianesthesia period and improve the safety of perioperative patients. Nurse anesthetists need to fully assess the risk of patients' own factors, surgical risks and anesthesia risks, among which the anesthesia nursing risk factors include: improper pre-anesthesia assessment, inadequate anesthesia nursing preparation, anesthesia nursing operation and anesthesia operation nursing coordination errors, improper anesthesia nursing management, anesthesia mechanical equipment failure, and lack of appropriate experience and technical level of anesthesia nursing staff.

Oral surgery is extensive, and anesthesia has its own unique features. The characteristics of oral surgery patients [3, 4] include: (1) the patients' age span is large and can occur at any age, with a high proportion of pediatric and elderly people, ranging from 1-week newborns to super senior citizens over 100 years old; (2) difficult airways are very common and serious, and at the same time, the oral and maxillofacial areas are adjacent to the respiratory tract, and surgical and anesthetic operations often interfere with each other; (3) patients not only have oral and maxillofacial malformations, but also may be accompanied by other important organ deformities and serious physiological disorders caused by these defects; (4) oral surgery diseases are closely related to psychological problems, and anesthesia requires smooth and complete analgesia. For this reason, before the start of anesthesia, the anesthesia nurse should make an accurate and comprehensive assessment and risk prediction, develop an effective anesthesia care plan, and make adequate pre-anesthesia preparations.

22.3.1 Preparation of Drugs Before Anesthesia

Before induction of anesthesia, the nurse anesthetist must prepare the relevant anesthetic drugs properly, which also ensures the safety of the whole anesthetic process. Usually the drugs before anesthesia for oral surgery are intravenous anesthetic drugs, muscle relaxant drugs, sedative and analgesic drugs, and antagonistic drugs, inhalation anesthetic drugs, and conventional resuscitation drugs, etc.

1. The operator must do a good job of checking and verifying the drugs, and maintain the principle of aseptic operation.
2. Reasonably draw and dilute the medicine according to the doctor's prescription, label the medicine with the corresponding label, indicate the dosage, keep the ampoule, fix it on the needle cap, and do "one person, one needle, one tube" with clear label, clear dosage and traceability.
3. After double-checking, place the drugs in the sterile treatment tray for backup, and pay attention to separate vasoactive drugs from sedative and analgesic drugs and muscle relaxants to avoid confusion.
4. Nurse anesthetists should be familiar with the usage, pharmacological effects, adverse reactions, and contraindications of commonly used anesthesia-related drugs. When using intravenous anesthetics, muscle relaxants, cardiac drugs, and vasoactive drugs, push them slowly, and closely observe changes in blood pressure and heart rate to ensure safety.
5. Syringes that need to be clamped on the microinjection pump should be connected to the extension tube and connected to the rehydration circuit to drain the air from the connection site and prevent air from entering the blood vessels.
6. Strictly implement the management of narcotic drugs and conduct regular training on the management of narcotic drugs. Strictly implement the norms for the storage of narcotic drugs and Class I psychotropic substances, and each link should be assigned to a person in charge, with clear responsibilities and shift handover records. The establishment of anesthesia induction room, the storage of narcotic drugs, Class I psychotropic substances should be equipped with the necessary anti-theft facilities in accordance with the norms. When dispensing narcotic drugs and Class I psychotropic substances for injection, empty ampoules should be retrieved, batch numbers and quantities should be checked and records should be kept. The remaining narcotic drugs and Class I psychotropic substances should be strictly implemented for the return procedures [5].

22.3.2 Preparation of Instruments and Tools Before Anesthesia

1. Difficult airway supplies: laryngoscope, guiding wire, fiberoptic bronchoscope, visual laryngoscope, laryngeal mask, etc.
2. Transnasal intubation: laryngeal nebulizer, lidocaine, intubation forceps, dental pads for backup, appropriate type of reinforced catheter or transnasal shaped catheter, etc.
3. Disposable items related to the respiratory tract, including breathing circuits, tracheal tubes, artificial noses, dental pads, tracheal fixators, suction tubes, oxygen masks, ventilation tracts, tracheal intubation replacement guidewires, etc.
4. Disposable items related to intravenous access, including central venipuncture kits, arterial indwelling needles, pressure monitoring sensors, analgesic pumps, tee, connecting tubes, etc.
5. Anesthesia equipment should be inspected before anesthesia, and it should be ensured that the anesthesia machine is in a standby state to ensure its normal operation during use, so as to guarantee the safety of patients. Focus on checking: (1) circulatory system; (2) inhalation evaporation system; (3) ventilator system; (4) flow meter, hand control and machine control; (5) main screen display; (6) monitoring and supervision system.
6. The working status of the monitors should be checked before the patient enters the room, and the time and parameters of the instruments and equipment should be checked and calibrated and recorded. The cardiac monitor includes heart rate, respiration, non-invasive blood pressure, body temperature, oxygen saturation, pulse rate; multi-functional monitoring instruments include invasive pressure, partial pressure of end-expiratory carbon dioxide, inotropic monitoring, EEG monitoring, etc.

22.3.3 Preparation of Patients Before Anesthesia

1. Check the information related to the patient, including: patient identification, anesthesia mode, surgical mode, surgical site, and related operations to be carried out; the patient brings the necessary emergency medicine, preoperative airway inflammation control, auscultation of bilateral lung breath sounds, airway assessment, etc. We also should provide psychological care to the patients.
2. Check the patient's vital signs, the presence of respiratory inflammation, ask the patient if there are any combined respiratory diseases, etc.
3. Evaluate the airway, mouth, and nasal cavity to see if the lesion affects intubation, and prepare intubation materials (materials related to difficult airway awake intubation or transnasal intubation) as required.
4. Establish a sense of mutual trust in pediatric patients so that anesthetic operations can be performed smoothly.

22.4 Monitoring Care During Oral Surgery Anesthesia

During the perianesthesia period, nurse anesthetists need to provide overall patient-centered care to patients throughout the entire process. The "Active-PATIENT evaluation and monitoring system" can be used to provide dynamic, circular, comprehensive, and efficient anesthesia evaluation and monitoring care for patients in real time, so that the workflow of nurse anesthetists can be more standardized, thus ensuring the safety of perianesthesia care.

22.4.1 Personnel Management and Responsibilities

The ratio of the configuration of anesthesia nurses in the operating room to the actual number of open operating rooms is $\geq 0.5:1$, and each nurse anesthetist is responsible for the management of the corresponding operating room, actively and closely observing the progress of surgical anesthesia and making relevant preparations for the implementation of the next anesthesia plan.

22.4.2 Key Points of Nursing Care During Anesthesia

22.4.2.1 P: Patient, Position, Protect

The nurse anesthetist needs to verify and confirm the basic information and physical condition of the patient under surgical anesthesia before each operation, including the history of drug allergy, the classification of physical condition, the patient's anesthesia duration, and the progress of surgery. The nurse anesthetist should work with the operating room nurse to keep the skin clean and remove blood from the face in a timely manner according to the patient's physical condition, nutritional status, skin condition, and position. Assess the patient and develop an individualized care plan for pressure injury prevention, e.g., oral surgery patients with more frequent transnasal tracheal intubation should be fully considered for protection against nasal pressure injury, and in addition, their care plan should also consider the impact of body position on the airway and the assessment of the impact on the maintenance period of anesthesia.

22.4.2.2 A: Airway

Keep the airway open to prevent hypoxia and carbon dioxide accumulation. Oral surgery patients have greater difficulty in maintaining airway patency due to the specificity of the disease or surgical site. Generally, the anesthetist is far away from the patient's head, the tracheal tube is fixed by the surgeon, and the tube is prone to displacement and bending during surgical operation, resulting in inadequate ventilation; induction of anesthesia and endotracheal intubation are both difficult and dangerous, which also increases the probability of dangerous airway occurrences during the anesthesia awakening period, and if there is bleeding, secretions or gastric contents reflux into the respiratory tract by mistake, it will easily lead to respiratory obstruction, asphyxia, aspiration pneumonia, atelectasis, and other complications. For this reason, airway patency and respiratory function monitoring care is of paramount importance throughout the perianesthesia period, including:

1. Timely observation of respiratory movement frequency, rhythm, amplitude, and mode (thoracic or abdominal breathing), etc.
2. Frequent monitoring of respiratory sounds for bilateral symmetry, presence of secretions, pharyngeal bronchospasm, and other abnormal respiratory sounds.
3. Skin, mucous membrane color, mouth, lips, nail color.
4. Perform arterial blood gas analysis collection as prescribed by the doctor and observe changes in values in a timely manner. The arterial partial pressure of oxygen was monitored for mild hypoxemia: arterial partial pressure of oxygen 50–60 mmHg; moderate hypoxemia: arterial partial pressure of oxygen 30–49 mmHg; severe hypoxemia: arterial partial pressure of oxygen <30 mmHg [6]. Meanwhile, oxygen saturation monitoring reflects the status of oxygen transport in blood and has a good correlation with arterial partial pressure of oxygen.
5. Commonly used monitoring indicators when controlling respiration under general anesthesia: tidal volume (VT), minute ventilation (MV), airway pressure (Paw), and end respiratory carbon dioxide partial pressure monitoring.
6. The normal value of end-breath carbon dioxide is 35–45 mmHg. The normal carbon dioxide waveform is divided into four segments: inspiratory phase baseline, expiratory ascending branch, expiratory plateau, and expiratory phase descending branch [7].

After successful placement of the tracheal tube, the catheter scale should be checked and fixed in time to ensure that the balloon pressure of the tracheal tube is effective, and the operator should be informed to fix the catheter with sutures if necessary to prevent accidental dislodgement of the tracheal tube during surgery. Patients undergoing oral surgery often need to fill the pharyngeal cavity with gauze strips to completely isolate the surgical area in the oral cavity from the respiratory tract to effectively prevent aspiration, but strict records and eye-catching reminder signs need to be made and removed in a timely manner after surgery; when there is a lot of secretions and blood leakage, adequate suction is applied and the catheter sleeve pressure should be sufficient to prevent inflow into the trachea. The nurse anesthetists should regularly monitor the normal and effective operation of the respiratory support equipment and the condition of the respiratory line to avoid twisting and bending of the catheter, and closely observe the airway obstruction and edema.

22.4.2.3 T: Temperature

The change of body temperature of patients during the maintenance period of anesthesia can be affected by many external factors, such as the change of climate and environment, drugs, blood transfusion and rehydration, low temperature anesthesia, intraoperative heat loss, cooling and warming measures during extracorporeal circulation surgery, etc. Therefore, nurse anesthetists need to do a good job of monitoring and managing body temperature during the perianesthesia period.

Nurse anesthetists should do preoperative assessment and pre-warming, monitor body temperature in time and formulate interventions to prevent hypothermia, and give effective insulation measures such as raising room temperature, using liquid warming devices, warming blankets and warming fans when necessary. Record body temperature every 30 min during the maintenance period of anesthesia and ensure that the patient's central body temperature is >36 °C. And an effective contingency plan for the occurrence of malignant hyperthermia should be established.

22.4.2.4 I: Inventions

1. Establish effective arterial and venous access and ensure its patency. The nurse anesthetist should strictly implement the operating procedures, strictly sterilize, regularly patrol, and pay attention to the infusion reaction and keep records. The nurse anesthetist should make the drug infusion plan according to the doctor's orders, ensure that the catheter is evaluated before each intravenous infusion, drug administration, and blood transfusion to make sure that it is in the blood vessel and observe whether there are abnormal manifestations such as redness, swelling, heat, and pain, and

always pay attention to the progress of surgery to adjust the drug infusion rate in accordance with the doctor's orders.
2. Closely observe the circulatory system indicators, including pulse rate, blood pressure, central venous pressure, pulmonary artery pressure, and pulmonary capillary pressure, cardiac output, blood loss, blood volume, and ECG changes; assess the patient's skin, lips, sclera, bulbar conjunctiva, conjunctiva, and mucous membrane color, at the same time, the nurse anesthetist should effectively grasp the preliminary judgment method of blood loss.
3. When monitoring invasive arterial pressure and central venous pressure, attention should always be paid to keeping the pipeline open, adjusting the position of the pressure sensor at the right time with the change of the surgical position; and ensuring that there is sufficient pressure in the pressurized bag. Standardize the technique of arterial blood specimen collection and flush the catheter with heparin dilution in a timely manner after the operation to avoid blockage or thrombosis; pay close attention to the results of arterial blood gas analysis with its commonly used indicators: blood pH, arterial blood carbon dioxide partial pressure, arterial blood oxygen partial pressure, standard carbonate and actual bicarbonate, base residual and standard base residual, and blood oxygenation and degree. After the arterial cannula is removed, the compression hemostasis time should be >5 min and closely observed [8].

22.4.2.5 E: Electric Care Monitor

The monitoring items of cardiac monitor include continuous monitoring of non-invasive/invasive blood pressure, changes of ECG, respiration, oxygen saturation, etc. Five-lead ECG monitoring is generally chosen for monitoring in surgical anesthesia. The nurse anesthetist should do the following.

1. Avoid the surgical sterilization region so as not to interfere with the surgery.
2. Ensure that the skin is intact and free of local inflammation, hard nodes, allergies, etc. before applying electrode pads.
3. Select the lead position according to the lead prompt to prevent abnormal waveforms caused by human factors; adjust the wave amplitude size to facilitate intraoperative observation.
4. In general, pulse and heart rate are consistent, but for certain heart diseases, both heart rate and pulse need to be monitored intraoperatively. Adjust the appropriate waveform amplitude to avoid excessive amplitude interfering with the instrument monitoring results; listen to the heart sounds or touch the carotid artery pulsation if the ECG monitoring is disturbed.
5. Choose the healthy side of the limb, or the lower limb if necessary.
6. Avoid rehydration access and blood oxygen monitoring side of the limb as much as possible; if rehydration access cannot be avoided, extend the interval of manometry appropriately; pad a sterile towel under the cuff to prevent subcutaneous bruising caused by long-term manometry.

For ECG monitor alarm first check the cause of the alarm, then check the source of the alarm failure in a targeted manner, and deal with the corresponding problems.

Myocardial monitor program: The effect of myocardial drugs is determined by measuring respiratory movements such as tidal volume, spirometry, ventilation per minute and the maximum negative pressure generated by inspiration.

Monitoring of depth of anesthesia monitoring: bispectral index (BIS) can determine the effect of anesthetic drugs on the brain, especially the hypnotic effect of anesthesia, to prevent intraoperative knowledge of the patient and avoid too deep anesthesia, BIS values range from 0 to 100, the greater the value, the more awake, and vice versa suggests that the more serious depression of the cerebral cortex [9].

22.4.2.6 N: Narcotics

The nurse anesthetist should clarify the pharmacological knowledge of anesthetic drugs, the sequence of drug use, proper suction, adverse reactions and treatment principles. For inhalation anesthetic drugs, know their clinical standard dosage and cooperate with the doctor for operation and examination. In case of drug leakage from the anesthesia machine, immediately check the performance of the anesthesia machine, whether the sodium-lime tank is in place and whether the seal is broken, and immediately reinforce the installation and replace the seal to ensure the normal operation of the anesthesia machine.

Configure the anesthetic drugs according to the doctor's prescription, make sure that the drugs are ready for use, master the usage and dosage of all kinds of intravenous anesthetic drugs, ensure the safety of medication, and make the patient pass the perianesthesia period smoothly.

22.4.2.7 T: Tubes

During the maintenance of anesthesia, all kinds of catheters should be kept open and prevented from twisting. The drainage of all kinds of catheters should be observed in time, including color, nature, and drainage flow. Particular attention should be paid to the status of indwelling catheter: (1) ensure that the urinary catheter is unobstructed and firmly fixed, and accurately record the time of insertion of the urinary catheter and the color of the urine volume in the urine bag for the first time; (2) combine with the in and out volume, arterial pressure, and central venous pressure during anesthesia to help determine the patient's internal circulation status.

22.5 Care During the Recovery Period of Oral Surgery Anesthesia

After general anesthesia for oral surgery, because the circulatory, respiratory, and metabolic dysfunction occurred during anesthesia has not been completely corrected, the residual effects of general anesthetic drugs have not disappeared, and the patient's protective reflexes have not been fully restored, various complications such as airway obstruction, hyperventilation, nausea and vomiting, aspiration, and unstable circulatory function may easily occur. Resuscitation should be performed in the post-anesthesia monitoring and treatment unit (PACU). In addition to continuing mechanical ventilation support for a period of time after surgery as required by the condition, early awakening after general anesthesia is conducive to the recovery of the patient's vital organ autoregulatory capacity and to the patient's rehabilitation postoperative care. Removal of endotracheal tube in oral surgery patients after general anesthesia is a risky moment, and it is necessary to decide whether to remove the tube according to the patient's condition and awakening situation, which is also a critical period requiring nursing cooperation.

22.5.1 Personnel Management and Responsibilities

On the basis of cooperation, medical and nursing personnel should clarify their respective professional scope and responsibilities. The ratio of the number of nurses in the PACU to the actual open beds in the recovery room should be ≥1:1 [10]. The nurse anesthetist is the main medical personnel in the PACU, responsible for providing monitoring and therapeutic care for patients, and should focus on bedside care. Job responsibilities include the following.

1. Surgeons and nurses in charge of PACU should provide continuous monitoring and care for patients in the anesthesia recovery period, and the PACU must be equipped with experienced and skilled high-quality nurse anesthetists and a nurse practitioner in charge of unified arrangement of nursing organization [11].
2. The transfer of patients to or from the PACU should be decided by the anesthetist. The nurse anesthetist assists the anesthetist to be responsible for the continuous monitoring and consultation of the patient's condition.
3. If the patient's awakening is unexpectedly prolonged, or the respiratory and circulatory functions are unstable, the cause should be actively investigated and dealt with in a timely manner, and consideration should be given to transfer to the postoperative intensive care unit to avoid delaying the condition.
4. When the patient is awake, muscle strength and respiration are restored, the Steward awakening score must reach 4, and the patient can leave the PACU only after the anesthetist has evaluated the decision.

22.5.2 Key Points of Anesthesia Recovery Care

1. Determine the person who regularly inventories the drugs, items and equipment in the PACU, and regularly check the performance of emergency equipment such as ventilator, monitor, defibrillator and negative pressure suction device to ensure that they are in standby condition.
2. Prepare all kinds of anesthesia recovery supplies in a timely manner according to the specific conditions of patients. After the patient enters the PACU, make timely assessment and, according to the patient's condition, give the patient oxygen or connect the ventilator to assist breathing if necessary in a timely manner according to medical advice.
3. The nurse anesthetist should record the patient's vital signs at least once every 5 min (automatically collected by the computer system), and record any changes in condition at any time; if not automatically collected by the computer system, the patient's vital signs during recovery from anesthesia should be recorded at least once every 15–30 min, and when there are special conditions, they should be recorded at any time and monitored more closely. Closely observe the changes in condition, report abnormalities to the anesthetist immediately and strictly implement medical advice.
4. After extubation of oral surgery patients, patients need to be further closely monitored for changes in consciousness, respiratory rate, heart rate, blood pressure, pulse oxygen saturation, body temperature, etc., and pain assessment should be performed and recorded in a timely manner, and the surgeon should be notified of any abnormalities in a timely manner. Early warning signs include risk factors for airway-related complications after extubation. Wheezing, bloody sputum, obstructive ventilatory symptoms, and agitation often indicate airway problems, while drainage, free flap blood supply, airway bleeding, and hematoma formation often indicate surgical problems. It is also important to note that pulse oximetry is susceptible to the surrounding environment and is not suitable as the sole indicator of ventilation monitoring.
5. Keep the bed unit flat and clean, ensure that all pipelines are smooth and effective, and that all drainage lines are clearly marked, not entangled with each other, placed in appropriate positions to avoid pressure on the catheter, observe the color, nature, and amount of drainage in a timely manner, and record them, and notify the doctor in a timely manner if there are any abnormalities. Encourage the patient to cough up sputum, inhale deeply, assist the patient to change position, and assist the anesthetist to treat the patient in a timely manner. Aspirate sputum according to medical advice and cooperate with extubation.

   Before extubation, the anesthetist and nurse should be alert to the pre-existing airway conditions and be fully prepared for the possible need to perform endotracheal intubation again. The nurse anesthetist should prepare all relevant supplies and effectively cooperate with the anesthesiologist for extubation. Before extubation, positive pressure ventilation, mask oxygen administration, monitor blood oxygen saturation, and estimate whether there are signs of airway obstruction or ventilation deficiency; closely observe the changes in condition during extubation, supply oxygen in time, attract secretions in the tracheal tube, in the mouth and pharynx, and cooperate with effective position placement, and do a good job of patient reassurance and psychological care [12].
6. Make good perioperative nursing handover of patients, nurse anesthetists need to know the relevant anesthesia records of patients; special reminders for important preoperative history, comorbidities and their management, difficult airway, indwelling catheter, intraoperative blood and fluid transfusion volume, special medications, etc.; observation of special surgical conditions such as drainage flow, etc., and make records of perioperative nursing record sheets; when patients leave the PACU, they should be escorted to the ward or postoperative intensive care unit, and strict handover, carefully fill in the electronic transfer handover record sheet.
7. Strictly implement the disinfection and isolation system, and do a good job in the prevention and control of hospital infection. Keep the PACU tidy and quiet.

22.6 Specification of Anesthesia Care Techniques for Oral Surgery

22.6.1 Tracheal Intubation Nursing Cooperation

Preparation before intubation	Prescription	Check the prescription
	Patient preparation	Make a good explanation for awake patients and provide psychological care
	Assessment	Airway assessment: patients are assessed for ease of intubation based on commonly used methods of difficult airway assessment (thyromental distance, Mallampati classification, etc)
		General examination: check the patient's nasal cavity, teeth, etc. If contraindications are found, communication should be made with the anesthetist to adjust the airway management plan in time
		History: any history of oral surgery, whether the normal structures in the oral cavity have been destroyed
		Patient's cooperation: assess the patient's cooperation
	Pre-operation preparation	Material preparation: anesthesia mask and anesthesia screw tube, oral (nasopharyngeal) airway, laryngoscope, suitable type of tracheal tube, endotracheal tube core, holding forceps, stethoscope, suction device, suction tube, saline, syringe, simple breathing balloon, dental pad, local anesthetic, sterile gloves, adhesive tape, eye protection patch, resuscitation supplies, etc
		Connect the cardiac monitor and do the monitoring of vital signs (heart rate, blood pressure, respiration, oxygen saturation, etc)
		Check the negative pressure suction device, in standby mode
	Choose the tracheal tube	Adult male: 7.0[a]–7.5[a]; adult female: 6.5[a]–7.0[a]; children: age/4 + 4 (prepare tubes of adjacent sizes)
	Examine the equipment	Check the performance of the anesthesia machine and its oxygen pressure is normal, check whether the suction device is in working condition, and check the brightness of the laryngoscope

Intubation cooperation	Position	Assist in positioning the patient in the position that is easiest to perform laryngoscopy, sniffing position is the most commonly used position with the atlantoaxial joint in extension
	Surface anesthesia	A 2% lidocaine spray was chosen for the root of the tongue, soft palate, hypopharynx, epiglottis, and oral surface anesthesia of the vocal tract
		For transnasal tracheal intubation, intranasal furosemide drops are used to prevent nasal bleeding
		Airway mucosal surface anesthesia can be achieved with the aid of a laryngoscope using a tracheal nebulizer extended into the glottis to spray local anesthetic into the airway, or by cricothyroid puncture
	Mask oxygen delivery	When the patient is awake, place the mask gently over the patient's mouth and nose, without sealing it to the face, to reduce the patient's nervousness
		After the patient's breathing decreases, tilt the head and lift the chin, and fasten the mask tightly over the patient's face
		Observe thoracic rise and fall, observe patient's vital signs
	Suction	The operator stands on the side of the patient's head, and the nurse cooperates with the appropriate time to attract the intraoral secretion suction
	Laryngoscope placement	Check the laryngoscope brightness again, pass it to the operator, who will place the laryngoscope into the mouth
	Glottic exposure	The operator places the laryngoscope, and when the patient's vocal fissure is poorly exposed, the nurse assists in exposing the vocal fissure by gently pressing the patient's cricoid cartilage with the hand
	Pass the tracheal tube	Evacuate the tube cuff
		Lubricate the stylet and place the tracheal tube
		Lubricate the tracheal tube and pass it to the operator
	Pull out the stylet	Orotracheal intubation: the tracheal tube is located in the vocal fissure, and the nurse assists in removing the stylet
		Nasotracheal intubation: when the tracheal tube is out of posterior nostril, the nurse assist in the extraction of the stylet
	Airbag inflation	The operator sends the tracheal tube to the second black line, removes the laryngoscope, and the nurse assists in inflating the balloon with an appropriate amount of air, 25–30 cmH_2O; transnasal tracheal intubation can be done with the aid of a tube holding clamp to send the tracheal tube
	Connection	Connect the ventilator to the tracheal tube
	Tube depth	Orotracheal intubation: incisors correspond to tube scale Adult male: 22–24 cm Adult female: 21–23 cm Children: Age/2 + 12 cm
		Nasotracheal intubation: Incisors correspond to tube scale Adult male:26–27 cm Adult female: 25–26 cm Children: Age/2 + 14 cm
	Check the tube	If the breath sounds are present but not symmetrical, the tracheal tube may enter the main bronchus on one side, deflate the air sac, re-adjust the position of the tracheal tube with the doctor, inflate the air sac again, assist the doctor in listening to the breath sounds of both lungs again, and fix the tracheal tube with adhesive tape after making sure the breath sounds of both lungs are symmetrical
		Observe the partial pressure curve of end-expiratory carbon dioxide with normal waveform, 35–45 mmHg
	Fixation	Orotracheal intubation: fix the dental pad and tracheal tube above the teeth with adhesive tape, fix firmly and not easily dislodged, pay attention to the pressure on the lips of the mouth
		Nasotracheal intubation: fix the tracheal tube on the bridge of the nose with Y-shape tape, pay attention to prevent pressure skin injury
Post-intubation procedure	Adjust parameters	Adjust ventilator parameters according to prescription
	Position	Place the patient in a comfortable position
	Disposal of items	Organize the tools used and sort the items

[a] mm (inside diameter, ID)

22.6.2 Fiberoptic Bronchoscopy Intubation Nursing Cooperation

Preparation before fiberoptic bronchoscopy intubation	Prescription	Check the prescription
	Assessment	Assess the patient with the anesthetist to confirm that tracheal intubation cannot be performed using conventional methods
		Assess patient's cooperation
		Detailed information about the patient's medical history, physical examination, X-rays, and other tests
	Preparation of the materials	Fiberoptic bronchoscope, paraffin oil, 2% lidocaine, 5 mL syringe, lidocaine topical spray, 1% ephedrine, syringe, pediatric suction tube or adult suction tube, suction device, tracheal tube, etc
	Choose the tracheal tube	Adult male: 7.0[a]–7.5[a]; adult female: 6.5[a]–7.0[a]; children: age/4 + 4 (prepare tubes of adjacent sizes) Nasotracheal intubation, tracheal tube selected 0.5 size smaller than the standard size
	Equipment examination	Check the expiration date of various items and medications, and whether the packaging is complete
		Check the performance of the anesthesia machine and its oxygen pressure to make sure it is normal
		Check if the suction is in standby
		Check the battery power and brightness of fiberoptic bronchoscope
	Fiberoptic bronchoscope preparation	Power on the fiberoptic bronchoscope and adjust the focal length and resolution
		Lubricate the front end of the fiberoptic bronchoscope to avoid excessive lubrication affecting the field of view
		Lubricate the front end of the tracheal tube, evacuate the cuff, and snap the tracheal tube along the fiberoptic bronchoscope at the root of the fiberoptic bronchoscope
	Patient preparation	Ask the patient to fast and abstain from food and water as prescribed by the doctor
		If the patient has a denture, he/she should be instructed to remove it to avoid accidental dislodgement when using the fiberoptic bronchoscope
		Sedation of the patient before fiberoptic bronchoscopy intubation as prescribed by the doctor
		Administering oxygen by mask as prescribed by the doctor
		In patients undergoing nasotracheal intubation, 1% ephedrine was administered in the nostril to reduce nasal bleeding

Fiberoptic bronchoscopy intubation cooperation	Position	Adjust the patient's position to a supine position with shoulder pads and head slightly tilted back
	Cardiac monitoring	Connect to the cardiac monitor for vital sign monitoring
	Surface anesthesia	A 5 mL syringe was used to draw 2 mL of 2% lidocaine and passed to the anesthesiologist for cricothyroid puncture, and surface anesthesia was administered to the tracheal mucosa
		Surface anesthesia of the mucosa around the glottis with lidocaine spray was performed as prescribed by the surgeon
	Fiberoptic bronchoscopy intubation	Nasotracheal intubation: pass the fiberoptic bronchoscope to the anesthesiologist, place it through the nasal cavity, and ask the patient to breathe calmly after placement
		Orotracheal intubation: gently lift the lower jaw to open the patient's mouth to facilitate the passage of the fiberoptic bronchoscope and to prevent the patient from biting the fiberoptic bronchoscope
		The operator places the fiberoptic bronchoscope by reorienting the fiberoptic bronchus, and when the fiberoptic bronchoscope reaches the epiglottis, the patient is instructed to take a deep breath through the nose
		The operator places the fiberoptic bronchoscope by reorienting the fiberoptic bronchoscope, and when the fiberoptic bronchoscope reaches the epiglottis, the patient is instructed to take a deep breath through the nose
		If mucous membrane or secretions obstruct the field of view, the operator returns or withdraws the fiberoptic bronchoscope and assists in cleaning the lens
		After completing tracheal intubation, assist the operator in withdrawing the fiberoptic bronchoscope
		The nurse assists in inflating the cuff of the tracheal tube with an appropriate amount of air, 25–30 cmH_2O
	Connection	Connect the ventilator to the tracheal tube
	Check the placement	Observe the partial pressure curve of end-expiratory carbon dioxide with normal waveform, 35–45 mmHg
	Induction	Administer intravenous medication as prescribed until the patient is under general anesthesia
	Fixation	Orotracheal intubation: fix the dental pad and tracheal tube above the teeth with adhesive tape, fix firmly and not easily dislodged, pay attention to the pressure on the lips of the mouth
		Nasotracheal intubation: fix the tracheal tube on the bridge of the nose with Y-shaped tape, pay attention to prevent pressure skin injury
Post-intubation procedure	Adjust parameters	Adjust ventilator parameters according to prescription
	Position	Place the patient in a comfortable position
	Disposal of items	Organize the tools used and sort the items.
		Check the battery of the fiberoptic bronchoscope, charge it make it in standby
		Sterilize the fiberoptic bronchoscope according to the hospital sterilization process

[a] mm (inside diameter, ID)

22.6.3 Deep Venipuncture Nursing Cooperation

Preparation before deep venipuncture	Prescription	Check the prescription
	Patient preparation	Verify patient information; explain to patients and families before operation, and do a good job of psychological care for patients
	Items preparation	Deep venipuncture kit, appropriate type of sterile central venous catheter, sodium lactate Ringer's solution, transfusion skin strip, infusion extension tube (long), sterile gloves, sterile patch, use of skin disinfectant (preferred chlorhexidine gluconate alcohol disinfectant cotton balls) in accordance with relevant national regulations, 2% lidocaine 5 mL (for patients under local anesthesia), syringes, etc
		Check that sterile items are within the expiration date and that the packaging is not damaged or wet
		Install infusion devices, check the expiration date of drugs, liquid for deterioration and carry out transfusion skin strip exhaust during the process
	Adjust the patient's position	Femoral vein puncture with the patient in a supine position, with the thigh on the punctured side flattened and externally rotated and abducted. For internal jugular vein puncture, the patient is placed in a supine position (20°–30°) with the patient's head turned to the opposite side. For subclavian vein puncture, the patient is placed in a supine head position with a small pillow to elevate the patient's right shoulder
Intraoperative coordination of deep venipuncture	Open the sterile kit	The nurse prepares all supplies and brings them to the patient's bedside and places them in the proper place
		Again check the sterile kit outer package cloth intact, no damage, no moisture, 3 m indicator tape discoloration, open the first layer of sterile kit, open the second layer of packing cloth with sterile holding forceps, check the 3 m indicator card has changed color, clamp to take three sterile cotton balls into the small medicine cup
		Open the central venous catheter to pass to the operator
		Remove the sterile patch to the operator
	Observe vital signs	During the puncture, closely observe the patient's vital signs and listen to the patient's complaints in a timely manner
	Local anesthesia	Open the package of 2% lidocaine, assist the operator to extract 3 mL, maintain sterility
	Connection	When puncture succeeds, connect the infusion, place the infusion bag at the low position of the puncture point, when the blood back out can be seen that is to confirm the deep vein catheter placed in the vessel, hang the rehydration fluid with the infusion rack, adjust the rehydration fluid drip rate
Procedure after deep venipuncture	Signs	Check the patch and sign puncture times
	Position	Place the patient in a comfortable position, arrange the bet, pay attention to keeping warmth for the patient
	Disposal of items	Organize the tools used and sort the trash
	Attention	Take care to enhance dressing changes and select appropriate sterile patches to avoid repeated punctures leading to injury
		Reduce retention time after puncture. Remove the deep venous catheter as soon as catheter-associated bloodstream infection is suspected or develops, and send the catheter tip for pathogenic culture of blood and/or secretions

22.6.4 Arterial Puncture Nursing Cooperation

Preparation for arterial puncture	Prescription	Check the prescription
	Patient preparation	Explain to patients and families before operation, and do a good job of psychological care for patients
	Items preparation	Arterial puncture kit, 22G trocar needle, sterile gloves, sterile patch, sterile cotton balls, positive pressure connector, sodium heparin, syringe, small cushion pillow, sodium lactate Ringer's solution, pressure transducer, pressurized bag
		Check the expiration date of all kinds of items, packaging for damage, moisture
	Solution preparation	Add 4200 IU of sodium heparin to 500 mL of sodium lactate Ringer's solution
	Install pressure sensors	Connect the pressure transducer, place the configured fluid into the pressurized bag and pressurize it, fix it in the saline rack and evacuate it, with the pressure transducer flat in the patient's fourth intercostal space, near the mid-axillary line
	Assess the patient	General examination: check the patient's skin at the puncture site for breaks and hard nodes; proximal artery for obstruction and vasculitis
		Past history: history of thrombosis or surgery on the punctured limb
		Laboratory tests: check the coagulation test report for coagulation disorders
	Puncture site selection	Radial artery: must check for positive Allen's test Dorsalis pedis artery: choose one side of the dorsalis pedis artery
	Positioning	Radial artery: place the patient's punctured arm in abduction, place a small round pillow under the wrist, and dorsiflex the wrist Dorsalis pedis artery puncture: expose the skin on the back of the patient's foot
Cooperation during the puncture	Puncture site confirmation	The operator determines the course of the artery and designates the point of strongest pulsation as the puncture point
	Open the sterile kit	The operator stands on the puncture side, the nurse opens the outer layer of the arterial puncture kit, opens the inner layer of the wrap with sterile forceps, unwraps the sterile gloves and hands them to the operator
		Clamp non-toxic cotton balls, pass cannula needles, positive pressure connectors, sterile patching film
	Sterilization	The operator with sterile gloves sterilizes the puncture site twice The first sterilization is performed with the puncture site as a circle with a 10 cm radius The second time, the puncture site is sterilized in a circle with a radius of 8 cm
	Lay fenestrated sheet	Lay the fenestrated sheet centered on the puncture point
	Puncture	With the needle tip beveled upward, the trocar needle is pierced from the puncture point, and when the blood is returned smoothly, the needle is stopped and the trocar needle is fixed
	Place the tube	Place the trocar needle horizontally, enter 2 mm again, place the trocar hose, withdraw the core, and in the case of non-positive pressure trocar needles, press the front end of the puncture needle to prevent bleeding
	Connection	Draw back arterial blood and connect to a positive pressure connector
	Fixation	Apply sterile patch to the puncture site to hold it in place and prevent the trocar needle from slipping out
	Connect to the pressure sensor	Evacuate the pressure sensor again and connect to positive pressure connector
	Zeroing	Adjust and fix the pressure sensor at the same height as heart position, close the patient arterial end of the pressure sensor, open the tee, press the zero button to adjust the zero, after the pressure value appears 0, close the tee, open the patient arterial end and check whether the arterial waveform is regular
Procedure after arterial puncture	Disposal of items	Organize the tools used and sort the items

22.6.5 Tracheal Tube Extubation Nursing Cooperation

Preparation for tracheal extubation	Patient assessment	Assess the patient's level of consciousness, whether the cough reflex and swallowing reflex are restored, and whether the patient can cooperate with the medical staff
		Whether the breathing pattern is normal, including whether it can breathe on its own, whether it is labored, whether the respiratory rate is greater or less than 30 times/min, tidal volume, etc
		Assess whether the patient can open the eyes and frown, and whether muscle strength is restored
		Presence of severe acid-base imbalance or hypoxia
		Circulatory stability: assess the presence of arrhythmias requiring urgent management, or high/low blood pressure requiring urgent management
		Assess the patient for upper airway obstruction due to the surgical site after extubation
		If the patient is eligible for extubation, the physician will give the order and the nurse will remove the tracheal tube under the direction of the physician
Cooperation during the extubation	Alert	Patient's pre-existing airway conditions should be alerted before extubation, and preparation for the possibility of reintubation of the endotracheal tube should be made
	Recording before extubation	Record the patient's consciousness, body temperature, heart rate, blood pressure and oxygen saturation, and arterial blood gas analysis before extubation
	Sputum suction	Choose a suitable type of suction tube, carry out negative pressure suction, be gentle, and suction the secretions left in the nasal cavity, mouth, throat, and trachea before removing the tube
	Preoxygenation	Provide preoxygenation
	Extubation	Evacuation of gas from the tracheal tube sleeve
		Patient's head is tilted to one side
		Remove tape fixation
		Retain the dental pad to remove the tracheal tube, which can prevent the teeth from closing after extraction and also facilitate the suction of oral secretions
		Remove oral, nasal, and airway secretions in a timely manner
	Oxygenation	After removal of the tracheal tube, the patient should continue to be given oxygen by face mask
	Observation	Observe the patient's consciousness, heart rate, blood pressure, respiration, oxygen saturation, and thoracic and diaphragmatic movements
	Precautions for extubation	The patient's oronasal, pharyngeal, and endotracheal secretions must be suctioned out before the tracheal tube is removed; after the tracheal tube is removed, suction should be continued to remove the secretions from the oronasal and pharyngeal cavities
		Be gentle in suction and closely observe the patient's heart rate, heart rhythm, blood pressure and oxygen saturation during suction
		Extubate the tracheal tube quickly and gently to minimize patient discomfort
		After removal of the tracheal tube, the patient must be promptly given oxygen by face mask or nasal cannula
	Recording after extubation	Record the time of extubation of the patient's tracheal tube and vital signs with the record sheet in a timely manner
Procedure after extubation	Disposal of items	Organize the tools used and sort the items
	Observation	Continue to observe the patient's vital signs (heart rate, rhythm, blood pressure, respiration, and oxygen saturation) after catheter removal, and observe and note the patient for the onset of respiratory distress

22.6.6 Airway Sputum Suction

Preparation before suction	Check	Check the prescription
		Check the patient's identity information
	Assessment	Know about the patient's condition, state of consciousness, sputum status, and assess the indication for suction
		Know about the ventilator's parameters setting
	Explanation	Explain to awake patient and get consent
	Auscultation	Breath sounds in both lungs
	Items preparation	Treatment tray (including two suction kits, two bottles of 0.9% sodium chloride 500 mL, balloon manometer, hand disinfectant, curved tray), cardiac monitor, negative pressure suction device
	Choose suction tube	The outer diameter of the suction (sputum) tube should not exceed 50% of the inner diameter of the artificial airway
	Check the items	Check the expiration date of the suction tube, packaging for damage and moisture
		Check the expiration date of 0.9% sodium chloride, the bottle has no breakage, cracks
	Adjust negative pressure	Check for negative pressure
		Negative pressure 80 mmHg–100 mmHg for children, 80 mmHg–150 mmHg for adults
	Double check	After washing hands and putting on a mask, bring supplies to the patient's bedside and check the patient's information again

Sputum suction	Oxygenation	Give the patient pure oxygen inhalation for 30s–60s and observe the change of oxygen saturation to prevent hypoxemia caused by aspiration
	Pipe arrangement	Organize the ventilator line and dump the condensate in the water collection cup
	Instruction	Instruct the patient to breathe deeply and cough effectively
	Wash hands	Seven-step hand washing technique
	Position	The patient's head tilted to one side
	Suction trial	Open the saline test suction bottle, tear open the front end of the outer package of suction package, take out the sterile gloves, put on sterile gloves on one hand, spread the sterile treatment sheet, pull out the suction tube in your hand, connect the root with the negative pressure tube and test suction in the suction test bottle
	Suction in the oral and nasal cavity	Oropharyngeal and/or nasopharyngeal suctioning should be performed first, followed by endotracheal suctioning
	Manual airway suction	When changing the suction site, the suction tube should be changed
		Disconnect the ventilator from the tracheal tube with ungloved hands and place the ventilator connector on a sterile sheet
		Quickly and gently feed the suction tube along the tracheal tube without negative pressure with sterile gloved hands, and if resistance is felt during placement or if the patient develops an irritated cough, withdraw the suction tube by 1–2 cm, give negative pressure, and gently rotate and pull the suction tube for 15 s to avoid lifting up and down in the trachea
		During suction, patients should be observed for sputum condition (color, quality, and quantity), oxygen saturation, vital signs, especially heart rate and rhythm changes
		If there's need for suction again, the suction tube must be changed
	Flushing	Flushing the suction tube in the saline flushing bottle in a timely manner after suction
	Assessment	Assessment of patient's facial color, respiration, oxygen saturation, heart rate/rhythm changes, blood pressure changes
	Connection	After suction, connect to the ventilator line immediately for mechanical ventilation
	Pure oxygen inhalation	Give the patient pure oxygen inhalation for 30s–60s
	Adjustment	Adjust the oxygen concentration to the original parameters after the oxygen saturation has risen to normal levels
	Wash hands	After the suction, remove the gloves and sterilize the hands
	Auscultation	Ascultate the patient's sound of breath in both lungs
	Confirm the position	Observe the tube's position and depth
	Pressure measurement	Measure tracheal catheter balloon pressure with a balloon pressure gauge
		Fill or deflate the airbag according to airbag pressure
	Assessment of effects	Changes in patient's face, respiration, oxygen saturation, heart rate/rhythm, blood pressure
		Whether there are changes in the mechanical ventilation curve and the sound of breath
		Low compression at the highest inspiratory plateau and reduced peak airway pressure to reduce airway resistance or increase dynamic compliance, and increase air delivery tidal volume in pressure control mode
		Improve blood gas analysis indicators or oxygenation status (oxygen saturation)
		Clear lung secretions
Procedure after suction	Position	Ask awake patient if it is needed
		Place the patient in a comfortable position
	Arrangement	Arrange the bed
		Arrange the ventilator line
	Recording	Record the color, nature, and volume of the suctioned matter in the nursing record
	Disposal of the items	Organize the tools used and sort the items

22.7 Common Complications and Care of General Anesthesia for Oral Surgery

With the development of modern anesthesiology, the incidences of anesthesia complications and mortality are gradually decreasing, but the current clinical anesthesia still cannot completely avoid the occurrence of serious complications and even the resulting death of patients. The following will introduce the common complications and care in oral surgery anesthesia clinic.

22.7.1 Complications of Endotracheal Intubation and Nursing Care

The common complications of endotracheal intubation include injury, bleeding, laryngeal edema, neuroreflex accidents, and vocal cord paralysis.

1. Injury is often caused by improper use of laryngoscope and rough intubation. It can cause upper front teeth loosening, lower lip cut and hematoma, pyriform sinus injury, and even subcutaneous emphysema of the neck, causing respiratory distress.
   (a) Standardize the operation, avoid exposing the vocal fossa with the laryngoscope when the masticatory muscles are not relaxed, or using the upper front teeth as the fulcrum to force the laryngoscope backward.
   (b) Pay attention to the protection of the lower lip when placing the laryngoscope.
   (c) Avoid putting the laryngoscope in too hard and too deep and using rough force during blind intubation.
   (d) If the patient has a subcutaneous cervical emphysema, cooperate with the physician to aspirate the hematoma by subcutaneous puncture of the patient's neck with a thick needle.
2. Bleeding is mostly caused by injury, especially in nasal intubation, which can cause severe nasal bleeding if resistance is encountered and still force to intubate.

   In case of nasal bleeding, the head should be lowered, a 1% ephedrine solution should be dripped into the nasal cavity, and a thinner tracheal tube should be replaced immediately for intra-catheter suction and oxygen administration. If the patient suffocates due to massive nasal bleeding before successful intubation, assist the physician to perform tracheotomy immediately, suction the airway secretions in a timely manner, administer oxygen and pay close attention to the changes in the patient's vital signs [13].

   The induction period of general anesthesia in oral surgery patients often takes a long time, and sometimes due to the patient's restricted mouth opening or partial upper airway obstruction before anesthesia, patients often have different degrees of hypoxia and carbon dioxide accumulation. Endotracheal intubation or extubation in such patients under shallow anesthesia may lead to laryngospasm, cardiac rhythm disturbance or even cardiac arrest due to excitation of the vagal nervous system.

   Before the induction of anesthesia begins, the nurse anesthetist needs to make adequate assessment and communication, and prepare all kinds of routine and emergency supplies; during the induction of anesthesia, the nurse anesthetist needs to actively cooperate with the doctor to provide the patient with effective oxygen in a timely manner, avoid the patient's hypoxia and carbon dioxide accumulation, keep the induction of anesthesia stable, monitor and inform the anesthesia doctor in real time, shorten the operation time through effective cooperation, and ensure the safe and effective operation. Once cardiac arrest occurs, perform cardiopulmonary resuscitation immediately.
3. Laryngeal edema and subglottic edema are particularly likely to occur in children. They usually have symptoms such as laryngeal stridor, hoarseness, and dyspnea within a short period of time after surgery, and in severe cases, inspiration is accompanied by the three concave sign, severe cyanosis, profuse sweating, and rapid heart rate. Oxygen should be

given immediately, and intravenous sedative drugs and nebulized inhalation should be given according to medical advice. When the symptoms of upper airway obstruction worsen, cooperate with the doctor to perform tracheotomy.

4. Vocal cord paralysis are most often seen in neck surgery, tracheal surgery or rough tracheal intubation. Vocal fold paralysis due to laryngeal nerve involvement may be transient, and laryngeal nerve severance may be permanent. Unilateral vocal cord paralysis can cause aspiration, and bilateral vocal cord paralysis is a serious complication that can lead to complete obstruction of the upper airway, commonly associated with laryngeal cancer or radical tracheal tumor surgery.

   Damage to the recurrent laryngeal nerve can be determined by whether the patient can effectively cough and occur. Assist the surgeon to perform endotracheal intubation if necessary, or tracheotomy and good airway care if it is permanent.

22.7.2 Upper Respiratory Tract Obstruction

Upper respiratory obstruction after oral surgery is a common complication, mostly due to posterior tongue drop, laryngeal spasm, edema or hematoma in the surgical area or surgical approach (such as cleft palate patients undergoing palatopharyngoplasty to reduce the original pharyngeal cavity), or over tightening of the compression bandage.

1. Glossoptosis due to incomplete recovery from general anesthesia and poor recovery of muscle strength, the tongue body obstructs part of the pharyngeal cavity backward and hinders the airway.

   Take the lateral or supine position to support the lower jaw, if the obstruction cannot be lifted, it is necessary to place the airway through the nose or mouth, and if necessary, insert a tracheal tube or laryngeal mask with the line.

2. Laryngospasm refers to the functional obstruction of the upper airway caused by spasm of the laryngeal muscles that closes the vocal cords. It mostly occurs in patients who have not recovered from upper respiratory tract infection before surgery, especially in pediatric patients. Laryngospasm may be induced by increased airway stress, pharyngeal congestion, and more postoperative intraoral secretions in the patient's oral cavity if the suction is not timely or over-stimulated.
   (a) Remove secretions and irritants from the patient's mouth or tracheal tube in a timely manner, take a chin lift or jaw lift to open the airway, apply a simple ventilator or 100% pure oxygen pressurized by the anesthesia machine to administer oxygen.
   (b) Deepen anesthesia (e.g., increase the concentration of inhalation anesthetics and sedation of anesthetics).
   (c) Use antispasmodics (such as aminophylline, salbutamol), glucocorticoids (such as dexamethasone, hydrocortisone, etc.) as prescribed by the surgeon.

3. Airway edema is common in pediatric patients with a history of upper airway infection, patients with allergic reactions and head, neck and oral surgery, followed by those with obesity, short neck, wide and short epiglottis, difficulty in revealing the voice box, and repeated tracheal intubation.

   Patients who have been extubated should be given pure oxygen by mask ventilation and head elevation, and if treatment is not effective, emergency tracheotomy should be prepared as soon as possible.

4. Surgical incision hematoma due to surgical site bleeding such as thyroid surgery, carotid lymphatic dissection, carotid endarterectomy, etc. Compression of neck hematoma can cause obstruction of venous and lymphatic reflux and severe edema.

   Neck hematoma must be treated immediately. Administer pure oxygen with a mask and intubate endotracheally while immediately notifying the surgeon and preparing the operating room for exploration. If tracheal intubation cannot be completed quickly, the incision must be opened immediately to temporarily relieve tissue pressure and congestion and improve airway patency.

5. Aspiration is a serious airway emergency. Foreign bodies (e.g., teeth, food), blood, and gastric contents are three common clinical misaspirations.

   Patients are given anticholinergic drugs before induction of anesthesia, and a gastric tube is placed postoperatively to suction gastric contents, and extubation is considered only after the patient's airway reflexes have fully recovered. Hypoxia, increased airway resistance, pulmonary atelectasis or pulmonary edema caused by aspiration require supportive therapy and care such as oxygen therapy, PEEP, CPAP, and mechanical ventilation [14].

22.7.3 Bronchospasm

Bronchospasm is caused by a spasmodic contraction of the bronchial smooth muscle, a sudden rise in airway resistance and expiratory dyspnea, resulting in severe hypoxia and carbon dioxide accumulation. If not corrected in time, it can cause hemodynamic changes in the patient and even cardiac arrhythmias and cardiac arrest [15].

Patients with previous respiratory disease should have a careful history, a preoperative respiratory function test, instruction to abstain from smoking for more than 2 weeks before surgery, and if there has been a recent acute inflammatory episode, elective surgery should be delayed for 2–3 weeks. After bronchospasm has occurred, the first step should be to identify the trigger and eliminate the irritant. If the anesthesia is too shallow, deepen the anesthesia and administer oxygen under positive pressure; promptly remove airway secretions and oozing blood; administer medication reasonably according to the prescription, and observe the reaction after medication until the condition is relieved.

22.7.4 Hypoxemia

Hypoxemia refers to the lack of oxygen in the blood, arterial partial pressure of oxygen is less than 60 mmHg, mainly manifested as a decrease in partial pressure of oxygen and blood oxygen saturation. Due to the effects of surgery and anesthesia, patients after oral surgery may have inadequate ventilation and ventilation function and a reduced ventilation blood flow ratio. Common causes include hypoventilation, upper respiratory obstruction, bronchospasm, pneumothorax, and pulmonary edema.

1. To prevent the occurrence of hypoxemia, postoperative oxygenation and oxygen saturation monitoring should be routinely performed in oral surgery patients when entering the PACU.
2. Keep the airway open and remove respiratory secretions in a timely manner.
3. Strengthen the management of intubated patients during general anesthesia, pay attention to the removal of mechanical faults in the anesthetic machine circuit and confirm the position and depth of the tracheal tube when handing over with other staff.
4. After removal of the tracheal tube, give the patient low oxygen flow (2 L/min–4 L/min) inhalation by mask to prevent central respiratory depression caused by anesthetic sedative and analgesic drugs.
5. Take arterial blood and perform blood gas analysis if necessary as prescribed by the doctor.
6. Administer postoperative analgesia to prevent the patient from refusing to breathe deeply due to wound pain.
7. Instruct and assist the patient in correct breathing, coughing, and coughing up sputum.

22.7.5 Hypotension

Hypotension is a common postoperative complication, mostly due to high intraoperative bleeding, absolute insufficiency of blood volume due to untimely blood volume replacement, or relative insufficiency of blood volume due to peripheral vasodilation caused by anesthetic drugs, or reduced cardiac output due to weakened cardiac function. A systolic and/or diastolic blood pressure below 20%–30% of the resting blood pressure is considered postoperative hypotension.

1. Notify the anesthetist promptly when hypotension is detected and administer medication as prescribed.
2. For excessive blood and fluid loss, speed up the rate of infusion, and if necessary, open another vein to increase the amount of fluids.
3. If hypoxia is present, increase the concentration of oxygen, identify whether ventilation is inadequate and deal with it promptly.
4. For hypothermia, adjust the air conditioning temperature, use warm blankets, cover with quilts and warm up the infusion.
5. Observe wound drainage and urine output and notify the surgeon immediately if there is any suspicion of continued postoperative bleeding.
6. Perform bedside ECG monitoring and consult a cardiologist if the patient has chest pain and dyspnea when there is no hemorrhage.

22.7.6 Hypertension

Most often occurs within 30 min after surgery, especially in patients with preoperative combined hypertension. Common causes include postoperative wound pain, discomfort due to tracheal catheter or catheterization, hypoxia, and hypercapnia, dilatory irritation of the bladder and gastrointestinal tract, etc. Postoperative hypertension is defined as systolic and/or diastolic blood pressure above 20%–30% of resting blood pressure. If left untreated and unattended, it can result in adverse consequences such as heart failure, myocardial ischemia, arrhythmias, and cerebrovascular accidents.

1. Bedside ECG and blood pressure monitoring.
2. Use sedative and analgesic drugs as prescribed to reduce postoperative pain.
3. Correct breathing problems and improve ventilation.
4. Suction gastric contents through a gastric tube prior to extubation or leave a gastric tube in place as prescribed to ensure effective gastrointestinal decompression.
5. Explain to patients with indwelling catheters to relieve anxiety and discomfort.
6. Use antihypertensive drugs as prescribed by the doctor to maintain blood pressure to normal range or preoperative level.

22.7.7 Arrhythmias

There are many causes of perioperative arrhythmias, including preoperative combined arrhythmias, the effects of anesthetic drugs, carbon dioxide accumulation, electrolyte disturbances, hypothermia, and pain. Common type of arrhythmias include sinus tachycardia, sinus bradycardia, paroxysmal supraventricular tachycardia, atrial flutter or atrial fibrillation, premature ventricular beats or ventricular tachycardia.

1. Perform electrocardiographic monitoring to assess the type of arrhythmia and provide symptomatic care.
2. Keep the airway open and administer oxygen to prevent hypoxemia.
3. Symptomatic management of the patient's complaints of wound pain, nausea and vomiting, urinary distention, etc.
4. Administer antiarrhythmic drugs as prescribed by the doctor, correct water-electrolyte disturbances, and maintain circulatory stability.
5. Use defibrillators if necessary.

22.7.8 Cerebrovascular Accident

Cerebrovascular accidents include ischemic strokes (about 80%) and hemorrhagic strokes (about 20%) [16]. They are difficult to detect intraoperatively and can only be detected postoperatively when there is a delayed awakening, impaired consciousness or specific signs in response to the cerebrovascular accident (e.g., coma, hemiparesis, aphasia, and pathological reflexes).

Assess the patient's level of consciousness, command completion, and extremity muscle strength prior to postoperative extubation and at handover to the ward in patients undergoing general anesthesia. If a cerebrovascular accident is suspected, keep the airway open, provide respiratory support, ask a neurosurgeon for a consultation and accompany the patient for imaging tests such as CT and MRI.

22.7.9 Hypothermia and Hyperthermia

22.7.9.1 Hypothermia

Hypothermia (body temperature below 36 °C) can be caused by low room temperature, intraoperative input of large amounts of unheated fluids, heat dissipation in the surgical field, flushing of surgical wounds with large amounts of fluid, and suppression of the thermoregulatory center by general anesthetic drugs. Hypothermia can delay anesthetic awakening, prolong bleeding time and, if chills occur, increase tissue oxygen consumption.

Patients are given prophylactic hypothermia during the perioperative period, maintaining an ambient temperature of at least 20 °C–24 °C, reducing body surface exposure, using warmed fluids or blood products, and providing equipment such as warm blankets and fluid warmers if available. Note the patient's symptoms and complaints of shivering and cold extremities during awakening and keep warm. Intraoperative and postoperative temperature monitoring should be performed for >3 h procedures such as oral surgery oncology or orthognathic surgery. If hypothermia occurs, prompt rewarming measures should be taken and heating equipment should be used, while the patient's urine output needs to be noted. Patients should not be transferred out of the PACU until their body temperature reaches 35 °C.

22.7.9.2 Hyperthermia

Hyperthermia can be caused by thick sterile sheets covering the body surface during surgery, atropine given before anesthesia to suppress sweating, transfusion reactions, infection, and malignant hyperthermia. Hyperthermia can lead to increased basal metabolism and oxygen consumption, as well as metabolic acidosis, hyperkalemia, and hyperglycemia. Convulsions may occur if the body temperature exceeds 40 °C.

The temperature should be monitored routinely during the perioperative period. If hypothermia is detected, physical cooling such as ice packs and alcohol baths should be used first, while symptomatic management of complications due to hypothermia, such as arterial blood gas collection and analysis, should be carried out according to medical advice. Patients should not normally be transferred out of the PACU until their temperature has dropped to 39 °C.

Malignant hyperthermia is a rare perianesthetic complication and, if not managed promptly, patients can die from circulatory or respiratory failure. The nurse anesthetist should closely monitor the patient's temperature, heart rhythm, skin changes, blood pressure and changes in end respiratory carbon dioxide, especially end respiratory carbon dioxide monitoring is of great value in the early diagnosis of malignant hyperthermia. The nurse anesthetist should, according to medical advice, (1) give sedative, antispasmodic, and diuretic drugs to rapidly lower the body temperature and correct the water-electrolyte imbalance; (2) establish invasive arterial pressure and central venous pressure monitoring as soon as possible; (3) use water beds with adjustable temperature, place ice packs and infuse large amounts of cold balance fluid to control the patient's body temperature; (4) give adequate oxygen to maintain ventilation and aeration.

22.7.10 Delayed Awakening

It is generally considered that if the patient's consciousness is not restored 2 h after the surgery, if he/she does not respond to calls, if he/she cannot open his/her eyes or raise his/her hands, and if there is no obvious response to painful stimulation, then the awakening is considered delayed. Reasons for delayed awakening may include excessive doses of sedative drugs, the effect of muscle relaxants, respiratory insufficiency, cardiovascular dysfunction, thermoregulatory dysfunction, metabolic disorders of water and electrolytes, and abnormal blood glucose, etc.

During awakening, patients should be closely monitored, with routine monitoring of ECG, blood pressure, oxygen saturation and body temperature, evaluation of the patient's state of consciousness and limb mobility, and early detection of potential nerve damage, such as hematoma and tight surgical dressings. For patients with delayed awakening, give further monitoring and care such as monitoring end-expiratory carbon dioxide, doing blood gas analysis, observing the patient's pupil size, reflex to light, recording urine output and various drainage fluids. Follow medical advice for etiological treatment, keep the patient's airway open or provide respiratory support; promptly correct glucose metabolism and water-electrolyte disorders, etc.; use antagonistic drugs reasonably and observe the patient's reaction to the drugs; rewarm patients with hypothermia.

22.7.11 Postoperative Delirium and Agitation

Delirium and agitation refer to the extreme disturbance of the patient's waking state, which affects his attention, orientation, perception and intelligence, and is accompanied by fear and anxiety. The clinical manifestations are the sudden onset of agitation, such as irritability and screaming, increased muscle tone in the limbs and trunk, trembling and writhing, followed by a return to calm and possibly a reoccurrence, with the duration of the delirium state varying. Both delirium and agitation are the result of altered neurological function, but the difference lies in the degree of difference.

The nurse should pay close attention to the patient's vital signs and state of consciousness, strengthen safety care, use the restraint belt appropriately during the awakening period, observe the patient's blood flow to the limbs and the IV site, and fix the drainage lines properly. If the patient becomes agitated, restraint and sedation are given and the tracheal tube is properly cared for to prevent the patient from being dislodged due to agitation. For patients with catheter intolerance, patiently explain the importance of postoperative indwelling catheterization and check for patency. For patients with other causes of agitation, such as hypoxia, hypothermia, postural discomfort, psychological tension and other discomforts, the principle of care is to remove the causative factors and symptomatic care, and not to blindly use mandatory restraint.

22.7.12 Pain

Patients do not feel pain during surgery due to the effect of anesthetic drugs, but at the end of surgery, as the effect of anesthetic drugs wears off, patients will gradually feel pain, which can interfere with normal physiological functions, such as affecting ventilation, limiting the elimination of respiratory secretions, increasing blood pressure, heart rate, nausea and vomiting, and urinary retention.

For patients using postoperative intravenous patient-controlled analgesia, patients should be properly instructed to use the analgesic device and have the effect of its use recorded in a return visit. If nausea and vomiting are severe due to painkillers, discontinue the analgesic pump as prescribed by the doctor and keep the mouth clean to prevent vomitus from causing accidental aspiration. If a patient complains of unbearable pain after surgery without the use of an analgesic pump, give analgesic drugs as prescribed by the doctor, record the changes in the patient's vital signs and evaluate the analgesic effect. In case of respiratory depression or cardiac arrest, immediately resuscitate the patient in situ and inform the physician.

22.7.13 Nausea and Vomiting

Oral surgery has a high incidence of postoperative nausea and vomiting due to gauze filling of the patient's intraoral wound, inability to swallow or excessive swallowing of blood and saliva, which also causes pain and anxiety to the patient.

Avoid patient nausea and vomiting and give anti-emetic medication as prescribed by the doctor. Assess the patient's risk and causes of nausea and vomiting, promptly remove secretions from the patient's mouth and aspirate the contents of the gastric tube. If nausea and vomiting occur, instruct the patient to tilt the head to one side, promptly suction to prevent inadvertent aspiration, give oxygen and psychological care.

References

1. Aana.com. 2022. [online]. https://www.aana.com/membership/become-a-crna. Accessed 1 Jun 2022.
2. National Center for Quality Assurance of Anesthesia, Standing Committee of the Chinese Society of Anesthesiology, Anesthesia Quality Management Group of the Chinese Society of Anesthesiology. 2021. Expert Consensus on Quality Control in Anesthesia [EB/OL]. http://www.csaqh.cn/guide/detail_1623.html.2021-09-30.
3. Atchison KA, Gironda MW, Black EE, Schweitzer S, Der-Martirosian C, Felsenfeld A, Leathers R, Belin TR. Baseline characteristics and treatment preferences of oral surgery patients. J Oral Maxillofac Surg. 2007;65(12):2430–7. PMID: 18022465; PMCID: PMC2763547. https://doi.org/10.1016/j.joms.2007.04.011.
4. Ji YD, Peacock ZS, Resnick CM. Characteristics of National malpractice claims in oral and maxillofacial surgery. J Oral Maxillofac Surg. 2020;78(8):1314–8. Epub 2020 Mar 23. PMID: 32305375. https://doi.org/10.1016/j.joms.2020.03.015.
5. Yesen Z, Hong J. Oral anesthesiology. Beijing: China Science Press; 2012.
6. Lai CC, Sung MI, Liu HH, Chen CM, Chiang SR, Liu WL, Chao CM, Ho CH, Weng SF, Hsing SC, Cheng KC. The ratio of partial pressure arterial oxygen and fraction of inspired oxygen 1 day after acute respiratory distress syndrome onset can predict the outcomes of involving patients. Medicine. 2016;95(14):e3333. https://doi.org/10.1097/MD.0000000000003333.
7. Anderson CT, Breen PH. Carbon dioxide kinetics and capnography during critical care. Crit Care. 2000;4(4):207–15. https://doi.org/10.1186/cc696.
8. Yun K, Jeon W, Kang B, Kim G. Effectiveness of a compressive device in controlling hemorrhage following radial artery catheterization. Clin Exp Emerg Med. 2015;2(2):104–9. https://doi.org/10.15441/ceem.14.018.
9. Baojaing L, Chuzhang C. Anesthesia nursing. Beijing: People's Medical Publishing House; 2013.
10. Weissman C, Scemama J, Weiss YG. The ratio of PACU length-of-stay to surgical duration: practical observations. Acta Anaesthesiol Scand. 2019;63(9):1143–51. Epub 2019 Jul 2. PMID: 31264209. https://doi.org/10.1111/aas.13421.
11. Chinese Society of Anesthesiology, Chinese Medical Association. Expert consensus on post-anesthesia monitoring treatment. J Clin Anesth. 2021;37(1):89–94.
12. Hongtao M, Wenjun H. Anesthesia nursing workbook. Beijing: People's Medical Publishing House; 2017.
13. Qin L, Linfeng D. Current status of peri-surge complications and care for patients undergoing tracheal intubation with general anesthesia. Nurs J Chin People's Lib Army. 2009;26(9):40–1.
14. Chinese Nursing Association. Endotracheal Suctioning in adults receiving invasive mechanical ventilation. Group Standards T/CNAS10–2020[EB/OL]. http://www.zhhlxh.org.cn/cnaWebcn/article/3239.2021-03-23.
15. Michelle H, Frances C. Complications of general anesthesia. Clin Plast Surg. 2013;40(4):503.
16. Morotti A, Poli L, Costa P. Acute stroke. Semin Neurol. 2019;39(1):61–72. Epub 2019 Feb 11. PMID: 30743293. https://doi.org/10.1055/s-0038-1676992.

Application of Artificial Intelligence in Oral and Maxillofacial Anesthesia

23

Ming Xia

23.1 Introduction

Artificial intelligence (AI) has been an attractive topic in medicine along with the rapid development of digital and information technologies. Nowadays AI has already made some breakthroughs in medicine. With the assistance of AI, more precise models were used in clinical prediction, diagnosis, and decision-making. Also, in the field of anesthesia, with the booming development of computer technology and techniques, the application of AI has become an attractive research direction that has great advantages and value for the future development of anesthesia. Predictive models can promptly indicate possible adverse events, and decision-making and diagnostic models can guide the corresponding clinical practice. In addition, intelligent monitoring and remote control technologies have greatly contributed to the development of remote anesthesia. The application and improvement of drug robots and operator-assisted robots will further automate clinical anesthesia.

This chapter is written to introduce the development and progress of AI applied in oral and maxillofacial anesthesia, and is divided into three sections: the first section introduces the definition of AI and other related concepts/terms, the second section summarizes and analyzes reported application of AI in oral and maxillofacial anesthesia, and the third section is an analysis of limitations and opportunities for development that could be concluded from all the existing cases of application.

M. Xia (✉)
Department of Anesthesiology, Shanghai Ninth People's Hospital Affiliated to Shanghai Jiao Tong University School of Medicine, Shanghai, China
e-mail: xiaming1980@xzhmu.edu.cn

23.2 Terminology

This section summarizes only main terms including artificial intelligence, machine learning, deep learning, big data, and their related terms since to include all terms related to AI and its application will be too much and blur the focus of this chapter. Other terms which are not included in this section are further explained when appearing in later sections.

23.2.1 Artificial Intelligence

In contrast to the natural intelligence display by humans or animals, artificial intelligence (AI) is a type of intelligence demonstrated by machines. An AI textbook defines this field as the study of "intelligent agents": any system capable of sensing its environment and taking action to maximize its chances of success [1]. Major AI researchers reject this definition of artificial intel-

H. Jiang, M. Xia (eds.), *Anesthesia for Oral and Maxillofacial Surgery*,
https://doi.org/10.1007/978-981-19-7287-4_23

ligence, which comprises machines that mimic the cognitive functions of the human brain, such as "learning" and "problem-solving," that humans typically associate with the human mind.

23.2.2 Machine Learning

The field of machine learning is a part of artificial intelligence. Automating the process of creating an analytical model is one of the features of this method of data analysis. A key characteristic of the system is its ability to identify patterns in data, and make decisions without requiring a lot of human intervention [2]. The study focuses on computer algorithms that can improve automatically over time based on experience and data.

A machine learning algorithm is a program that allows computers to discover how to perform tasks without being explicitly programmed. During this process, computers learn from data provided so that they can carry out certain tasks. Algorithms can be programmed to instruct computers how to solve simple problems; computers do not need to learn to solve problems of this nature. Creating algorithmic solutions can be challenging for humans, especially for more advanced tasks. A machine that develops its own algorithm is often more effective than having a human programmer specify every necessary step [3].

23.2.3 Training Data Set, Validation Data Set, Test Data Set

The study and construction of algorithms is a common task in machine learning, and such algorithms function by making data-driven predictions or decisions through building a mathematical model from input data. These input data are usually divided into three data sets and are used in different stages of the creation of the model, they are training data set, validation data set, and test data set.

A training data set is also known as a sample date set. It is a set of examples used to fit the parameters of the model. In practice, it often consists of pairs of an input vector and the corresponding output vector, and the answer key is commonly denoted as a target (or label) here [4].

The fitted model is then used to predict the responses for the observation. This process is realized in the second data set, the validation data set [4]. The validation data set provides an unbiased evaluation of a model fit on the layer widths—in a neural network.

Finally, an unbiased evaluation of a final model fit on the training data set is provided using the test data set [5].

23.2.4 Deep Learning

An artificial neural network with representation learning is the basis of deep learning (also known as deep structured learning). There are three types of learning: supervised, semi-supervised, and unsupervised [6].

In essence, deep learning is a combination of three or more layers of neural networks. The neural networks simulated here are far from being able to mimic the human brain's ability to process large amounts of data, but they are able to "learn" from it. Adding hidden layers to a neural network can help refine and optimize the predictions made by a single layer [7].

23.2.5 Artificial Neural Network

An artificial neural network (ANN), also known as a neural network (NN) or a neural circuit, is a computing system that is inspired by the biological neural networks in animal brains. The neural network is built using artificial neurons, which are connected units modeled loosely after the neurons in a biological brain. An individual connection can transmit a signal to another neuron, similar to synapses in a biological brain [8].

23.2.6 Big Data

In terms of traditional data processing methods, it refers to data that is so large, fast, or complex that it would be impossible to process it. For decades, large amounts of information have been accessed and stored for analytics. The traditional 3V basic characteristics of Big Data are Volume, Variety, and Velocity. Volume stands for large amount of data, Variety stands for many types of data (each type of sensor records a different type of data, sound data, image data, location data, etc., also, with the development of IoT, there will be more and more types of data), and Velocity stands for fast data processing speed (for example, the same visual sensor, the human eye cannot distinguish changes in less than 0.1 s, while the current high-speed camera can capture changes in 0.001 s, its efficiency in data acquisition is 100 times more than the human) [9].

23.2.7 Support Vector Machine (SVM)

The support vector machine (SVM) is one of the key algorithms. In collaboration with colleagues, Vladimir Vapnik developed SVM at AT&T Bell Laboratories. Generally, it is used for solving binary classification problems within the field of pattern recognition as a supervised learning algorithm. A statistical learning framework called VC theory was proposed by Vapnik (1982, 1995) and Chervonenkis (1974), making SVM one of the most robust prediction methods. The SVM training algorithm builds a model by analyzing a set of training examples that have been categorized into two categories. This is a non-probabilistic binary linear classifier (although Platt scaling can be used to make it a probabilistic classifier). To maximize the width of the gap between the two categories, SVM maps training examples to points in space. According to which side of the gap new examples fall, they are predicted to belong to a specific category. SVM aims to find the best hyperplane in multidimensional space which makes the interval between positive and negative samples maximum [10].

23.2.8 Decision Tree

The decision tree is a tree structure, in which each decision node represents a judgment rule based on attributes, each branch represents the output result of the judgment, and eventually, each leaf node represents a terminal classification result [11]. Every decision node can be divided into two or multiple branches. The top level of the decision tree is the root node, which represents the whole set of training data samples. An optimal feature would be selected and the root node would be split into different subsets according to this feature so that each subset gets the best classification under the current conditions. If these subsets can complete the correct classification, then the leaf nodes are constructed; if they cannot be classified correctly, then we continue to select new optimal features to construct the decision nodes until all subsets are constructed as leaf nodes so that the decision tree is established. Decision trees are fast and can quickly classify large data sources. However, decision trees are prone to overfitting, and pruning or random forest methods are needed to avoid overfitting.

23.2.9 Random Forest

Random forest is a highly flexible novel ML algorithm that integrates multiple unrelated decision trees to construct a forest in a random way for regression or classification [12]. The basic unit of random forest is the decision tree and the essence is the idea of ensemble learning—a bunch of ML. Intuitively, each decision tree is a classifier that can output one classification result, while the random forest integrates all classification results and designates the category with the highest number of votes as the final output result. Ensemble learning solves a single problem by building a combination of several models, which is better than any other single classification. This makes the random forest less prone to overfitting and has better noise immunity.

23.2.10 Fuzzy Logic

Fuzzy logic is a classic concept in the history of AI development. It is widely known that the basis of a computer program is typical Boolean logic with the basic values of "0" and "1," which mean "no" or "yes." Boolean logic enables the computer to make automatic judgments and decisions, but it still has limitations and defects. Usually, human beings won't deal with problems by the simple way of a clear judgment of "yes" or "no." Thus, fuzzy logic is proposed to imitate human thinking patterns and allow for the input of uncertain variables rather than explicitly classified variables. In fuzzy logic, there is no strict boundary between certain classifications while the variable is measured by the degree of membership. Compared with probability theory, it is a probability belonging to a certain classification [13]. Fuzzy logic transforms the input value into the degree of membership of each set through fuzzification and puts out a defuzzied value by a preset program to solve practical problems. It is recognized as an ideal and feasible model for computerized decision-making systems.

23.2.11 Summary

The foundation of AI is big data, whereas the core is analysis and algorithms. Although physicians are not obliged to gain insight into complex algorithms, general knowledge of some basic algorithms helps understand ML and AI better.

Nowadays, ANN is widely used in ML and AI as a mathematical model parallel to the human nervous system to discern inherent connections in nonlinear data patterns instead of common linear models [14]. It provides a relatively effective and simple method for solving complex problems in the area of AI. The basic structure of a neural network consists of an input layer, an output layer, and one or more hidden layers. Each node of the input layer corresponds to a variable and each node of the output layer corresponds to a target variable. Between the input layer and the output layer is the hidden layer, which is invisible to the users. The number of hidden layers and the number of nodes in each layer determine the complexity of the ANN. Each node of the neural network is connected with many nodes in front of it, which are called the input nodes of this node, and each connection corresponds to a weight. The output value is obtained by taking the total value of all its input nodes and the corresponding connection weight as the input of an activation function. Adjusting the weight of the connection between nodes in the work of training when constructing ANNs. The typical structures widely used in neural networks mainly include multilayer perceptron networks and error backpropagation.

With the increasing number of hidden layers, the concept of deep learning rises from ANN for more intricate problems. Deep learning is a bunch of ML. The essence of deep learning is to learn more intrinsic features by ML models with numerous hidden layers and massive training data, to improve the accuracy of classification or prediction ultimately [15]. Instead of multilayer perceptron network and error backpropagation, deep learning adopts a very different training mechanism from that of a traditional neural network. The difficulty of deep neural network training can be overcome by "layer-wise pre-training" [16]. The convolutional neural network is a kind of deep learning and has become a research hotspot in the field of speech analysis and image recognition in recent years.

23.3 Application of AI in Oral and Maxillofacial Anesthesia

In perioperative medical practice, anesthesiologists keep an eye on the patient's assessment to keep track of the dynamics and guide the follow-up treatment, making rapid decisions accordingly to reduce risk and mortality. In particular, some advanced machine models may even give valuable recommendations for clinical decision-making. Due to the inexactness in many medical concepts and their relationships, Fuzzy logic (FL) provides an approximate inference method that allows the input of fuzzy and inexact variables and is widely used to develop intelligent decision-making systems and medical expert systems.

Most clinical real events are diverse, variable, and heterogeneous. Based on multiple criteria decision analysis (MCDA), Sobrie et al. developed a probabilistic model called "MR-Sor" to assess preoperative ASA classification by multiple parameters with a prediction accuracy of up to 96%. Belton and Stewart defined multi-criteria decision analysis as a decision-making approach that gives the most optimal recommendation by considering multiple approaches. For example, Hancerliogullari et al. used the Fuzzy Analytic Hierarchy Process (FussyFuzzy-AHP) and the Technique for Order Preference by Similarity to an Ideal Solution (TOPSIS) to create a multi-criteria decision analysis model to determine the best anesthesia for pediatric circumcision. Patrick Tighe et al. [17] created machine learning used to assess the necessity of femoral nerve blocks in ACL reconstruction surgery to provide advisory value for clinical decision-making. Intelligent decision systems enabled by AI influence and improve the practice of medicine through rational computation and application of data, helping physicians to make better clinical decisions and also enabling them to focus more on the patients themselves.

23.3.1 Prediction for Hypotension and Hypoxemia

Hypotension and hypoxemia are common clinical adverse events during general anesthesia and can even have a negative prognostic impact. Hypotension refers to the status where patient's blood pressure is more than 30% lower than the resting blood pressure, which is commonly caused by bleeding, reflexes, heart failure, etc., and can be solved with infusion or vasoconstrictor like catecholamine. Hypoxemia, on the other hand, could be a result caused by respiratory complications such as airway obstruction and bronchospasm.

Although clinical anesthesiologists try their best to avoid these adverse events, it is difficult to make very accurate judgments by relying solely on their existing experience. The application of AI in the prediction for hypotension and hypoxemia also benefits anesthesiologists and clinicians who work in the field of oral and maxillofacial anesthesia.

There are already some examples of the application of AI in the prediction of hypotension and hypoxemia. In the study of Lin et al. [18], they developed an artificial neural network model with high reliability and credibility to predict the occurrence of hypotension after induction. The purpose of the study was to develop ANN models to identify patients at high risk for post-induction hypotension during general anesthesia. The ANN model developed in this study had good discrimination and calibration and would provide decision support to clinicians and increase vigilance for patients at high risk of post-induction hypotension during general anesthesia.

In the study by Kendale et al. [19], the algorithm of the machine model was trained by eight models and the one with the best fit was selected to predict the occurrence of post-induction hypotension, while more satisfactory results were obtained in the sensitivity analysis. They hypothesized that machine learning methods can provide a prediction for the risk of post-induction hypotension, and found that the success of this technique in predicting post-induction hypotension demonstrates the feasibility of machine learning models for predictive analytics in the field of anesthesiology, with performance dependent on model selection and appropriate tuning. However, both the training and testing sets of the models in this study were retrospective studies based on data from existing electronic medical records and lacked prospective validation in real clinical situations.

Lundberg et al. [19] developed a "prophetic" system by training a gradient-enhanced machine model to provide an initial and real-time prediction of perioperative hypoxemia for timely intervention by anesthesiologists and validated the model during surgery. The results show that the model can better improve anesthesiologists' clinical awareness and prediction of hypoxemia risk.

A review by van der Ven et al. [20] describes the development and validation of one of the first machine learning prediction algorithms for the operating room setting, the Hypotension Prediction Index. The review cites two randomized controlled trials demonstrating that the algorithm can reduce intraoperative hypotension by predicting impending hypotensive events in real time and, as a result, anesthesiologists can act in a timely manner. Van der Ven et al. conclude that although HPI can predict hypotension, it still has some limitations, for example, it may not be generalizable to cardiac surgery and intensive care patient populations because it was developed from records of non-cardiac surgery and intensive care patients; furthermore, the algorithm does not require a dynamic learning process that evolves from the use of clinical patient care, which means that the algorithm is fixed.

23.3.2 Prediction for PONV

Postoperative nausea and vomiting (PONV) is a common complication after general anesthesia procedures, including oral and maxillofacial surgeries. The identification and prophylactic treatment of patients at high risk for PONV can improve patient satisfaction, reduce the occurrence of adverse events such as misaspiration, and reduce healthcare costs.

Numerous machine models have been developed to predict postoperative nausea and vomiting. Traeger M. et al. [21] in Germany used the ANN algorithm for machine learning to predict the incidence of PONV and showed a higher clinical relevance compared to the currently used Apfel score (0.66; 95% CI: 0.61–0.71) and Koivuranta score (0.69; 95% CI: 0.65–0.74) discriminatory ability (0.74; 95% CI: 0.70–0.78).

PONV is still a frequent and subjectively very unpleasant side effect of anesthesia. Nevertheless, antiemetic prophylaxis should only be given to patients at risk, who have to be identified by appropriate prediction models. All traditional risk scores are based on the results of logistic regression analyses. Alternatively, however, an artificial neural network (ANN) can be used for such predictions, which can be used to model complex and nonlinear relationships well. The development of such an ANN for PONV prediction is presented and its prediction accuracy with that of two simplified risk models (Apfel Score and Koivuranta Score).

Researchers at Suhre et al. [22] conducted a retrospective machine learning casual analysis to investigate the relationship between cannabis use and PONV. A total of 27,388 adult ASA 1–3 patients receiving general anesthesia for non-obstetric, non-cardiac procedures and receiving postoperative care in the PACU were analyzed in this study, and 16,245 patients were analyzed in the external validation dataset. According to the chart, patients reported using cannabis in any form during the pre-anesthesia evaluation was the strongest predictor of post-anesthesia complications. Prior to PACU discharge, there must be documentation of PONV of any severity, including the administration of rescue medications. As a consequence, the study concluded that cannabis use is associated with a small increase in the marginal probability of PONV.

More accurately speaking, study mentioned in the previous paragraph is not an example of machine learning in the prediction of PONV—it is used as a tool of data analysis in this study. However, it still proves the great potential of ML application in medical field.

An analysis of 1086 in-patients under general anesthesia, without antiemetic prophylaxis, was conducted by Peng et al. [23]. In the process of ANN training, the estimation of ×2 statistic and information gain with respect to PONV was used to select the predictors. The ANN was configured using a software tool. Following that, an ANN was trained using data from a training set ($n = 656$). In case the ANN did not know how the remaining 430 patients would fare regarding PONV, testing validation was conducted. For estimating predictive performance, the receiver operating characteristic (ROC) curves were used. Naive Bayesian classifiers, logistic regression models, simplified Apfel scores, and Koivuranta scores were compared with ANN performance.

23.3.3 Prediction for Difficult Airway

Tracheal intubation is the gold standard for securing the airway, and it is not uncommon to encounter intubation difficulties in intensive care units and emergency rooms. Difficult airway management has always been one of the main causes of adverse events related to anesthesia, especially oral anesthesia, and has the potential for life-threatening complications, and the prediction of difficult airways before surgery has been a topic of concern for anesthesiologists.

There are more and more reports on methods to predict difficult airway, mainly including some routine physical examinations, imaging, and scale assessment, but all of them have some limitations and cumbersome procedures. Gabriel Louis Cuendet from Switzerland et al. [24] developed a method for rapid prediction of the difficult airway by fully automated face scanning. The face data was obtained from a patient database, facial feature points were fitted according to an algorithm, and an algorithmic model was built using artificial intelligence to automatically predict difficult airways. In the validation dataset, this automated facial scanning method was similar to the level of manual assessment of difficult airway. This study provides an idea for the development of a more intelligent and convenient prediction model that can predict difficult airways more accurately with a simple facial scan alone. However, due to the small sample size of this study, the prediction method of the difficult airway by face scanning still needs to be further investigated and validated.

A deep learning artificial intelligence model was created by Hayasaka et al. [25] for classification of intubation difficulty. In their study, patients scheduled for surgery at Yamagata University Hospital with altered facial appearances, altered neck range of motion, or intubation performed by a physician with less than 3 years of anesthesia experience were excluded. In the first day after surgery, they received 16 different facial images from the patients. In order to create a deep learning model that links the facial image of the patient with the difficulty of intubation, all images were judged as "easy"/"difficult" by an anesthesiologist. In order to compute sensitivity, specificity, and area under the curve (AUC), receiver operating characteristic curves were developed for both the actual intubation difficulty and the AI model. AI model classification of intubation difficulties was visualized using heat maps of class activation. A supine-side-closed mouth-base position was found to be the most effective location for generating the best artificial intelligence model for identifying intubation difficulties. According to the results, the majority of the heat map's activation was concentrated around the neck regardless of background; the AI model recognized facial contours and identified difficulty in intubating regardless of background; the AUC was 0.864; and the 95% confidence interval was [0.731–0.969], indicating that the heat map's activation was concentrated around the neck, regardless of background. Using deep learning and an artificial intelligence model, this study is the first to classify intubation difficulties using deep learning. Under general anesthesia or emergency situations, the AI model developed in this study may be useful for tracheal intubation by inexperienced medical staff.

23.3.4 Artificial Intelligence in Perioperative Management and Remote Control

Anesthesiologists need to provide comprehensive management of all aspects of the patient in the anesthetized state, including airway and respiratory system, basic vital signs, depth of anesthesia, and pain monitoring and management, among others. Despite good clinical training, anesthesiologists occasionally feel flustered and anxious when faced with multiple tasks at the same time, which increases the workload and psychological stress of anesthesiologists and even generates burnout. According to a research study by Cooper JB et al. [26], most of the unplanned events during anesthesia are related to human negligence and instrument malfunction, which can be actively prevented and controlled. On the other hand, too many false alarms can interfere with the judgment of anesthesiologists and increase unnecessary work. The development of AI may free anesthesiologists from their burdensome tasks. In addition, continuous and comprehensive monitoring, more accurate electronic recording, and timely recognition of emergencies using machines may reduce human accidents and ensure patient safety in the perioperative period.

In recent years, there have been major breakthroughs and developments in intelligent monitoring and alerting technologies. Mylrea K C. et al. [27] used artificial neural networks for integrated monitoring from multiple variables to identify unexpected situations and effectively reduce false alarms. Gohil Bhupendra et al. [28] developed RT-SAAM intelligent monitoring and alerting system using the fuzzy logic approach to identify clinical events such as intraoperative hypovolemia, low cardiac output, malignant hyperthermia, etc., which is better for multiple problems. Similarly, based on this, Mirza Mansoor et al. [29] introduced the Fuzzy logic monitoring system (FLMS) for better supervision of the anesthesia process. Also with the popularization of smartphones and medical apps, smartphones can be used for measurement, monitoring, and recording of vital signs and may become a common medical tool for physicians and patients in the future.

Unlike blood pressure, pulse rate, and heart rate, which are vital signs that can be directly measured by physical or chemical means, methods of assessing depth of anesthesia have always been controversial. BIS, E entropy, and auditory evoked potentials are common clinical measurements based mainly on the analysis of EEG and evoked potentials, but still have limitations. With the increasing computational power of machines to handle large amounts of data and problems, intelligent models have been further applied for the analysis of anesthesia depth. Liu Quan et al. [30] used neural networks combining multiscale entropy (MSE) and independent entropy for effective and reliable monitoring of anesthesia depth and evaluated the performance of the method, and More satisfactory results were obtained. Benzy et al. [31] developed a new intelligent anesthesia depth assessment index using a neuro-fuzzy intervention system. Effective EEG biometrics for guiding precise sedation can also be further explored by machine learning algorithms.

Telemedicine technology is also currently receiving a lot of attention from clinicians, and remote control can be applied to anesthesia outside the operating room, anesthesia management in remote areas and extreme environments, and some remote medication guidance. In their study, Kamata Kotoe et al. [32] reported the use of remote anesthesia detection technology in pediatric gamma knife radiosurgery. The use of remote monitoring under general anesthesia is feasible, keeping the anesthesiologist outside the operating room to prevent radiation hazards while also being able to ensure the safety of the patient. Telemedicine allows real-time dialogue and collaborative communication between specialists across regions, regardless of regional limitations or shortage of medical resources, and Stephen W. et al. [33] have experimented with the use of a remote control system for communication during anesthesia with satisfactory results.

In addition, postoperative analgesia, a common concern for most patients, can benefit from remote management for timely adjustment of individualized medication regimens. One study reported a remote operating system for postoperative continuous peripheral nerve blocks (CPNB) pump setup [34]. Patient data and requirements can be immediately transmitted to the competent anesthesiologist via the Internet, and the anesthesiologist can make timely and remote changes to the pump settings. In addition to the advantages of allowing real-time feedback and addressing postoperative pain, the system reduces the workload of the physician who subsequently follows up with the patient. "Manage My Pain (MMP)" is a mobile application launched by ManagingLife in 2011 that remotely tracks patients' pain fluctuations [35]. Moreover, data mining and machine learning from the database created by MMP will help clinical providers explore new ways to measure pain as well as predict pain fluctuations [36].

23.3.5 Application of Automation and Robotic Assistance

Although robotic-assisted surgical operating systems are now more common in clinical practice, providing better views and more dexterity and refinement in minimally invasive surgery, there is still much room for the development of robotic-assisted technology and automated operations in anesthesia. The concept of automated anesthesia was developed to assist anesthesiologists in some routine daily tasks, and the two most important issues are automated anesthetic drug delivery systems and machine-assisted operating systems.

Schwilden and Schuttler proposed a classical anesthetic drug delivery system, the target controlled infusion push pump (TCI) [37], based on a three-compartment model of drug pharmacokinetics in 1990, but one of the limitations of this system is that it ignores the actual anesthetic effect. In contrast to the TCI system, the closed-loop system (CLS) selects specific parameters that reflect the effect of the drug as a reference for the automatic infusion of the anesthetic drug [38]. The central control system allows the pump to adjust the drug infusion rate based on the analysis of target variables. Some studies have reported successful clinical applications of closed-loop systems in sedation control and neuromuscular blockade [39–43]. The McSleep system is a closed-loop automatic drug delivery system that combines consciousness, analgesia, and muscle relaxation assessment, three elements considered to be the most essential for general anesthesia. In addition to automatic infusion delivery of anesthetic drugs, the system is equipped with an intelligent voice prompting system for routine steps in anesthesia, providing the anesthesiologist with the necessary cues and keeping him or her focused [44]. The safety and stability of these automated drug delivery systems have also been demonstrated in comparison to manual operations, and better results have been obtained with the application of the system even in elderly people undergoing cardiac surgery. These satisfactory findings suggest that automated drug delivery systems might be widely adopted and promoted in the future.

On the other hand, robotic-assisted operating systems have some prospects for routine anesthesia operations such as intubation, arteriovenous puncture, nerve block, or intravertebral block. The Kepler intubation system (KIS) was the first robotic system for tracheal intubation developed by Hemmerling T. M. et al. [45]. The anesthesiologist can adjust the position of the mechanical manipulator arm at three different speeds through the control of the manipulator lever and easily observe the operation through a real-time picture display on an external screen. Following relevant tests on airway manikins, a small study used the KIS operating system in a real clinical setting and achieved a more satisfactory intubation success rate [46]. However, the current lack of studies with large sample data limits the further clinical application of KIS. Also, KIS systems are semi-automated operating systems, and the implementation of fully automated operations has not yet been reached.

In the last decade or so, several new robotic-assisted systems have also been used in the operation of regional anesthesia. Tighe P. J. et al. first used the S-type Da Vinci surgical system (DVS) to achieve the assisted operation of peripheral nerve blocks on ultrasound body models [47]. The Magellan nerve robotic block system (Magellan robotic nerve block system), the first robotic-assisted system for clinical nerve block manipulation, was created in 2013 to identify the nerve by ultrasound and enhanced imaging system, then insert a needle into the target nerve sheath and inject local anesthetic around the nerve [48]. All 13 patients enrolled in this study successfully underwent a Magellan system-assisted nerve block within an average of 3 min. Compared with manual ultrasound-guided nerve blocks, the operator acquired the nerve block skills faster and reduced the number of repeated probe punctures with the guidance of the robotic system [49, 50].

Robotic-assisted systems can also be applied in intravertebral anesthesia. Conventional blind localization methods rely on anatomical landmarks and breakthrough sensation for probe localization, resulting in higher rates of repositioning, mispenetration, and associated complications [51]. Real-time ultrasound imaging systems can visualize the optimal location and depth of the probe, but the lack of clarity of the ultrasound image display due to interference from acoustic clutter or artifacts, as well as the difficulty in understanding ultrasound images for young anesthesiologists, limit the application of ultrasound systems [52, 53]. Several intelligent systems have been proposed in several studies to improve the visualization and utility of ultrasound imaging systems. In one study [54], researchers developed a user-friendly ultrasound system interface that included three image windows for raw ultrasound images, anatomical images, and probe movement direction schematics to output images more intuitively and facilitate probe guidance. Other studies have designed novel ultrasound imaging methods for three-dimensional image presentation [55, 56] or have automatically positioned the target location of the probe through machine learning algorithms [57] to assist clinical operators for more convenient observation and manipulation.

The use of hyperspectral imaging (HIS) can improve early oral cancer diagnosis, in-depth monitoring and reduced cancer-related mortality and morbidity by detecting tumors in different depths using near infrared (NIR) and visible spectrum lights. DL methods are suitable for processing the extensive spectral-spatial cube information efficiently and automatically. In order to assess the status of complex, pathologically altered oral mucosa, it is crucial to understand the spectral characteristics of its main components (oral mucosa, muscle, and fat). According to HIS data from a representative number of fresh surgical, ex vivo oral tissue samples, Thiem et al. used 316 fresh surgical ex vivo oral tissue samples to categorize their reflectance values into fat, muscle and mucosa. An ordinary and time-saving deep learning (DL) strategy achieved an overall accuracy score of 87% using common optimization techniques. The clinical use of non-invasive, automated oral mucosal changes could be feasible and tangible if more patient data and a hyperspectral database of dozens of samples come together. With non-pre-processed hyperspectral cube data, future studies will use convolutional neural networks (CNNs) to determine whether tissue samples are healthy, dysplastic, or cancerous [58].

23.4 Limitations and Challenges

Although AI has shown great advantages in terms of improving the quality of care, increasing patient satisfaction, and reducing the burden on anesthesiologists, some controversies and challenges are still inevitable.

First, for most clinicians, there are difficulties regarding the understanding of machine learning and algorithmic language, thus hindering further interdisciplinary communication and interaction. This also implies that we need more training and the introduction of medical-industrial crossover talents. However, in routine clinical applications, because models and algorithms are usually not publicly available, clinicians also do not need a rigorous understanding of the models and principles of machine learning. Another challenge is the reliability and validity of artificial intelligence systems. When a computer provides a recommendation that is inconsistent with clinical experience, physicians should carefully consider whether to adopt the recommendation. In addition, the security of AI systems is threatened by the high risk of intentional intrusion and control of electronic medical devices. Privacy concerns due to massive data collection and sharing have also received increasing ethical attention, which requires a high level of confidentiality and reliable precautions to be taken. In addition to security, the application of AI in medicine is further subject to ethical challenges. Screening and risk assessment of specific populations may bring about some discrimination and bias, or even inequitable distribution of medical resources. At the same time, developers of some decision systems can easily increase desired gains and profits through programming. It can even bring some challenges to the doctor-patient relationship and the trust between patients and machines. Finally, AI devices are usually expensive to develop and maintain, and patients may not be able to afford the high costs, which can also limit further clinical applications of AI.

23.5 Summary

The rapid advances in artificial intelligence indicate that we are at the beginning of a whole new field of information technology development. Artificial intelligence applications in anesthesia can improve medical safety and accuracy, reduce anesthesiologists' workload, and increase patient satisfaction. On the other hand, we should strive to address the shortcomings and challenges in the current development of artificial intelligence. The proportion of difficult airways in oral surgery is high, so how to accurately predict difficult airways through AI and intelligently navigate intubation through AI technology and even apply it to the whole perioperative management should be the future development direction. We believe that through further exploration and research, artificial intelligence will be a powerful tool in clinical anesthesia practice.

References

1. Poole D, Mackworth A, Goebel R. Computational intelligence: a logical approach. New York: Oxford University Press; 1998; ISBN 978-0-19-510270-3. Archived from the original on 26 July 2020. Retrieved 22 August 2020.
2. Mitchell T. Machine learning. New York: McGraw Hill; 1997; ISBN 0-07-042807-7. OCLC 36417892.
3. Alpaydin E. Introduction to machine learning. 4th ed. Cambridge, MA: MIT; 2020. p. xix, 1–3, 13–18. ISBN 978-0262043793.
4. James G. An introduction to statistical learning: with applications in R. New York: Springer; 2013. p. 176; ISBN 978-1461471370.
5. Brownlee J. What is the difference between test and validation datasets? 2017. Accessed 12 Oct 2017.
6. Bengio Y, Courville A, Vincent P. Representation learning: a review and new perspectives. IEEE Trans Pattern Anal Mach Intell. 2013;35(8):1798–828. https://doi.org/10.1109/tpami.2013.50; arXiv:1206.5538.
7. Education I. What is deep learning? 2021. [online] Ibm.com. https://www.ibm.com/cloud/learn/deep-learning. Accessed 13 Sept 2021.
8. Education I. What are neural networks? 2021. [online] Ibm.com. https://www.ibm.com/cloud/learn/neural-networks. Accessed 13 Sept 2021.
9. Sas.com. 2021. Big Data: what it is and why it matters. [online]. https://www.sas.com/en_us/insights/big-data/what-is-big-data.html#:~:text=Big%20data%20is%20a%20term,day%2Dto%2Dday%20basis.&text=It's%20what%20organizations%20do%20with,decisions%20and%20strategic%20business%20moves. Accessed 13 Sept 2021.
10. Uddin S, Khan A, Hossain ME, et al. Comparing different supervised machine learning algorithms for disease prediction[J]. BMC Med Inform Decis Mak. 2019;19(1):281.
11. Cruz JA, Wishart DS. Applications of machine learning in cancer prediction and prognosis. Cancer Inform. 2007;2:59–77.
12. Zhao X, Wu Y, Lee D L, et al. IForest: interpreting random forests via visual analytics. IEEE Trans Vis Comput Graph. 2018.
13. Hashimoto DA, Witkowski E, Gao L, et al. Artificial intelligence in anesthesiology: current techniques, clinical applications, and limitations. Anesthesiology. 2020;132(2):379–94.
14. Pergialiotis V, Pouliakis A, Parthenis C, et al. The utility of artificial neural networks and classification and regression trees for the prediction of endometrial cancer in postmenopausal women. Public Health. 2018;164:1–6.
15. Hinton G. Deep learning-a technology with the potential to transform health care. JAMA. 2018;320(11):1101–2.
16. LeCun Y, Bengio Y, Hinton G. Deep learning. Nature. 2015;521(7553):436–44.
17. Lin CS, et al. Application of an artificial neural network to predict postinduction hypotension during general anesthesia. Med Decis Mak. 2011;31(2):308–14.
18. Kendale S, et al. Supervised machine-learning predictive analytics for prediction of postinduction hypotension. Anesthesiology. 2018;129(4):675–88.
19. Lundberg SM, et al. Explainable machine-learning predictions for the prevention of hypoxaemia during surgery. Nat Biomed Eng. 2018;2(10):749–60.
20. van der Ven W, Veelo D, Wijnberge M, van der Ster B, Vlaar A, Geerts B. One of the first validations of an artificial intelligence algorithm for clinical use: the impact on intraoperative hypotension prediction and clinical decision-making. Surgery. 2021;169(6):1300–3.
21. Traeger M, Eberhart A, Geldner G, et al. Vorhersage von Ubelkeit und Erbrechen in der postoperativen Phase durch ein künstliches neuronales Netz [Prediction of postoperative nausea and vomiting using an artificial neural network]. Anaesthesist. 2003;52(12):1132–8. https://doi.org/10.1007/s00101-003-0575-y.
22. Suhre W, O'Reilly-Shah V, Van Cleve W. Cannabis use is associated with a small increase in the risk of postoperative nausea and vomiting: a retrospective machine-learning causal analysis. BMC Anesthesiol. 2020;20(1):115.
23. Peng S, Wu K, Wang J, Chuang J, Peng S, Lai Y. Predicting postoperative nausea and vomiting with the application of an artificial neural network. Br J Anaesth. 2007;98(1):60–5.
24. Cuendet GL, et al. Facial image analysis for fully automatic prediction of difficult endotracheal intubation. IEEE Trans Biomed Eng. 2016;63(2):328–39. https://doi.org/10.1109/TBME.2015.2457032.
25. Hayasaka T, Kawano K, Kurihara K, Suzuki H, Nakane M, Kawamae K. Creation of an artificial intelligence model for intubation difficulty classification by deep learning (convolutional neural network) using face images: an observational study. J Intensive Care. 2021;9(1):38.
26. Cooper JB, Newbower RS, Long CD, et al. Preventable anesthesia mishaps: a study of human factors. BMJ Qual Safety. 2002;11:277–82.
27. Mylrea KC, Orr JA, Westenskow DR. Integration of monitoring for intelligent alarms in anesthesia: neural networks--can they help? J Clin Monit. 1993;9:31–7.
28. Bhupendra G, Hamid G, Harrison Michael J, et al. Intelligent monitoring of critical pathological events

during anesthesia. Conf Proc IEEE Eng Med Biol Soc. 2007;2007:4343–6.
29. Mansoor M, Hamid G, Harrison Michael J. A fuzzy logic-based system for anaesthesia monitoring. Conf Proc IEEE Eng Med Biol Soc. 2010;2010:3974–7.
30. Quan L, Yi-Feng C, Shou-Zen F, et al. EEG signals analysis using multiscale entropy for depth of anesthesia monitoring during surgery through artificial neural networks. Comput Math Methods Med. 2015;2015:232381.
31. Benzy VK, Jasmin EA, Cherian KR, et al. Relative wave energy-based adaptive neuro-fuzzy inference system for estimation of the depth of anaesthesia. J Integr Neurosci. 2018;17:43–51.
32. Kotoe K, Motohiro H, Osamu N, et al. Initial experience with the use of remote control monitoring and general anesthesia during radiosurgery for pediatric patients. Pediatr Neurosurg. 2011;47:158–66.
33. Cone Stephen W, Lynne G, Russell H, et al. Remote anesthetic monitoring using satellite telecommunications and the internet. Anesth Analg. 2006;102:1463–7.
34. Macaire P, Nadhari M, Greiss H, et al. Internet remote control of pump settings for postoperative continuous peripheral nerve blocks: a feasibility study in 59 patients. Ann Fr Anesth Reanim. 2014;33:e1–7.
35. ManagingLife Inc. Manage my pain. https://www.managinglife.com.
36. Rahman QA, Janmohamed T, Pirbaglou M, et al. Defining and predicting pain volatility in users of the manage my pain app: analysis using data mining and machine learning methods. J Med Internet Res. 2018;20(11):e12001.
37. Schwilden H, Schuttler J. The determination of an effective therapeutic infusion rate for intravenous anesthetics using feedback-controlled dosages. Anaesthesist. 1990;39:603–6.
38. Ngai L, Morgan LG, Fatima B-L, et al. Feasibility of closed-loop titration of propofol and remifentanil guided by the spectral M-entropy monitor. Anesthesiology. 2012;116:286–95.
39. Hemmerling TM, Charabati S, Zaouter C, et al. A randomized controlled trial demonstrates that a novel closed-loop propofol system performs better hypnosis control than manual administration. Can J Anesth. 2010;57:725–35. https://doi.org/10.1007/s12630-010-9335-z.
40. Liu N, Chazot T, Hamada S, Landais A, Boichut N, Dussaussoy C, Trillat B, Beydon L, Samain E, Sessler DI, Fischler M. Closed-loop coadministration of propofol and remifentanil guided by bispectral index: a randomized multicenter study. Anesth Analg. 2011;112:546–57.
41. Cédrick Z, Hemmerling Thomas M, Stefano M, et al. Feasibility of automated Propofol sedation for transcatheter aortic valve implantation: a pilot study. Anesth Analg. 2017;125:1505–12.
42. Eleveld DJ, Proost JH, Wierda JM. Evaluation of a closed-loop muscle relaxation control system. Anesth Analg. 2005;101(3):758–64.
43. Mendez JA, Leon A, Marrero A, et al. Improving the anesthetic process by a fuzzy rule based medical decision system. Artif Intell Med. 2018;84:159–70. https://doi.org/10.1016/j.artmed.2017.12.005.
44. You're Getting McSleepy, So Very McSleepy.... McGill Alumni. Available from: https://mcgillnews.mcgill.ca/s/1762/news/interior.aspx?sid=1762&;gid=2;pgid=1187.
45. Hemmerling Thomas M, Mohamad W, Cedrick Z, et al. The Kepler intubation system. Anesth Analg. 2012;114:590–4.
46. Hemmerling TM, Taddei R, Wehbe M, et al. First robotic tracheal intubations in humans using the Kepler intubation system. Br J Anaesth. 2012;108:1011–6.
47. Tighe PJ, et al. Robot-assisted regional anesthesia: a simulated demonstration. Anesth Analg. 2010;111(3):813–6.
48. Hemmerling TM, et al. First robotic ultrasound-guided nerve blocks in humans using the Magellan system. Anesth Analg. 2013;116(2):491–4.
49. Morse J, Terrasini N, Wehbe M, et al. Comparison of success rates, learning curves, and inter-subject performance variability of robot-assisted and manual ultrasound-guided nerve block needle guidance in simulation. Br J Anaesth. 2014;112:1092–7.
50. O'Donnell BD, et al. Robotic assistance with needle guidance. Br J Anaesth. 2015;114(4):708–9.
51. de Filho GR, Gomes HP, da Fonseca MH, Hoffman JC, Pederneiras SG, Garcia JH. Predictors of successful neuraxial block: a prospective study. Eur J Anaesthesiol. 2002;19(6):447–51. https://doi.org/10.1017/s0265021502000716.
52. Conroy PH, Luyet C, McCartney CJ, McHardy PG. Real-time ultrasound-guided spinal anaesthesia: a prospective observational study of a new approach. Anesthesiol Res Pract. 2013;2013:525818.
53. Karmakar MK, Li X, Ho AM-H, Kwok WH, Chui PT. Real-time ultrasound-guided paramedian epidural access: evaluation of a novel in-plane technique. Br J Anaesth. 2009;102(6):845–54.
54. Leng Y, Shuang Y, Tan KK, et al. Development of a real-time lumbar ultrasound image processing system for epidural needle entry site localization. Conf Proc IEEE Eng Med Biol Soc. 2016;2016:4093–6.
55. Belavy D, Ruitenberg MJ, Brijball RB. Feasibility study of real-time three−/four-dimensional ultrasound for epidural catheter insertion. Br J Anaesth. 2011;107:438–45.
56. Parmida B, Paul M, Abtin R, et al. Three-dimensional ultrasound-guided real-time midline epidural needle placement with Epiguide: a prospective feasibility study. Ultrasound Med Biol. 2017;43:375–9.
57. Mehran P, Victoria L, Purang A, et al. Automatic localization of the needle target for ultrasound-guided epidural injections. IEEE Trans Med Imaging. 2018;37:81–92.
58. Thiem D, Römer P, Gielisch M, Al-Nawas B, Schlüter M, Plaß B, Kämmerer P. Hyperspectral imaging and artificial intelligence to detect oral malignancy – part 1 - automated tissue classification of oral muscle, fat and mucosa using a light-weight 6-layer deep neural network. Head Face Med. 2021;17(1):38.

Batch number: 10732801

Printed by Printforce, the Netherlands